MRI for Radiotherapy

Gary Liney · Uulke van der Heide
Editors

MRI for Radiotherapy

Planning, Delivery, and Response Assessment

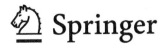

Editors
Gary Liney
Department of Medical Physics
Ingham Institute
Sydney
New South Wales
Australia

Uulke van der Heide
Department of Radiation Oncology
Netherlands Cancer Institute
Amsterdam
Noord-Holland
The Netherlands

ISBN 978-3-030-14441-8   ISBN 978-3-030-14442-5 (eBook)
https://doi.org/10.1007/978-3-030-14442-5

© Springer Nature Switzerland AG 2019
This work is subject to copyright. All rights are reserved by the Publisher, whether the whole or part of the material is concerned, specifically the rights of translation, reprinting, reuse of illustrations, recitation, broadcasting, reproduction on microfilms or in any other physical way, and transmission or information storage and retrieval, electronic adaptation, computer software, or by similar or dissimilar methodology now known or hereafter developed.
The use of general descriptive names, registered names, trademarks, service marks, etc. in this publication does not imply, even in the absence of a specific statement, that such names are exempt from the relevant protective laws and regulations and therefore free for general use.
The publisher, the authors, and the editors are safe to assume that the advice and information in this book are believed to be true and accurate at the date of publication. Neither the publisher nor the authors or the editors give a warranty, expressed or implied, with respect to the material contained herein or for any errors or omissions that may have been made. The publisher remains neutral with regard to jurisdictional claims in published maps and institutional affiliations.

This Springer imprint is published by the registered company Springer Nature Switzerland AG
The registered company address is: Gewerbestrasse 11, 6330 Cham, Switzerland

MRI in Radiotherapy: Introduction

As radiotherapy delivery has increased in terms of conformity and precision, so too has the need for accurate imaging in order to plan these treatments. MRI has much to offer as the imaging technique of choice; the soft-tissue contrast provides exquisite visualisation of both the tumour target and organs at risk improving the simulation and planning; it allows functional parameters to be measured in the same examination providing physiological information about tumour response or tissue toxicity. Furthermore, because MRI is a nonionising modality, it lends itself to repeat imaging offering the prospect of using this information frequently during treatment and adapting the radiation dose as needed on an individual patient basis.

The benefits of MRI for radiotherapy were first recognised as early as the 1980s, and subsequent work went on to quantify geometrical accuracy and demonstrate bulk density correction for MR-only planning. However, clinical practice changed little over the ensuing decades; CT remained the gold standard modality, and the perceived difficulties associated with MRI persisted. There are perhaps two good reasons for this; the fields of radiotherapy and MRI are large and different enough for these subjects to remain distinct in terms of training and education; access to MRI is a perennial problem and is typically limited to the ad hoc use of radiology scanners further restricting development for all but the larger research centres. These factors have all too often been a barrier to implementing MRI routinely in the clinic.

Nevertheless, in recent years, there has been a drive to see 'MR in RT' become a specialism in its own right, and there are a couple of initiatives worthy of mention. In 2010, ESTRO introduced its 'imaging for physicists' course with a focus on MRI. This course is now in its tenth year and remains consistently popular all across Europe. A second big step has been the creation of the dedicated 'MR in RT Symposium'. What began as a local workshop between James Balter and a few colleagues in 2013 has since grown into an important fixture on the international calendar. The Symposium has been held across the USA, Europe and Australia with attendance continuing to rise each year.

At the same time, MRI vendors have recognised this growing interest and developed RT solutions for treatment-position imaging and MR-only planning. More importantly, radiotherapy centres have begun installing their own MRI systems. Throughout all of this, there has been the exciting development of hybrid MRI treatment devices. We are now starting to see the long-term follow-up from the early pioneering MRI-cobalt machines with results showing the benefit of MR-guided adaptation. In 2017, the first ever patients were treated on commercial MRI-Linac systems.

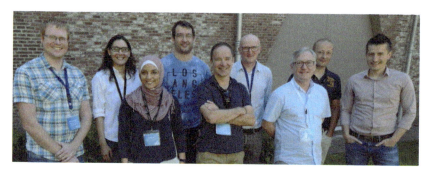

Photograph taken during the 6th International MR in RT Symposium in Utrecht July 2018, featuring some of the book contributors: (left to right) Richard Speight, Neelam Tyagi, Robba Rai, Brad Oborn, Gary Liney, Uulke van der Heide, Michael Barton, Rob Tijssen and Teo Stanescu

The emergence of MR in RT is also clear through an increasing body of published literature. Journals in the field of radiation oncology are including more and more MRI articles, with both a technical and clinical scope. While for some new developments, such as clinical treatments on MR-guided systems, experience is still limited, in other areas, the field is maturing, and a consensus on utilisation is building. Nonetheless, a comprehensive overview of the issues and opportunities of MRI in radiotherapy is still lacking. Against this backdrop, the time seemed overdue for writing (or rather editing!) such a textbook. In doing so, we have brought together colleagues who are recognised experts in this field, all of whom actively participate in the professional development of 'MR in RT'. Each of the authors represent the multiple disciplines involved in our field, namely, physics, radiography and oncology, and the text is aimed at an equally wide audience.

The book is divided into five parts showing how MRI is being used in the clinic in a logical progression from simulation through to real-time guidance. Part I begins with treatment planning, and Chap. 1 covers image acquisition from patient set-up to image protocols. MRI registration with CT is then described followed by quality assurance with a particular emphasis on geometric distortion. The final chapter in this part goes through the clinical sites of importance. Part II deals with the role of MRI as a tool during treatment; functional imaging techniques are introduced, and then studies in response assessment are considered. This part concludes with the use of MRI for motion management. MR-only radiotherapy is the focus of Part III, and both the dosimetry requirements and the techniques used to replace CT are covered here. The book then moves into the newest area of development, namely, in-room guidance; the chapters here review the first results obtained on ViewRay's cobalt system and go on to discuss the technical challenges and current status of MRI-Linac systems. To conclude, there is a discussion on the future roles for MRI with one eye towards proton therapy.

We hope you agree that the end result has been an outstanding first edition of what is sure to become a must-read in the field of MRI in radiotherapy. We would like to end by acknowledging each of the contributing authors for their time and commitment to this project and to Springer for backing the initial proposal.

Sydney, New South Wales, Australia	Gary Liney
Amsterdam, The Netherlands	Uulke van der Heide

About the Editors

Gary Liney is the senior medical physicist at the Ingham Institute for Applied Medical Research and Liverpool Cancer Therapy Centre, Sydney, Australia. He is providing the scientific lead into the MRI-simulator and MRI-Linac programs at Liverpool. Gary is a recognised expert in the use and integration of MRI techniques into radiotherapy planning and published over 70 scientific papers and three textbooks. He has taught on the ESTRO 'imaging for physicists' course since its inception in 2010. He is currently leading the investigations on the Australian phase 2 MRI-Linac system using a dedicated split bore open magnet to provide real-time MRI-guided therapy.

Uulke van der Heide works as a medical physicist and group leader at the Netherlands Cancer Institute in Amsterdam, the Netherlands. He holds a chair as professor of imaging technology in radiotherapy at the Leiden University. He was the course director on the ESTRO 'imaging for physicists' course until 2017. His research group works on the improvement of target definition in radiotherapy by application of MRI and the development and validation of quantitative imaging methods for tumour characterisation for radiotherapy dose painting. He further leads the MR-guided radiotherapy program at the Netherlands Cancer Institute.

Contents

Part I   MRI for Planning

1 **Implementation and Acquisition Protocols** 3
Rob H. N. Tijssen, Eric S. Paulson, and Robba Rai

2 **MRI to CT Image Registration** 21
Richard Speight

3 **Quality Assurance** 43
Teo Stanescu and Jihong Wang

4 **Clinical Applications of MRI in Radiotherapy Planning** 55
Houda Bahig, Eugene Koay, Maroie Barkati,
David C. Fuller, and Cynthia Menard

Part II   MRI During Treatment

5 **Functional MR Imaging** 73
Marielle Philippens and Roberto García-Álvarez

6 **Response Assessment** 95
Ines Joye and Piet Dirix

7 **Motion Management** 107
Eric S. Paulson and Rob H. N. Tijssen

Part III   MRI-Only Radiotherapy

8 **Challenges and Requirements** 119
Neelam Tyagi

9 **MR-Only Methodology** 131
Jason A. Dowling and Juha Korhonen

Part IV   MRI for Guidance

10 **MRI Linac Systems** 155
Brendan Whelan, Brad Oborn, Gary Liney, and Paul Keall

11 MRI at the Time of External Beam Treatment 169
Michael Roach and Carri K. Glide-Hurst

Part V Future Direction

12 Will We Still Need Radiotherapy in 20 Years? 191
Michael B. Barton, Trang Pham, and Georgia Harris

13 Real-Time MRI-Guided Particle Therapy 203
Bradley M. Oborn

Part I
MRI for Planning

Implementation and Acquisition Protocols

Rob H. N. Tijssen, Eric S. Paulson, and Robba Rai

1.1 Introduction

The past decade has shown that magnetic resonance imaging (MRI) is increasingly being utilised in the radiation therapy setting not only for radiation therapy planning (RTP) purposes but also in assessment of treatment response and online MR-guidance on hybrid MR-linac systems. Because of the ever-growing use of MRI in radiation therapy, it is inevitable that more departments will be looking to move forward and use MRI as a complementary imaging modality in their RTP protocols or as a sole imaging modality in MR-only workflows.

There are many requirements for the effective utilisation of MRI in radiation therapy including screening and safe scanning of common devices used in oncology, reproducible and comfortable setup for patients, and specific scanning protocols required to meet the needs for RTP. Additional education and training will be required to ensure that centres harness the full potential of MRI.

1.2 Implementing MRI for Treatment Planning

1.2.1 Site Planning and Installation

1.2.1.1 Room Design

Modern MRI scanners are designed to have a small footprint. However, there are various considerations that need to be accounted for when setting up an MRI suite in radiation therapy including shielding, equipment storage, and room safety.

An MRI suite requires (active) shielding to ensure that the magnetic fringe field does not encroach on sensitive equipment that may be in the vicinity of the area such as linear accelerators. In addition to shielding the magnetic fringe field of the scanner, the room needs to be shielded against radio frequency (RF) as RF from external sources distorts the MR signal and the RF produced by the scanner may interfere with other surrounding medical devices. Finally, building vibrations may introduce image artefacts.

R. H. N. Tijssen (✉)
Department of Radiotherapy, University Medical Center Utrecht, Utrecht, The Netherlands
e-mail: R.Tijssen@umcutrecht.nl

E. S. Paulson
Department of Radiation Oncology, Medical College of Wisconsin, Milwaukee, WI, USA

Department of Radiology, Medical College of Wisconsin, Milwaukee, WI, USA

Department of Biophysics, Medical College of Wisconsin, Milwaukee, WI, USA

R. Rai
Liverpool and Macarthur Cancer Therapy Centres, Liverpool, NSW, Australia

Ingham Institute for Applied Medical Research, Liverpool, NSW, Australia

South Western Sydney Clinical School, University of New South Wales, Liverpool, NSW, Australia

© Springer Nature Switzerland AG 2019
G. Liney, U. van der Heide (eds.), *MRI for Radiotherapy*,
https://doi.org/10.1007/978-3-030-14442-5_1

Vibration levels in the scanner room need to be low and comply with the system's requirements provided by the vendor.

A modern MRI requires a lot of equipment such as gradient and radio-frequency cabinets, power cabinets, helium compressor, and a chiller. These system components are stored in separate cabinets and must be accessible to medical physics and engineering staff for routine servicing and preventative maintenance. Access to these system components must be restricted to prevent tampering by the public and untrained staff.

The American College of Radiology Expert Panel on MRI safety (Kanal et al. 2013) has defined geographical MRI safety zones. The MRI control area is included in Zone III, and access to Zone III should be restricted to MRI-trained staff only (see Sect. 1.2.3.1). Various doors can be implemented that lead to the control room such as a single sliding door that can only be accessed by patients under the supervision of MRI-trained staff. All members of the general public and untrained oncology staff should not have access to Zone III.

Zone IV is defined as the MRI scanner room. Some departments with dedicated MRI simulators in oncology will include an obvious demarcation in their floor design to indicate where the 30 gauss fringe field line is in relation to the MRI (Fig. 1.1) (Xing et al. 2016).

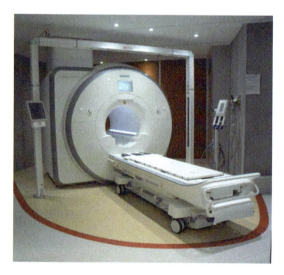

Fig. 1.1 Example of a MRI simulator with 30 G line marked on the floor

1.2.1.2 RT Immobilisation Equipment

A major difference between radiation therapy and radiology is the heavy use of immobilisation equipment. Prior to using RT immobilisation devices in the MRI room, equipment needs to be compatible for both safety and image quality. It is important to note that carbon fibre is often used in RT equipment and this has the potential to cause RF heating and attenuation of MR signal (Juresic et al. 2018; Jafar et al. 2016). The MRI compatibility of devices and equipment used in Zone IV should be designated with MRI safety labels (e.g. MR safe, MR conditional, MR unsafe). However, in the event that an unlabelled device or equipment is to be used, in-house testing for MRI compatibility should be performed prior to releasing the device for clinical use.

Immobilization devices should also be tested to ensure that they fit within the MRI bore. RT immobilisation devices are traditionally designed for large bore CT simulators and open table linear accelerators, so ensuring these devices are compatible with a MRI closed-bore scanner is essential.

It is also important to note that RT immobilisation equipment can have a severe impact on the overall image quality of MRI simulation scans and this should be quantitatively assessed with phantom studies. This will be addressed in further detail in Sect. 1.2.4.1.

1.2.2 Training

To introduce an MRI into the radiation therapy workflow in a safe and effective manner, training is essential. MR imaging requires specialised expertise, which is very distinct from kV-based imaging. Training is a multidisciplinary effort in which the radiation technologists (RTT), as well as the radiation oncologists (RTO), and medical physicists (MP) must be involved. The obvious common ground here is MRI safety as discussed below, but also the quality of the images is something that needs to be reviewed periodically in order to assure that the image quality remains of high standard. Continuing education is extremely important as imaging protocols and the use of the images (e.g. MR-only and 4D-MRI) continue to evolve. A good collaboration with radiology is therefore extremely beneficial when setting up an MRI for RT.

For departments that share resources with radiology, the collaboration is prerequisite as the logistics need to be aligned. Scan slots for radiotherapy, for example, need to be longer than a regular diagnostic scan slot as patient setup takes more time (e.g. due to accurate laser alignment and the use of positioning devices). Even when a radiation therapy department owns dedicated MRI-RT systems, it is advisable to maintain a close collaboration with radiology. The experienced radiology staff may contribute in setting up safety procedures and assist in protocol development and quality assurance. Furthermore, the established relationship between the radiology department and the MRI vendor can be very useful when service is required or when purchasing new equipment.

1.2.3 MR Safety

1.2.3.1 Safety Certification and Scanner Access

Departmental safety training for all staff in oncology will ensure that staff who require access to Zones III or IV are made aware of the most recent information regarding both international and local safety standards. Access to the MRI room should be strictly monitored, preferably with smart card or key access only granted to staff that are abreast of MRI safety standards. The American College of Radiology recommends that all individuals working in Zone III should have successfully attended MRI safety lectures and live presentations and that these should be repeated annually and documented to confirm ongoing educational efforts (Kanal et al. 2013).

1.2.3.2 Safety Screening

All staff involved in the day-to-day scanning of patients in MRI departments should be screened prior to working in this section of the department. There are many examples of MRI screening questionnaires available, including online sources (Shellock 2017a) or adapted versions from established radiology departments. The screening form should be completed and reviewed by the Principal Physicist or MRI safety officer in charge of the area to ensure staff are safe to work in the area prior to commencement.

Patients should complete a safety questionnaire prior to MRI simulation, to assess their suitability for the procedure and detect any potential contraindications to the MRI. This should be completed with a trained MRI technician or the RTO at time of consultation for radiation therapy. The screening questionnaire should be completed with ample time to review and ensure any potential devices that the patient may have implanted are checked for compatibility with the MRI simulator.

For patients with implantable medical devices, the Medicines and Healthcare products Regulatory Agency (MHRA) recommends that a risk assessment should be undertaken with involvement of a multidisciplinary team including the MR responsible person (radiation therapist or diagnostic MRI technician), MR safety expert (MRI Physicist) and relevant specialist clinician (radiologist or oncologist) (Medicines and Healthcare products Regulatory Agency (MHRA) 2007). They advise that the following should be considered:

- Alternative imaging modalities.
- Imaging on an MRI with a lower static and/or gradient field.
- Advise from implant manufacturer.
- Locally available advice and recommendation from professional organisation.
- Published evidence of scanning the device.
- Available data about the device.
- Assessment of MRI artefacts arising from the device.
- MRI device parameters.

The decision to image a patient with an implantable medical device should be decided by local departmental protocol based on recommendations and advice from your local governing professional organisation.

1.2.3.3 Vascular Devices In Situ

Patients undergoing concurrent chemoradiotherapy (CRT) may have vascular devices inserted such as port-a-caths (ports) and peripherally inserted central catheters (PICCs) at time of their MR imaging. Ports and PICCs are common in situ vascular devices used in oncology with specific safety restrictions for scanning in MRI. Patients with these devices should be scanned under particular conditions, and the technician staff needs to ensure that specific absorption rate (SAR) levels are strictly controlled.

Considerations

Prior to MR scanning, the referring physician is responsible for managing the patient relative to the use of MRI and ensures that the following information regarding the device is considered:

- *Compatibility of device at specific field strength.*
  Before a patient with a vascular device is scanned in the MRI, the MRI compatibility of the device should be confirmed for the field strength of the scanner.
- *Safe spatial gradient field recommendations as defined by the device manufacturer.*
  Individual scanners will have a unique spatial gradient field map (i.e. change in B0 field with proximity to bore), and this should be used as a guide to determine where the strongest spatial gradient field is in relation to the device.
- *MRI-related heating using normal and first level SAR limits.*
  Scan modes typically include normal (2 W/kg) and first level (3 W/kg) modes (vendor neutral). The modes determine the tolerance for SAR levels during a single examination. Manufacturers of these devices will usually include safe scan mode recommendations based on their own independent testing, and this should be followed in the clinical setting to ensure safe scanning of patients with these devices.

1.2.3.4 Cardiac Pacemakers and Defibrillators

Cardiac pacemakers and implantable cardioverter defibrillators (ICDs) are devices implanted into patients to help control abnormal heart rhythms by using electrical pulses to ensure the heart beats at a normal rate. For patients with these devices, the MRI compatibility of the devices must also be confirmed with manufacturer guidelines prior to the MR simulation exam.

Legacy pacemaker's and ICD devices have traditionally been contraindicated in MRI as the risks to the patient outweigh the benefits. Potential problems include (Shellock 2017b):

- Movement of the device or leads.
- Potential adverse modification of function of the device.
- Unavoidable triggering or activation of the device.
- Heating in the leads.
- Induced currents in the leads.
- Electromagnetic interferences.

These effects often pertain to older cardiac pacemakers and ICDs; consequently patients with devices implanted prior to the year 2000 are at greatest risk during MRI scanning (Ahmed et al. 2013). Therefore, the risk versus benefits need to be weighed when considering MRI for patients with older cardiac pacemakers and ICDs, even if they are safe for radiation therapy. Some manufacturers of modern cardiac pacemakers and ICDs (post-2000) have developed MRI-conditional devices that can be scanned under particular conditions (e.g. 1.5 T or less). Manufacturer guidelines should be followed strictly to ensure that the patient is safe during the MRI exam. This includes monitoring the performance and functionality of the device before, during and after scanning.

It is also important to note that patients who have MRI-compatible devices must also have the leads checked for compatibility. Some leads may not be MRI compatible and can have potential to heat or induce current during the MRI scanning process.

1.2.3.5 Safe Administration of Gadolinium

Gadolinium-based contrast agents (GBCAs) are commonly used to enhance T_1 images in areas of abnormality by shortening the T_1 relaxation properties of the local microenvironment. These agents are filtered through the kidneys. There are two types of GBCAs based on their chemical structure: linear and macrocyclic. Mounting evidence demonstrates that linear GBCAs are retained in the body longer compared to macrocyclic GBCAs, with higher levels of gadolinium remaining in the body after administration of linear GBCAs (U.S. Food and Drug Administration 2017). Both the FDA and European Medicines Agency recommend the suspension of linear GBCAs except for liver-specific agents such as gadoxetic and gadobenic acids as they are taken up in the liver only and its benefits outweigh the risks.

Prior to administration of contrast, appropriate blood analysis including eGFR (estimated glomerular filtration rate) and creatinine should be assessed in the patient to ensure that kidney function is optimal for filtration of GBCAs' post administration. The patient should be counselled on possible side effects of gadolinium based on local departmental guidelines.

Clinically, the usefulness of contrast-enhanced MR imaging should be weighed against contrast-enhanced CT. There is little evidence in the literature to suggest the optimal waiting time between administration of iodine and GBCAs. However, Golder et al. recommend that "it is advisable to wait longer than one day to perform the second iodine or gadolinium-enhanced test" (Golder 2012). Although GBCAs can be safely administered within a short period of iodinated contrast, the burden to the patient having double contrast within a short period of time should be considered in the planning process.

1.2.4 Integrate MRI into the RTP Workflow

MRI datasets can be used for both registrations to CT to assist in tumour and organs at risk (OAR) delineation in radiotherapy planning and also to be used solely for the purposes of MR-only planning.

Scans acquired in the radiology setting are used to investigate where the disease is and deduce a differential diagnosis based on its imaging features (Devic 2012). Although diagnostic acquired MRI does not consider the treatment position of the patient, these datasets may still be useful for registration to CT to assist with planning so long as there is an indicator of the geometric fidelity of the diagnostic MR images.

The following section will address various scenarios where MRI can be used in conjunction with CT and can be used as a guide for the effective use of MRI in individualised clinical settings based on Fig. 1.2.

1.2.4.1 MRI Acquired in Radiotherapy Position

Immobilisation devices are used to minimise the risk of movement and improve overall reproducibility for fractionated treatments (Devic 2012). Figure 1.3a shows various immobilisation devices used for radiation therapy setup including a flat table overlay with indexing, thermoplastic mask secured to the flat table as well as knee and ankle fixation devices.

For imaging in the treatment position, there are a number of considerations when using RT immobilisation equipment including:

- Flat table overlay.
  - In-house built tables as well as commercially available devices should be tested to ensure the materials do not cause any heating.
  - The thickness of the table should be measured to assess signal-to-noise ratio (SNR) loss resulting from the increased distance between the patient and the integrated RF coils under the bed.
- Thermoplastic masks, knee, and ankle fixation.
  - All devices should be tested to ensure the materials do not cause any heating and are compatible with flat table overlay and indexing system.

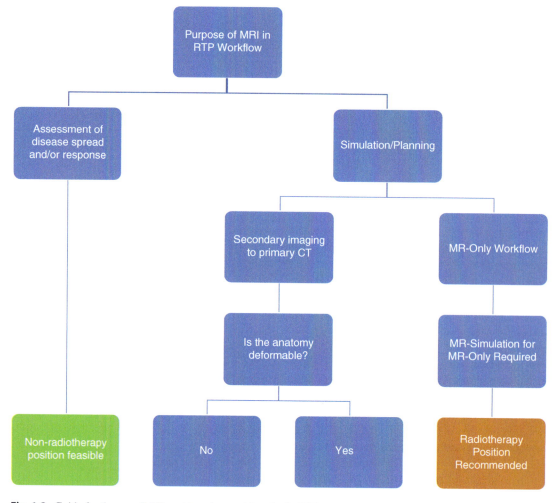

Fig. 1.2 Guide for the use of different imaging positions in the RTP workflow

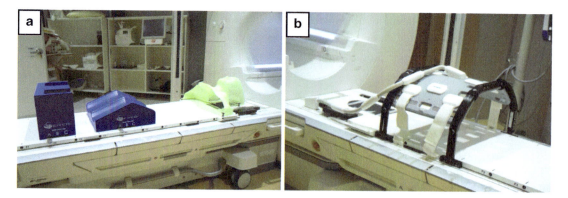

Fig. 1.3 Various RT-specific immobilisation devices that can be used in MRI for reproducible setup to improve registration to CT in the planning process including (**a**) thermoplastic masks, flat table overlays, and knee and ankle fixation devices and (**b**) RF coils attached to bridges to minimise deformation of external body contours

- RF coil bridges.
  - Similar to the flat table overlay, the addition of RF coil bridges (Fig. 1.3b) may increase the distance between the region being scanned and the coil elements. Imaging protocols may have to be adjusted accordingly.

Figure 1.4 shows an example of a head and neck setup using a thermoplastic mask and vacuum bag. These setups will often require the use of flexible coils arranged to cover the anatomy of interest. Signal to noise ratio should be taken into consideration with individual coil arrangements and sequences required for planning.

In the case that the MRI will be used as a secondary imaging modality to the primary CT, coils can be placed directly over the patient anatomy to improve the overall image quality as long as the region of interest is not deformed by the weight of the coil.

External lasers can be useful in aligning patients to reproduce their CT simulation position. In complex setups such as extremities (Fig. 1.5a), care should be taken to try to position target volumes as close to MR isocentre as possible. This may require the patient be offset laterally in the MRI bore (Fig. 1.5b) but will reduce residual geometric distortions. For modern MRI scanners where closed-bore systems are becoming the norm, the use of RT immobilisation devices may pose positioning challenges due to size restrictions, and this should be taken into consideration for radiotherapy planning positions.

1.2.4.2 MRI Acquired in Non-radiotherapy Position

For anatomical regions where deformation and variation in position of targets and OARs are prevalent, such as the abdomen, head, and neck, MR images acquired with a non-radiotherapy position may be difficult to co-register to planning CT images for RTP. In regions where deformation of the anatomy is not an issue, such as the brain, scans acquired with diagnostic RF coils and non-radiotherapy position may still be useful for registration to CT (Fig. 1.6). These aspects of image registration will be covered in Chap. 2.

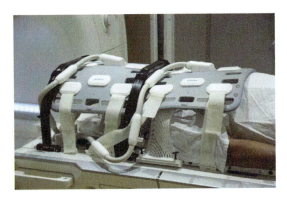

Fig. 1.4 Example of a head and neck setup with the patient immobilised using a thermoplastic mask and vacuum bag

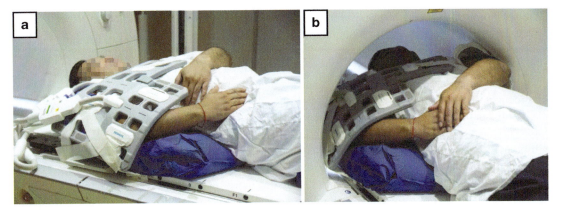

Fig. 1.5 Example of upper extremity setup using a tailored coil arrangement (**a**). The participants was offset laterally to position the arm closer to the isocentre of the MRI to improve image quality (**b**)

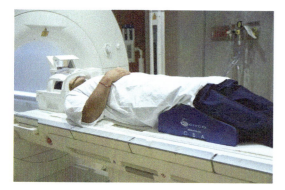

Fig. 1.6 Positioning for brain imaging using a dedicated head and neck coil in a diagnostic MRI setup

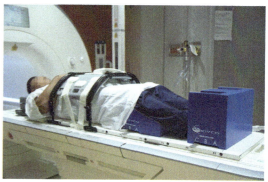

Fig. 1.7 Example of a pelvis setup in the radiotherapy position. The coil is suspended above the subject's pelvis and secured with Velcro to coil bridges to minimise deformation of the external body contour

The advantages of using a non-radiotherapy position with dedicated anatomical coils include (1) improvement in image quality due to increased SNR, (2) greater comfort for the patient as immobilisation devices do not need to be used, and (3) minimisation of the risk of motion artefacts.

1.2.4.3 MR-Only Planning

MR-only planning workflows require specific sequences for synthetic CT generation and are discussed in detail in Chaps. 8 and 9.

In regard to setup, patients should be positioned in their treatment position, ideally in an MRI simulator or diagnostic department equipped with RT-specific immobilisation, external laser positioning, and marking system for alignment. In comparison to MRI acquisition as a complimentary modality to CT, care needs to be taken when placing RF coils over the anatomy of interest. Coils should not be directly placed over the anatomical regions as any added weight from the coil on the anatomy can deform the external body contours, leading to a potential variation in dose (Fig. 1.7).

High-resolution large field-of-view imaging is a prerequisite for MR-only workflows, and coverage of the entire treatment volume is essential. For anatomical sites in which fiducial markers will be used for registration, such as in prostate, MRI examinations should include sequences that will assist with the visualisation of these markers such as gradient echo or proton density-weighted turbo spin echo. These sequences will enhance the paramagnetic susceptibility effects of these fiducials as they are often made of gold or polymer with a stainless steel core.

1.3 Acquisition Protocols for RTP

MRI for RTP requires dedicated imaging protocols to ensure high imaging standards for RTP including high resolution with minimal geometric distortions. This section covers the basic MR theory needed for protocol development and will detail recommended parameters for MR simulation for RTP.

1.3.1 Image Contrast

MRI is an extremely versatile imaging modality. Unlike any other modality, MRI offers a vast array of image contrasts. A typical exam for radiotherapy treatment planning therefore includes a number of contrasts that offer complementary information.

1.3.1.1 Anatomical Imaging: T1 and T2 Contrast

The most fundamental properties that MRI makes use of are T1 and T2 relaxation (Table 1.1) (De Bazelaire et al. 2004; Stanisz et al. 2005; Wansapura et al. 1999). Since the relaxation phenomenon is described in much detail in all textbooks on MRI physics (King et al. 2004; Haacke

Table 1.1 T1 and T2 relaxation times at 1.5 and 3 T

Tissue	1.5 T T1 (ms)	1.5 T T2 (ms)	3 T T1 (ms)	3 T T2 (ms)
Subcutaneous fat	343	58	382	68
Liver	586	46	809	34
Pancreas	584	46	725	43
Spleen	1057	79	1328	61
Muscle	856	27	898	29
Prostate	1317	88	1597	74
White matter	600	80	830	80
Grey matter	900	100	1330	110
CSF	3500	2200	4000	2000

et al. 2014; McRobbie et al. 2006), we suffice here by reminding the reader that T1 relaxation describes the realignment of the proton spins towards the direction of the magnetic field, while T2 relaxation refers to the loss of coherence in transverse magnetization. The different tissues in the human body all have their own characteristic T1 and T2 relaxation rates (Table 1.1). These differences in relaxation are at the basis of contrast generation. Contrast is generated by setting the RF flip angle and the sequence timing parameters in such a way that differences in signal intensity between species with different relaxation parameters are maximized. Relaxation rates at 3 T are different than those at 1.5 T, so the sequence parameters required to generate optimal contrast will also vary for the different field strengths.

T1 Contrast

The timing parameter that determines T1 contrast is the repetition time (TR). By increasing the TR, more time is allowed for the longitudinal magnetization (M_L) to recover to its equilibrium state. The amount of longitudinal magnetization determines the amount of signal that is available for the next readout. Figure 1.8a shows the longitudinal relaxation after a 90° RF pulse. It takes about five times the T1 for the longitudinal magnetization to fully recover. By choosing a shorter TR (denoted by the dotted line), the magnetization will only partly recover, but, more importantly, the amount of recovery will be different between different tissues. Tissues with a short T1 (e.g. liver tissue) will thus provide higher signal than tissues with a long T1 (e.g. muscle or CSF). T1 contrast is optimized by finding the right combination of RF flip angle and TR. Additionally, T1 weighting can be amplified by placing an inversion pulse in front of the sequence, which inverts the longitudinal magnetization of both species to be antiparallel with the main magnetic field (Fig. 1.8c). By carefully choosing the inversion time (TI: the time between the inversion pulse and the regular excitation pulse), one could null (i.e. suppress) the signal of one of the two species as described in more detail in Sect. 1.3.1.2.

T2 Contrast

T2 contrast is determined by the echo time (TE), which is the time between the RF excitation pulse and the actual collection of the data. Immediately after the RF pulse, the spins start to dephase, which causes a reduction of the transverse magnetization (M_T), and thus signal (Fig. 1.8b). The rate of dephasing is different for each tissue and determined by the different T2 values. Again, the contrast is optimized by choosing the timing parameter (in this case the TE) in such a way that the difference between species A and B is maximized. For sequences that acquire multiple lines of k-space per TR, for example, turbo spin echo (TSE), the TE is defined as the time at which the central line in k-space is collected.

The Effect of Gadolinium

Because of its paramagnetic properties, gadolinium shortens both the T1 and the T2 relaxation times. Which effect dominates depends on the baseline relaxation times of the tissue under investigation and gadolinium concentration, but for most anatomical imaging, gadolinium is administered to enhance T1 contrast. By shortening the T1 of the nearby hydrogen protons, the signal is enhanced in areas where the contrast agent is present. Especially for brain tumours that have leaky vessels, contrast-enhanced imaging is very useful to distinguish between active tumour tissue and the necrotic core. An example showing the effect of contrast enhancement is shown by Fig. 1.8d.

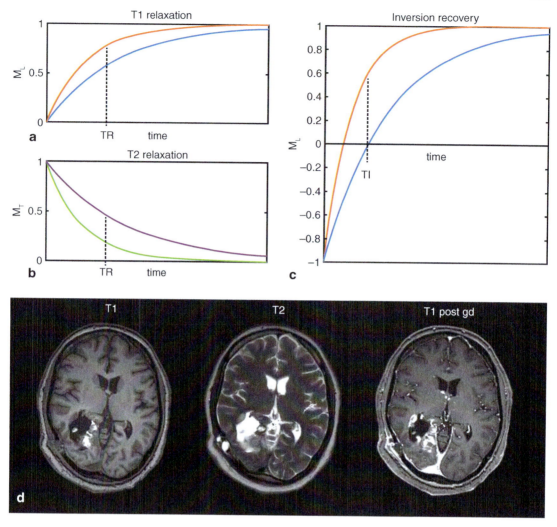

Fig. 1.8 Panels **a**–**c** show T1 and T2 relaxation curves with optimal timing parameters (TR, TE, and TI) denoted by the dotted lines. Panel **a** shows the longitudinal relaxation after a 90° RF pulse, while panel **c** simulates a 180° inversion pulse. Panel **d** shows examples of T1-weighted, T2-weighted, and post contrast T1-weighted images

1.3.1.2 Anatomical Imaging: Fat Suppression

Due to its short T1 and due to T2 elongation effects (Hardy et al. 1992; Stables et al. 1999), fat appears very bright on both T1-weighted (T1w) and T2-weighted (T2w) TSE imaging. The bright signal of fat can obscure pathology and hamper delineation of tumours that are bordering or invading fatty tissue. Examples are breast tumours, head and neck tumours, or mediastinal lymph nodes in oesophageal or advanced lung cancer. Fortunately a number of methods exist to suppress the bright signal of fat to enhance the contrast.

STIR. Short tau inversion recovery (Fleckenstein et al. 1991) is a fat suppression technique that relies on the short T1 relaxation of fat. The sequence consists of an inversion recovery pulse, followed by a specific inversion time (TI) that corresponds to the time at which the longitudinal magnetization of fat crosses zero. At that time the 90° excitation pulse, which puts the (non-zero) longitudinal magnetization of all other tissues into the transverse plane, is applied, and the data is collected. The technique is insensitive to off resonance, but the non-selective inversion causes a drop in SNR as it also partially saturates the longitudinal magnetization of other tissues (Fig. 1.8c). By changing the TI, other species such as cerebral spinal fluid (CSF) can also be nulled. This technique is utilized by the fluid-attenuated inversion recovery (FLAIR) sequence (De Coene et al. 1992; Hajnal et al. 1992).

SPIR. Spectral presaturation with inversion recovery (Oh et al. 1988). This technique differs from STIR in the sense that the inversion pulse is a spectrally selective pulse. As a result only fat signal is inverted. The benefit compared to STIR is the improved SNR due to the fact that the longitudinal magnetization of the other tissues is unaffected by the inversion. The spectral-selective inversion, however, makes SPIR sensitive to B0 inhomogeneities and may therefore be less effective in regions like the thorax.

SPAIR. Spectral adiabatic inversion recovery (King et al. 2004). This technique is very similar to SPIR, except that the inversion pulse is changed to an adiabatic pulse, which makes the sequence insensitive to B1 inhomogeneities. SPAIR preparation usually takes a little longer than SPIR, leading to increased total scan duration. Figure 1.9c provides an example of SPAIR fat suppression.

DIXON imaging. The DIXON method (Dixon 1984) takes advantage of the resonance frequency offset between water and fat. Due to the difference in precession frequency between water and fat, a phase difference is introduced, which is a function of TE. For a frequency offset of 220 Hz (the frequency offset at 1.5 T), water and fat will be out of phase at TE = 2.3 ms and in phase at TE = 4.5 ms. When water and fat are out of phase, their signal will cancel, and the resulting signal will thus be reduced in voxels that contain both water and fat. The DIXON technique takes advantage of this phenomenon by acquiring multiple images with different TE. By solving a set of linear equations, the amount of water and fat can be calculated, and separate water and fat images can be produced. This technique has the advantage of high SNR and reduced sensitivity to B0 inhomogeneities, although at large field offsets, water-fat swaps can occur in the reconstructed images. In many cases DIXON is the preferred fat suppression technique.

1.3.1.3 Applications

The use of T1 and T2 with or without fat saturation is heavily dependent on the anatomical site and the type of tumour. T1-weighted imaging is often performed in conjunction with contrast enhancement. For H&N T1 pre- and post-contrast with fat saturation is used for GTV delineation and to assess tumour invasion into fat. In the prostate T1 Dixon is used to identify abnormalities, such as haemorrhages due to biopsies or fiducial marker implantation, as these lesions may look similar to tumour foci on T2w scans (Philippens 2016). T2-weighted imaging with fat saturation is used in H&N for the identification of oedema, delineation of salivary glands, and detection of metastatic lymph nodes. For rectum cancer, the GTV as well as the mesorectum and bladder are delineated on T2w scans, while in the lung, T2w-fatsat can be used to identify metastatic mediastinal lymph nodes (Cobben et al. 2015). T2w-FLAIR imaging is used to visualise oedema in the brain.

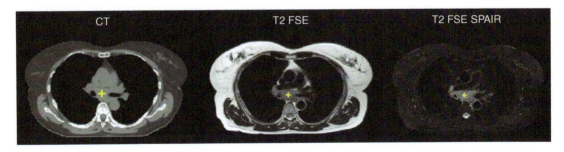

Fig. 1.9 Example of effective fat saturation in a stage III lung cancer patient. The T2-TSE with SPAIR fat saturation highlights a large positive mediastinal lymph node (N7). The T2 without fat saturation is acquired to define surrounding anatomy

Table 1.2 RT-specific parameters for MRI acquisition for the purposes of RTP

Parameter	Recommendation	Purpose
Field of view (FOV)	At least one scan with full FOV covering the entire radiation window (including skin contours)	Full FOV needed for MR-to-CT registration and MR-only workflows
In-plane resolution	≤1 mm (Paulson et al. 2016; Liney et al. 2013)	Detailed view of tumour and organ boundaries
Slice thickness	1–2 mm (CNS including stereotactic) 2–3 mm (body and extremity imaging)	Detailed view of tumour and organ boundaries and improves digitally reconstructed radiograph image quality for MR-only workflows (Paulson et al. 2014)
Slice gaps	0 mm	Zero slice gap maintains true slice resolution
Readout bandwidth	≥440 Hz/mm at 3 T ≥220 Hz/mm at 1.5 T (Allow ≤1 mm fat-water shift)	High bandwidth minimises chemical shift and susceptibility-induced spatial distortions (Paulson et al. 2014; Liney and Moerland 2014)
Gradient non-linearity correction	3D is a minimum requirement (Paulson et al. 2016). 2D can be used if a 3D option is unavailable[a]	Correction of in-plane (2D and 3D) and through-plane (3D) distortions induced by gradient non-linearities (Walker et al. 2015)
B0-induced distortion correction (field map)	Optional	Can be used to correct B0-susceptibility distortions

[a]Availability is based on vendor and availability for certain sequences

Chapter 4 provides a comprehensive overview of the literature supporting the use of planning MRI across all these sites.

1.3.2 Image Acquisition Strategies

Unlike diagnostic MRI, RT requirements are more stringent and require close monitoring to ensure both geometric integrity of imaging and optimal image quality for target delineation. Table 1.2 outlines a summary of recommendations to improve the geometrical and positional accuracy of MR imaging acquired for the purposes of RTP.

1.3.2.1 Resolution and Field-of-View Requirements

The acquisition of multiple scans with different contrasts often results in lengthy exams. To reduce the overall scan time, the FOV is usually limited as much as possible. It is, however, required that at least one sequence is acquired at full FOV that covers the entire radiation window, to aid in the registration from MR to CT. This sequence, which should be acquired with geometric accuracy as an absolute prioritization, serves as a link between the other MR images and planning CT in a CT-based workflow. In an MRI-only workflow, this full-FOV sequence will provide the source data for the synthetic CT generation.

In terms of resolution, the requirements for RT treatment planning are higher than in diagnostic imaging. Whereas diagnostic MRI is optimized to provide high detectability of lesions, the purpose of pretreatment imaging is accurate demarcation of the target area (i.e. lesion) and/or organs at risk. For radiotherapy purposes the in-plane resolution must be around 1 mm. Slice thickness can either be 1–2 mm for CNS applications and up to 3 mm for body and extremity imaging. The achievable resolution depends on two other factors that are key in MRI: the image SNR and available scan time. The relation between these three factors is informally referred to as the Holy Trinity of Image Quality. Depending on the other two factors, the resolution requirements may sometimes not be entirely met for each sequence in the exam.

1.3.2.2 2D Multi-slice

The process of image formation starts with a selective-excitation RF pulse that restricts the excitation to a two-dimensional plane or slab of interest within the patient. A selective excitation is achieved by applying a field gradient *during* the excitation pulse. By changing the centre frequency of the RF pulse, one can alter the location of the excited slice along the applied gradient. Once the slice or slab is excited, imaging gradients are played out to sample a 2D k-space and ultimately form a 2D image via a Fourier transform (detailed information on MR image formation can be found in the following text books (King et al. 2004; Haacke et al. 2014; McRobbie et al. 2006)). This technique, in which a single line of k-space is acquired with each RF pulse, is referred to as 2DFT imaging. In order to collect volumetric imaging data, one could repeat the acquisition for multiple slice locations. For each slice the location is adjusted by changing the centre frequency of the RF pulse. In theory one is free to choose the order in which the slices are collected, but on most scanners, the ordering is limited to sequential (one after another, in subsequent order: 1, 2, 3, ..., n) or interleaved (first the even slices, followed by the odd slices: 2, 4, 6,..., n, 1, 2, 3 ..., $n − 1$). Normally interleaved would be preferred to mitigate slice crosstalk caused by the imperfect slice excitation profile: due to imperfections in the slice excitation pulse, a portion of the spins experiences excitation twice when adjacent slices are excited directly after one another. The thinner the slice, the more difficult it is to produce a rectangular slice profile. Also, SNR is linearly dependent on the slice thickness, where thinner slices produce lower SNR. For these reasons, a slice thickness < 3 mm usually very hard to achieve in 2D multi-slice imaging.

1.3.2.3 3D Volumetric Imaging

A solution that overcomes the problem of slice profile imperfections is to acquire a 3D volume instead of multiple 2D slices. The advantage of 3D versus 2D acquisitions is that 3D imaging allows isotropic high-resolution imaging, since the slice thickness is not limited by the slice excitation profile. Because the entire volume is excited with every RF pulse (and hence is contributing to the signal), the SNR is higher for scans with an equivalent slice thickness. The disadvantage of 3D acquisitions is that the TR is typically short, which limits the use of prepulses (e.g. fat saturation or T1 enhancement pulses) in combination with some imaging contrasts. Also, a 3D readout is longer than a 2D readout, which makes 3D acquisition more sensitive to motion than 2D acquisitions. The short TR in 3D imaging makes GRE the most natural contrast for 3D acquisitions. This includes spoiled sequences, such as SPGR (or FLASH), that provide pure T1 contrast as well as steady-state sequences, such bSSFP, that provide a T2/T1 contrast. More recently, however, 3D T2-TSE is becoming more mainstream due to the advances in echo train design, which enable acquisitions with very long echo trains. Due to the long echo trains, 3D T2-TSE typically has a stronger T2 weighting compared to 2D T2-TSE acquisitions.

1.3.2.4 Non-Cartesian Readouts

During the acquisition, k-space is sampled via a path defined by the applied gradients. There are many trajectories possible. Most clinical exams sample k-space along a Cartesian (i.e. rectilinear) grid. A Cartesian readout is a very robust acquisition scheme, since errors in gradient timing, off-resonance effects, or other imperfections only have an effect along a single direction in k-space. The artefacts are therefore either small or predictable. This is the main reason why Cartesian readouts are often the method of choice in clinical exams. A disadvantage of Cartesian readouts is that geometric distortions, caused by field inhomogeneities, also manifest in a single direction, causing a systematic offset (Sect. 1.3.3). Non-Cartesian readouts are defined as readouts that do not follow the Cartesian grid. By applying a combination of gradients, any path through k-space can be traversed. Examples that are offered by most vendors are radial or spiral trajectories. Non-Cartesian readouts are often used to overcome some of the limitations of Cartesian imaging. Radial readouts, for example, have the advantage that the centre of k-space is sampled by every readout line, which makes it very robust against intraview motion (i.e. motion during acquisition). Due to the rotating readout direction, field inhomogeneities manifest as image blur rather than a geometric offset. Another benefit of non-Cartesian imaging is the fact that undersampling artefacts are incoherent in imaging space, which is beneficial for iterative reconstruction techniques, like compressed sensing, that allow higher acceleration factors compared to the traditional parallel imaging techniques (Sect. 1.3.2.6).

1.3.2.5 Echo-Planar Imaging

Echo-planar imaging (EPI) requires special mentioning in imaging for radiotherapy. EPI was developed in 1977 by Sir Peter Mansfield and is still one of the fastest readout methods to date (Mansfield and Pykett 1978). EPI differs from 2DFT imaging in the sense that multiple phase-encode lines are acquired after a single RF excitation. In EPI the readout gradients are quickly reversed multiple times to generate a series of gradient echoes. Interspersed phase-encode gradients are applied to spatially encode each gradient echo such that multiple k-space lines are sampled after a single excitation. This significantly increases acquisition speed. For this reason EPI was also referred to as snapshot imaging. The property that an entire 2D k-space can be collected after a single excitation is extremely important for diffusion-weighted imaging (DWI), which requires all the k-lines to be acquired with the same motion sensitization. For this reason EPI is the main workhorse for DWI. A downside of EPI that does not match well with the high geometric accuracy required in radiotherapy is the increased sensitivity to geometric distortions. Geometric distortions in EPI are an order of magnitude higher due to the relatively low bandwidth along the phase-encode axis (typically 30 Hz/px). The poor geometric fidelity of EPI-based DWI is something that should be taken into consideration when using this type of imaging for treatment preparation.

1.3.2.6 Image Acceleration Methods

Most clinical exams use standard acceleration methods such as partial Fourier and parallel imaging to reduce scan time. Partial Fourier can be applied effectively to speed up the acquisition by up to 40% without considerable loss in image quality. In partial Fourier (PF) only a portion of k-space (5/8 or more) is collected. PF methods rely on the property of the Fourier transform that real functions have conjugate symmetry in k-space. The simplest PF reconstruction fills the missing lines with zeros, whereas other methods synthesize the uncollected lines in k-space by exploiting conjugate phase symmetry in k-space. Downsides of partial Fourier are reduced SNR and potential image blur (in the case of zero filling).

Parallel imaging can be employed to further accelerate the acquisition. Parallel imaging methods use the spatially varying coil sensitivity profiles in multichannel receiver coil arrays to subsample k-space (e.g. by skipping every other line) (Roemer et al. 1990; Sodickson and Manning 1997; Pruessmann et al. 1999; Griswold et al. 2002). Various accelerated parallel imaging reconstructions have been implemented by the vendors that either work in the image domain or in k-space. While SENSitivity encoding for fast MRI (SENSE) (Pruessmann et al. 1999) operates in the image domain, generalized autocalibrating partially parallel acquisitions (GRAPPA) (Griswold et al. 2002) operates in the k-space domain. The amount of acceleration depends on the coil geometry and undersampling pattern. In general higher acceleration factors can be achieved for 3D acquisitions, as the undersampling (and thus resulting aliasing) can be spread over two dimensions. Typical acceleration factors for current clinically available multichannel (e.g. 32 channels) arrays range between $R = 3$ for 2D and $R = 6$ (2×3) for 3D acquisitions.

A more recent development is compressed sensing (CS) MRI (Lustig et al. 2007). CS MRI is an approach to image acceleration that is founded on the notion that all medical images can be compressed by finding an appropriate transform domain, in which the image can be sparsely represented (e.g. spatial finite differences or wavelet domain). This, together with a random sampling pattern in k-space, allows images to be reconstructed from far fewer data than prescribed by the Nyquist-Shannon sampling theorem (Liu and Saloner 2014). CS has allowed up to 20-fold image acceleration, far higher than any parallel imaging technique (Lustig et al. 2007). Several vendors are now offering CS MRI as product to further accelerate clinical exams. The iterative nature of the reconstruction, however, results in reconstruction times that are considerably longer than conventional linear reconstruction methods.

1.3.3 Geometric Distortions

Geometric fidelity is absolutely essential in image-guided RT. In contrast to projection imaging (i.e. CT), the geometric fidelity in MRI is not guaranteed and may be unacceptable if the acquisition parameters are set incorrectly. In MRI geometric distortions may arise from three distinct sources: (1) system B0 inhomogeneity, (2) gradient non-linearities, and (3) patient-induced susceptibility effects as depicted in Fig. 1.10. Fortunately, all these effects are measurable, reproducible, and predictable, which is described in detail in Chap. 3. With the appropriate measures, the geometric distortions can be largely mitigated and reduced to levels that are well within clinically acceptable levels.

1.3.3.1 Mitigating Geometric Distortions

Although geometric distortions can be potentially large when not taken into account appropriately, a number of effective methods exist to minimize the distortions and to assure a geometric fidelity that is adequate for radiation therapy planning. System B0 inhomogeneity can be reduced by careful placement of shim irons during the installation phase of the magnet, while gradient non-linearities are also corrected for adequately by the vendor-provided implementations. To further minimize the effects of gradient non-linearities, the prescribed imaging volume should be shifted to the scanner isocentre. In addition, several methods have been proposed that correct for the residual geometric distortion (Baldwin et al. 2007; Doran et al. 2005), although these corrections have not yet made it to routine clinical use. Patient-induced field offsets, as well as system B0 inhomogeneities, are best mitigated by increasing the readout bandwidth. The resulting displacement is inversely linear with the readout bandwidth, so doubling the readout bandwidth halves the effective distortion. Note, however, that the SNR will also be reduced by a factor of $\sqrt{2}$. Single-shot EPI readouts are particularly prone to distortions due to the low bandwidth along the phase-encode direction (Jezzard and Balaban 1995). To reduce distortions the echo train length can be shortened by combining partial Fourier and parallel imaging or segmentation (i.e. changing the sequence to a multi-shot acquisition), adjusting the readout bandwidth to minimize the spacing between gradient echoes and using the minimum TE. Another solution is to acquire a B0 field map, which measures magnetic field across the image. Using the information of the local magnetic field, the distorted images can be corrected retrospectively (Jezzard and Balaban 1995; Andersson et al. 2001; Hutton et al. 2002; Jenkinson 2003).

1.3.3.2 Water-Fat Shift

A separate, but related spatial displacement error is the well-known water-fat shift. The water-fat

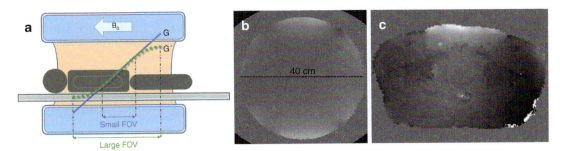

Fig. 1.10 Different sources of geometric distortion: (**a**) gradient-non-linearities depicted by the green dotted line, (**b**) system B0 inhomogeneities measured with a large spherical phantom, and (**c**) patient induced susceptibility effects shown by the in vivo acquired B0 map

shift refers to the relative shift of fat compared to water and is caused a difference in resonance frequency between the protons in fat and in water. Due to the different chemical compositions of fat, the resonance frequency of protons in fat molecules is slightly slower than the protons in water molecules. This difference is referred to as the chemical shift and has been determined to be approximately 3.5 ppm. This corresponds to an absolute difference of approximately 220 and 440 Hz at 1.5 and 3 T, respectively. Due to this shift, fatty tissue will appear shifted compared to water. Particularly in readouts with low bandwidth (e.g. the phase-encode direction in EPI), the water-fat shift can be severe (Jezzard and Clare 1999). It is advisable to keep the water-fat shift <1 mm to prevent errors in image registration arising from structures dominated by unsuppressed fat.

1.3.4 Field Strength

3 T offers higher SNR and thus allows scanning at higher resolution. Susceptibility effects, however, are also stronger, which may introduce higher image distortions if not mitigated by reducing the readout duration (e.g. by choosing a higher readout bandwidth). The choice between 1.5 and 3 T is therefore a balance between the required image resolution and geometric distortion, which might be different between anatomical sites and applications. For example, pelvic regions are less susceptible to field inhomogeneities and will benefit from the increased SNR at 3 T with manageable increase in image distortions, while thoracic imaging (e.g. oesophagus and lung) is not recommended due to the large tissue-air interfaces (Bainbridge et al. 2017). For the brain, a site that is easily shimmed, the trade-off is made based on the application. For large tumours and gliomas, patients are recommended to be scanned at 3 T to benefit from the improved contrast and SNR, while SRS patients are scanned in thermoplastic mask on a 1.5 T to guarantee optimal geometric accuracy (Philippens 2016).

References

Ahmed FZ, Morris GM, Allen S, Khattar R, Mamas M, Zaidi A. Not all pacemakers are created equal: MRI conditional pacemaker and lead technology. J Cardiovasc Electrophysiol. 2013;24(9):1059–65. https://doi.org/10.1111/jce.12238.

Andersson JLR, Hutton C, Ashburner J, Turner R, Friston K. Modeling geometric deformations in EPI time series. NeuroImage. 2001;13(5):903–19.

Bainbridge H, Salem A, Tijssen RHN, et al. Magnetic resonance imaging in precision radiation therapy for lung cancer. Transl Lung Cancer Res. 2017;6(6):689.

Baldwin LN, Wachowicz K, Thomas SD, Rivest R, Fallone BG. Characterization, prediction, and correction of geometric distortion in MR images. Med Phys. 2007;34(2):388–99.

Haacke ME, Thompson MR, Venkatesan R, Brown RW, Cheng YN. Magnetic resonance imaging: physical principles and sequence design. Hoboken, NJ: Wiley-Blackwell; 2014.

Cobben DCP, de Boer HCJ, Tijssen RH, et al. Emerging role of MRI for radiation treatment planning in lung cancer. Technol Cancer Res Treat. 2015;15(6):NP47–60.

De Bazelaire CMJ, Duhamel GD, Rofsky NM, Alsop DC. MR imaging relaxation times of abdominal and pelvic tissues measured in vivo at 3.0 T: preliminary results. Radiology. 2004;230(3):652–9.

De Coene B, Hajnal JV, Gatehouse P, et al. MR of the brain using fluid-attenuated inversion recovery (FLAIR) pulse sequences. Am J Neuroradiol. 1992;13(6):1555–64.

Devic S. MRI simulation for radiotherapy treatment planning. Med Phys. 2012;6701(2012):6701–11. https://doi.org/10.1118/1.4758068.

Dixon WT. Simple proton spectroscopic imaging. Radiology. 1984;153(1):189–94.

Doran SJ, Charles-Edwards L, Reinsberg SA, Leach MO. A complete distortion correction for MR images: I. Gradient warp correction. Phys Med Biol. 2005;50(7):1343.

Fleckenstein JL, Archer BT, Barker BA, Vaughan JT, Parkey RW, Peshock RM. Fast short-tau inversion-recovery MR imaging. Radiology. 1991;179(2):499–504.

Golder W. Combined use of contrast media containing iodine and gadolinium for imaging and intervention: a hitherto widely ignored topic in radiological practice. Radiology. 2012;52(2):167–72. https://doi.org/10.1007/s00117-011-2279-7.

Griswold MA, Jakob PM, Heidemann RM, et al. Generalized autocalibrating partially parallel acquisitions (GRAPPA). Magn Reson Med. 2002;47(6):1202–10.

Hajnal JV, Bryant DJ, Kasuboski L, et al. Use of fluid attenuated inversion recovery (FLAIR) pulse sequences in MRI of the brain. J Comput Assist Tomogr. 1992;16:841.

Hardy PA, Henkelman RM, Bishop JE, Poon ECS, Plewes DB. Why fat is bright in RARE and fast spin-echo imaging. J Magn Reson Imaging. 1992;2(5):533–40.

Hutton C, Bork A, Josephs O, Deichmann R, Ashburner J, Turner R. Image distortion correction in fMRI: a quantitative evaluation. NeuroImage. 2002;16(1):217–40.

Jafar MM, Reeves J, Ruthven MA, et al. Assessment of a carbon fibre MRI flatbed insert for radiotherapy treatment planning. Br J Radiol. 2016;89(1062):1–7. https://doi.org/10.1259/bjr.20160108.

Jenkinson M. Fast, automated, N-dimensional phase-unwrapping algorithm. Magn Reson Med. 2003;49(1):193–7.

Jezzard P, Balaban RS. Correction for geometric distortion in echo planar images from B0 field variations. Magn Reson Med. 1995;34(1):65–73.

Jezzard P, Clare S. Sources of distortion in functional MRI data. Hum Brain Mapp. 1999;8:80–5.

Juresic E, Liney GP, Rai R, et al. An assessment of set up position for MRI scanning for the purposes of rectal cancer radiotherapy treatment planning. J Med Radiat Sci. 2018;65(1):22–30. https://doi.org/10.1002/jmrs.266.

Kanal E, Barkovich AJ, Bell C, et al. ACR guidance document on MR safe practices: 2013. J Magn Reson Imaging. 2013;37(3):501–30. https://doi.org/10.1002/jmri.24011.

King KF, Bernstein MA, Zhou XJ. Handbook of MRI pulse sequences. Amsterdam: Elsevier; 2004.

Liney GP, Moerland MA. Magnetic resonance imaging acquisition techniques for radiotherapy planning. Semin Radiat Oncol. 2014;24(3):160–8. https://doi.org/10.1016/j.semradonc.2014.02.014.

Liney GP, Owen SC, Beaumont AKE, Lazar VR, Manton DJ, Beavis AW. Commissioning of a new wide-bore MRI scanner for radiotherapy planning of head and neck cancer. Br J Radiol. 2013;86(1027):20130150. https://doi.org/10.1259/bjr.20130150.

Liu J, Saloner D. Accelerated MRI with CIRcular Cartesian UnderSampling (CIRCUS): a variable density Cartesian sampling strategy for compressed sensing and parallel imaging. Quant Imaging Med Surg. 2014;4(1):57.

Lustig M, Donoho D, Pauly JM. Sparse MRI: the application of compressed sensing for rapid MR imaging. Magn Reson Med. 2007;58(6):1182–95.

Mansfield P, Pykett IL. Biological and medical imaging by NMR. J Magn Reson. 1978;29(2):355–73.

McRobbie DW, Moore EA, Graves MJ, Prince MR. MRI: from picture to proton. Cambridge: Cambridge University Press; 2006.

Medicines and Healthcare Products Regulatory Agency (MHRA). Safety Guidelines for Magnetic Resonance Imaging Equipment in Clinical Use. London: MHRA; 2007.

Oh CH, Hilal SK, Cho ZH. Selective partial inversion recovery (SPIR) in steady state for selective saturation magnetic resonance imaging (MRI). In: Proceedings seventh annual meeting of the society of magnetic resonance in medicine (SMRM). San Francisco, CA: ISMRM; 1988.

Paulson ES, Erickson B, Schultz C, Allen Li X. Comprehensive MRI simulation methodology using a dedicated MRI scanner in radiation oncology for external beam radiation treatment planning. Med Phys. 2014;42(1):28–39. https://doi.org/10.1118/1.4896096.

Paulson ES, Crijns SPM, Keller BM, et al. Consensus opinion on MRI simulation for external beam radiation treatment planning. Radiother Oncol. 2016;121(2):187–92. https://doi.org/10.1016/j.radonc.2016.09.018.

Philippens MEP. Approaches for including MRI in radiation therapy planning. In: Philips, editor. Field strength. Best: Philips; 2016.

Pruessmann KP, Weiger M, Scheidegger MB, Boesiger P. SENSE: sensitivity encoding for fast MRI. Magn Reson Med. 1999;42(5):952–62.

Roemer PB, Edelstein WA, Hayes CE, Souza SP, Mueller OM. The NMR phased array. Magn Reson Med. 1990;16(2):192–225.

Shellock F. Screening form – MRI. 2017a. Safety.com. http://www.mrisafety.com/GenPg.asp?pgname=ScreeningForm. Accessed 6 Feb 2018.

Shellock F. Cardiac pacemakers, implantable cardioverter defibrillators (ICDs), and cardiac monitors. 2017b. http://www.mrisafety.com/SafetyInfov.asp?SafetyInfoID=167. Accessed 26 Mar 2018.

Sodickson DK, Manning WJ. Simultaneous acquisition of spatial harmonics (SMASH): fast imaging with radiofrequency coil arrays. Magn Reson Med. 1997;38(4):591–603.

Stables LA, Kennan RP, Anderson AW, Gore JC. Density matrix simulations of the effects of J coupling in spin echo and fast spin echo imaging. J Magn Reson. 1999;140(2):305–14.

Stanisz GJ, Odrobina EE, Pun J, et al. T1, T2 relaxation and magnetization transfer in tissue at 3T. Magn Reson Med. 2005;54(3):507–12.

U.S. Food & Drug Administration. Gadolinium-based contrast agents (GBCAs): drug safety communication – retained in body; new class warnings. USFDA Silver Spring, MD 2017. https://www.fda.gov/Safety/MedWatch/SafetyInformation/SafetyAlertsforHumanMedicalProducts/ucm589580.htm. Accessed 26 Mar 2018.

Walker A, Liney G, Holloway L, Dowling J, Rivest-Henault D, Metcalfe P. Continuous table acquisition MRI for radiotherapy treatment planning: distortion assessment with a new extended 3D volumetric phantom. Med Phys. 2015;42(4):1982.

Wansapura JP, Holland SK, Dunn RS, Ball WS Jr. NMR relaxation times in the human brain at 3.0 Tesla. J Magn Reson Imaging. 1999;9(4):531–8.

Xing A, Holloway L, Arumugam S, et al. Commissioning and quality control of a dedicated wide bore 3T MRI simulator for radiotherapy planning. Int J Cancer Ther Oncol. 2016;4(2):1–10. https://doi.org/10.14319/ijcto.42.1.

MRI to CT Image Registration

Richard Speight

2.1 Introduction

This chapter is broken down into three sections. The first covers an introduction of why MRI to CT registration is important in radiotherapy and the challenges of using it in the clinic. Methods for performing image registration will be detailed in Sect. 2.2. Methods to commission and verify image registration accuracy on a per patient basis will be covered in Sect. 2.3.

2.1.1 Motivation of MRI to CT Image Registration

To use MRI information in a CT-based radiotherapy workflow, there is a requirement to accurately propagate the MRI delineated structures onto the planning CT. This is done using a process referred to as image registration, in which a mathematical transformation is used to align points in the MRI onto the same geometry as the CT. Once the MRI and CT are aligned, then structures can be delineated on the MRI and transferred onto the CT. Image registration is often referred to as fusion by users or manufacturers, but there is an important distinction between these terms: image registration is the process of applying a transform to align the two images, whereas fusion is the process of merging and displaying information from the aligned voxels post registration (Brunt 2010; Brock et al. 2017).

This chapter aims to give an overview of what image registration is, how it is used in the radiotherapy clinic and how to quality assure image registration for radiotherapy. As the aim of this book is to inform the reader on techniques for introducing MRI into the radiotherapy treatment pathway, only MRI to CT registration for the purpose of defining structures on the MRI will be discussed. From herein image registration will refer to MR to CT registration.

Other overviews of image registration for radiotherapy treatment planning can be accessed for further information if required. These include but are not limited to:

- Brock and Dawson in 2014 discussed the technical challenges and solutions of multi-modal image registration (Brock and Dawson 2014).
- Brunt produced a detailed overview of the topic and review of the literature up to 2010 (Brunt 2010).
- Devic reviewed all aspects of using MRI simulation for radiotherapy (Devic 2012).
- The Swedish National Group, Gentle Radiotherapy, published a book on the use of MRI in radiotherapy offering practical advice on how to perform rigid registration using

R. Speight (✉)
Leeds Cancer Centre, Leeds, UK
e-mail: Richard.speight@nhs.net

© Springer Nature Switzerland AG 2019
G. Liney, U. van der Heide (eds.), *MRI for Radiotherapy*,
https://doi.org/10.1007/978-3-030-14442-5_2

RayStation and eclipse radiotherapy treatment planning systems (TPSs) (Gustafsson et al. 2016).
- Viergever et al. (2016) reviewed how image registration in the medical field has evolved in the previous 20 years.

2.1.2 Challenges with Image Registration

Registering images acquired at different times is an imperfect process, and potential sources of error need to be both understood and accounted for to avoid treatment incidents (Mutic et al. 2001). One of the main sources of potential error is that each modality creates images in different ways, by mapping signal from protons in MR and electron density in CT. Hence the visibility of tissues between modalities can be inherently different, even if registration is perfect (Brock and Dawson 2014). It is important to note that image registration is often optimised over a region of interest (ROI) that requires MRI for contouring, and therefore registration results should not be used clinically outside of this ROI. The ROI can be the whole image if MRI is required to delineate multiple structures (referred to as *global registration*) or it can be over a small volume to contour a single structure on MRI (referred to as *local registration*). The decision on whether to use local or global registration should be defined at the beginning and be guided by the oncologist who will use the registered MRI for contouring.

Image registration accuracy is partly dependent on factors that are covered elsewhere in this book. These include:

- Image acquisition parameters for both MRI and CT images.
- Image quality for both MRI and CT images, including artefacts.
- Time between MRI and CT acquisition (which affects internal anatomy).
- Similarity of patient position during acquisition of MRI and CT images.

This last point can be partly addressed by using the same immobilisation devices and couch on both MRI and CT to match the physical external position of the patient. Figure 2.1 shows an

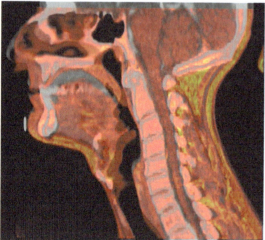 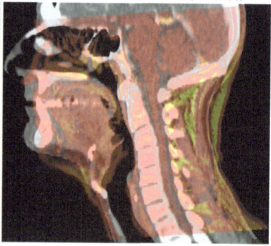

Fig. 2.1 Images of a patient with an oropharyngeal squamous cell carcinoma, grey overlay images are CT, and lava overlay are MRI. MRI images acquired in the treatment position and a diagnostic position show significant variations in neck and chin position

example of this for a head and neck patient where the MRI was acquired in both a treatment position and a diagnostic position. It is clear that in the diagnostic position MRI, the patient's neck and chin are in a very different position than in the treatment planning CT. Physiological changes in the patient's internal anatomy can also affect image registration results as variations between MRI and CT challenge the registration algorithm by creating potentially significant differences between images, e.g. rectal or bladder filling (van Herk et al. 1995), and this can lead to image registration not being sufficient in regions with large anatomical changes. Registration results can however be improved if there is an attempt to match the internal anatomy by following strict patient preparation protocols on both MRI and CT (Brunt 2010).

2.1.3 The Need for Deformable Image Registration

Problems with patient preparation highlight an important factor for image registration accuracy, namely, that tissue is deformable in nature. Therefore even if the external contours match exactly between MRI and CT, this is no guarantee that structures within the patient are also appropriately registered. This was illustrated for head and neck patients by Fortunati et al. (2014), and an example in the pelvis can be seen in Fig. 2.2. The ability to match internal structures between MRI and CT acquired at different times is dependent on the clinical site. For example, within the brain it is likely the tissue between MRI and CT will match well due to a lack of deformation within the skull; however in the pelvis it is less likely they will match well due to changes in organ filling such as the rectum and bladder.

To accommodate for different tissues within the human body, different registration types can be used. Registration techniques can be broken down into three techniques:

- *Rigid registration* which is global in nature and constrained to allow only 6 degrees of freedom, namely, translations in three orthogonal planes and rotations of pitch, yaw and roll.
- *Affine transformation* which is more comprehensive and accounts for global gross distortion, achieved via three rotations, three translations, three stretches and three shears (Devic 2012).
- *Deformable* (or non-rigid) *registration* which is non-global in nature and allows different local regions to be registered in different ways, mimicking the deformable nature of tissue. This is achieved by defining a deformation vector field (DVF) that describes mathematically how voxels from one image are deformed so that they correspond to another image.

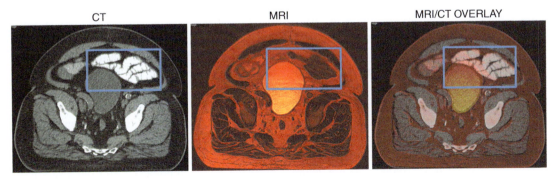

Fig. 2.2 Images of a patient with a rectal carcinoma showing that despite the same external immobilisation being used and the patient external contours being well matched, the internal anatomy had changed between MRI and CT image acquisition (bladder and bowel filling differences highlighted in blue box)

2.1.4 Registration Accuracy and Its Validation

It is important that operators of image registration in the clinic understand the limitations of the techniques used in their department and how the variation of registration accuracy across images impacts treatments. Assessing multimodal image registration (assumed throughout the rest of this chapter to be registration of MRI and CT) accuracy is non-trivial because a ground truth registration (i.e. the correct answer) cannot be known (Loi et al. 2008; Nix et al. 2017). Therefore it is important that image registration is adequately tested to ensure accuracy and safety of using MRI to contour structures in a GTV-based radiotherapy workflow (Brunt 2010; Kim et al. 2015).

Multimodal image registration is complex, and its validation for treatment planning in the clinic hadn't been adequately addressed in 2016 (Viergever et al. 2016). This problem was at least partly addressed in 2017 with the publication of the AAPM TG132 report (Brock et al. 2017), which offers key recommendations on how to perform and validate image registration in the radiotherapy clinic. However there are tools that are required for validation of image registration that are still not routinely available in the clinic.

2.1.5 Registration in the Clinic

Radiotherapy treatment planning systems (TPSs) generally have some form of registration algorithm available as standard (Brock et al. 2017; Brock and Dawson 2014). Often radiotherapy TPSs only have access to rigid registration algorithms, and deformable image registration algorithms are typically only available within imaging-specific software. Deformable registration for treatment planning is currently limited in its use in the clinic, which is thought to be due to current algorithms: not being robust to image acquisition parameter variations and not being constrained correctly, thus producing unrealistic deformations (Fortunati et al. 2014).

2.2 Techniques for Image Registration

2.2.1 General Overview

It is beyond the scope of this chapter to give a full description of all image registration techniques as it is a large and fast-moving field. This work will give a brief overview of image registration techniques that are currently employed in the clinic. Further information can be found in the review articles by Hill et al. (2001), Viergever et al. (2016) and Maintz and Viergever (1998).

When registering two images, one of the images is defined as static (or a reference) and the other as a moving image. The moving image is transformed in the image registration process to match the geometric frame of reference of the static image. In this case CT is the static image, and MRI is the moving image as the MRI is being transformed onto the frame of reference of the CT.

2.2.1.1 Manual and Automatic Registration Overview

Image registration can be classified as *manual* where an operator has full control over the registration process or *automatic* where no operator interaction is required to perform the registration. Manual registration between MRI and CT for radiotherapy is subject to potentially large inter- and intra-operator errors due to human error (Khoo et al. 1997). Due to this and the time-consuming nature of manual registration, automated methods are appealing in the clinic.

Manual image registrations in clinical software usually involve tools that allow the application of translations/rotations in three dimensions by manually transforming the moving image guided only by a visualisation of the image fusion in the software. In practice in the clinic, often a hybrid of manual/automatic registration methods are used with manual registration being used to align images before automatic registration. This gives the best seed point (i.e. starting position of the MRI and CT images) for registration and allows the operator the opportunity to manually

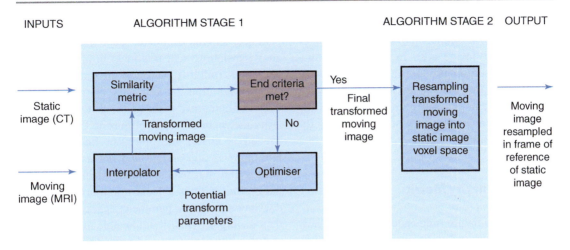

Fig. 2.3 Schematic of the automatic image registration process

edit automatic registration results if they are not deemed accurate.

The process of *automatic image registration* is more complicated and involves multiple steps, as shown in Fig. 2.3. Static and moving images can have different resolutions, meaning intensity information from voxels from each image may not align. To get around this problem, registrations can be performed in 'real space', e.g. independent from the static or moving images, and once registered the moving image is resampled onto the static image voxel space. The resampling process requires interpolating the values in the moving image to estimate the values that would have been measured at the static image voxel locations. If MRI voxel size is larger than CT, or the MRI is acquired in a non-transaxial plane, then interpolation in the resampling process is increased. This can have the effect of degrading image quality. It is therefore recommended that MRI for radiotherapy is acquired transversely with slice thickness similar to that of the CT.

The automatic registration process is performed by an algorithm consisting of an interpolator, similarity metric and optimiser (further detail given in Sects. 2.2.2–2.2.4). End criteria are defined in the algorithm and are often based on a maximum number of iterations (so registrations do not continue indefinitely), a property of the similarity metric such as its rate of change from the previous iteration (so registrations stop if they converge) or a mixture of the two. The algorithm iterates around the loop shown as algorithm stage 1 in Fig. 2.3 until the end criteria are met, and then the transformed moving image is resampled into the static image voxel space.

If registrations are performed locally to improve results in a small region, then registration is driven by an operator-defined ROI on the static image (sometimes referred to as a clip box or bounding box (Brunt 2010)). Careful choice of the ROI is important as it improves computational efficiency and registration results (Hamdan et al. 2017). If the ROI is too large, then irrelevant information not required for MRI contouring is accounted for in the registration. Whereas using a ROI to drive the local registration that is too small may lead to too little information being present to find a successful solution.

2.2.2 Interpolator

The interpolator applies the current candidate transformation to the moving image. On the first iteration, the raw moving image is the input, and the interpolator converts that image into the static image voxel space for comparison to the static image by computing the similarity metric (the measure of how similar the moving MRI image and static CT image are). In subsequent iterations, the optimiser produces a test transformation for the interpolator to apply to the raw moving image to generate a transformed moving image for comparison to the static image by the similarity metric.

2.2.3 Similarity Metric

The similarity metric is designed to quantify how well the moving and static images are registered. There are many options for similarity metrics, and a brief overview is given here, but they are well covered in the literature (Brock et al. 2017). Similarity metrics can generally be broken down into three groups:

1. Point based which aims to minimise the distances between operator-selected anatomical points on the two images, this is user dependent and leads to inter- and intra-operator variability.
2. Surface based which matches features in images such as bones, often referred to as chamfer matching. Chamfer matching is based on edge detection and minimising the difference between the edges on both images.
3. Intensity based which aims to minimise differences in intensity such as root mean square error or mutual information. Mutual information measures how well one image describes the other by using the concept of relative entropy, a measure of the degree of randomness in a system. It has recently become the most commonly used similarity metric in the clinic (Brunt 2010; Viergever et al. 2016; Torresin et al. 2015).

2.2.4 Optimisers

The goal of the optimiser is to obtain a candidate transformation that describes the best image alignment by optimising the similarity metric. Optimisers are iterative and vary transformation parameters in the parameter space (i.e. iteratively alter translations and rotations) in order to converge the similarity metric to the optimal value. At each iteration the similarity metric is calculated and compared to the previous iteration similarity metric in order to optimise it. Great care is needed to ensure the optimiser finds a global minimum as appropriate and not a local minimum as this may lead to a nonoptimal solution. If the optimiser finds a local minimum value and does not sample the parameter space adequately, then the algorithm will not be able to distinguish that this has happened and will converge to this incorrect solution.

2.2.5 Rigid Registration

Rigid registration is possible on clinical software using landmark-based similarity measures, requiring the operator to define the location of landmarks on both images. At least three points must be defined, but increasing the number of landmarks defined theoretically increases accuracy as any error in defining a single landmark will have less of an effect. It is vital when selecting landmark points that they are widely spaced and in different planes in order to increase accuracy of registrations. Once the points have been defined, the process of registration can be automated by reducing the least square difference between points defined on both images (Jaradat et al. 2003).

Landmark-based registration for most patient groups has been superseded in the clinic by voxel intensity-based techniques (often mutual information based). This is because results are generally as good without having the need for manually placing landmarks, thus making the registration process quicker and less operator dependent.

An example of landmark-based rigid registration that is still used in the clinic is fiducial marker matching in the prostate (Hanvey et al. 2012; Seppälä et al. 2015). In this technique markers are defined on both images, and an automated algorithm is used to minimise the difference between the defined points.

2.2.6 Deformable Registration

A brief overview of how deformable image registration works is given here, but further details can be found in the literature (Brock et al. 2017; Kim et al. 2015). The aim of deformable registration is to find the spatial transformation that best transforms the moving image into the frame of reference of the static image. The spatial transformation can be parameterised by a DVF or another model such as basis spline (or B-spline). When using another model, the DVF must be calculated from the transformation in order to produce the transformed moving image, e.g. for B-spline the DVF is calculated by interpolating control point displacements. Transformations can be produced using a variety of algorithms, and many options have been explored in the literature in a research environment, but as these are not used clinically, they will not be covered here in detail. However further information can be found in the literature for the following algorithms:

- Demons (Bricault et al. 1998; Guimond et al. 2001; Pennec et al. 1999; Thirion 1998; Vercauteren et al. 2007, 2009).
- Optical flow (Zhang et al. 2008a, b).
- Finite element modelling (Brock et al. 2006; Ferrant et al. 2001; Xuan et al. 2006; Zhong et al. 2007).
- Free form deformation (Jacobson and Murphy 2011; Kybic and Unser 2003; Rueckert et al. 1999).

The main choice of transformation algorithms used clinically is based on B-splines which utilise grids of control points with basis points that can be constrained globally or locally dependent or whether deformations are desired to be driven globally or locally.

Deformable image registration algorithms have the same components as for rigid registration (shown in Fig. 2.3) with two main differences. The first is that the optimiser produces a more complicated transformation parameter which could be the DVF or the B-spline control point displacements. The second main difference is that the optimiser also applies regularisation to the DVF. This process constrains the DVF to ensure it has only clinically plausible deformations, for example, smoothly varying and non-folded. Regularisation can be achieved by applying constraint penalties in a cost function during optimisation or applied to smoothen the DVF after it is updated at each iteration. It is important that this process is optimised as any over-smoothing of the DVF can lead to local errors in the registration in regions of high deformation (Nix et al. 2017).

Practically, deformable registration is often done hierarchically (Hamdan et al. 2017):

- Starting with automatic rigid registration.
- Followed by manual rigid registration editing, if required, this step can be very important as the results of the deformable registration are improved by having the best possible seed point to avoid the optimiser getting trapped in a local minima.
- Finally using automated deformable image registration.

These steps, and the potential error if the optimal seed point is not selected, are shown in the clinical head and neck example in Fig. 2.4.

Treatment position MR images reduce the need for deformable registration; however limitations in MRI access mean this isn't always possible. Deformable image registration algorithms can be successfully used in the clinic to register nontreatment position MRI scans with treatment position CT for both the prostate (Hamdan et al. 2017; Hanvey et al. 2012; Sabater et al. 2016) and head and neck (Chuter et al. 2017). However, using deformable image registration to register diagnostic position MRI must be done with care.

2.2.7 Clinical Examples of Image Registration

2.2.7.1 Brain

One of the most common sites for rigid registration is the brain. Often MRI images are acquired

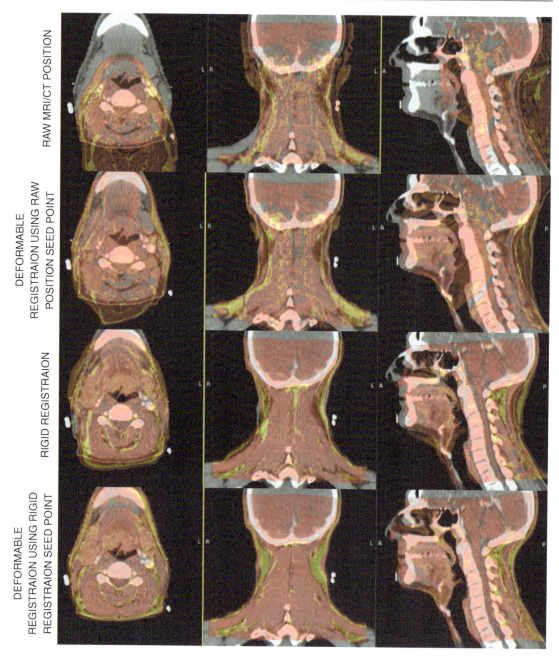

Fig. 2.4 Screenshots showing different stages of deformable image registration. CT (grey) and MRI (lava) acquired in treatment and diagnostic position, respectively. Top: raw images showing a large translational offset. Second: deformable image registration using raw position as a seed point; registration results are poor. Third: rigid registration between raw images, approximately aligning images. Fourth: deformable image registration using the MRI from the third row as a seed point; registration is improved compared to the second row

in the diagnostic position as the current generation of MRI receiver coils are optimised for this position. Due to difference in patient set-up between MRI and CT, it is important that local registration is used with a ROI including only the region within the skull, e.g. not the neck or mandible. An example registration including the suggested ROI to drive local registration is shown in

2 MRI to CT Image Registration

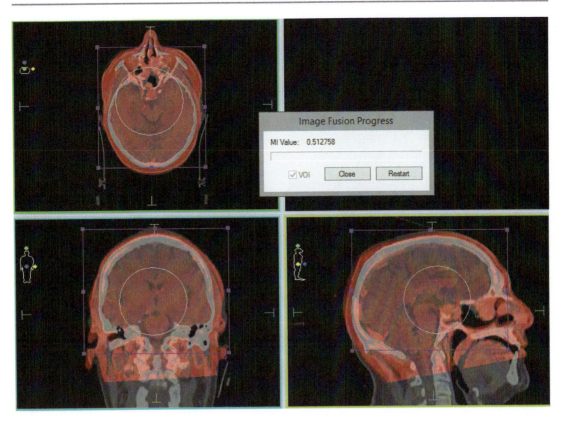

Fig. 2.5 Local intensity-based rigid registration using mutual information for a patient with a benign neoplasm of the pituitary gland, grey overlay images are CT and lava overlay are MRI. ROI used to drive local registration is shown in purple

Fig. 2.5. One important thing to note for brain patients is that they can receive surgery that significantly alters anatomy both at the time of surgery and post-surgery due to swelling. Therefore it is important that both the MRI and CT to be used for registration are acquired both post-surgery.

2.2.7.2 Head and Neck

If MRI is acquired in the treatment position in the same immobilisation mask used for CT acquisition, then rigid registration can be used successfully to register the two, although it has been shown that deformable registration can improve results in this case (Fortunati et al. 2014). As long as the patient is adequately immobilised, then for the majority of patients, global registration can be used. However, in some cases global registration may not be acceptable if the patient anatomy varies between MRI and CT scans, e.g. due to tumour change or if the tumour is near mobile anatomy such as the tongue. An example registration is shown in Fig. 2.6.

2.2.7.3 Prostate

In the clinic prostate image registration is often based on landmark matching of implanted fiducial marker. In this case it is recommended to acquire at least two MRI scans, one optimised to visualise the fiducial marker and the other optimised to visualise the anatomy of interest. The MRI optimised for fiducial marker visualisation should be registered to the CT with fiducial marker centroids used as landmarks for point-based registration, an optional pre-step of local intensity-based registration driven by a ROI including mainly soft tissue around the prostate may improve results if necessary. Once this registration is deemed acceptable, the transformation should be applied to the MRI optimised to visualise the anatomy of interest to put this in the frame of reference of the CT. As the two MRI scans are

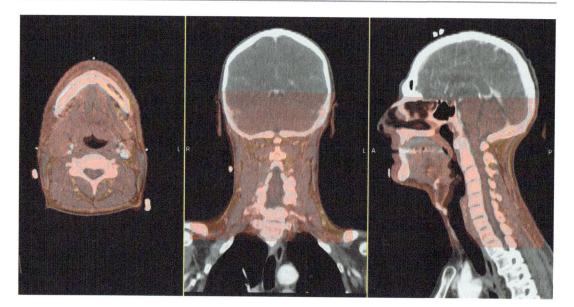

Fig. 2.6 Global rigid intensity-based registration using mutual information for a patient with an oropharyngeal squamous cell carcinoma, grey overlay images are CT and lava overlay are MRI

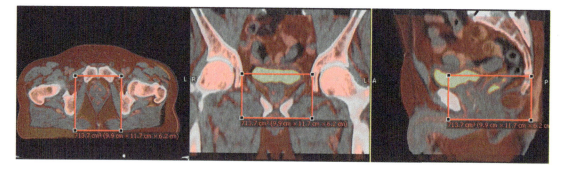

Fig. 2.7 Local intensity-based rigid registration using mutual information for a patient with a prostate carcinoma, grey overlay images are CT and lava overlay are MRI. ROI used to drive local registration is shown in red

acquired at different times, there is the potential for patient movement between scans. Therefore the soft tissue match must be assessed around the anatomy of interest on this final registration.

If fiducial markers are not available and intensity-based registration is used, then it is important that local registration is performed, driven by a ROI that includes mainly soft tissue around the prostate. An example ROI is shown in Fig. 2.7.

2.2.7.4 Liver

The liver is subject to breathing motion which can result in motion artefacts or images being acquired in different phases of the breathing cycle. In order to reduce the effect of breathing motion on registration, it is recommended that all imaging is acquired in breath hold (Høyer et al. 2012) and effort is made to ensure the breath hold is matched on both CT and MRI. In order to reduce the risk of deformation, it is recommended that a ROI including just the liver is used to drive local registration, even when acquiring both MRI and CT in the same immobilised position. If deformation is still present and affecting registration accuracy, then a smaller ROI including the region around the GTV or particular OAR of interest can be used. An example showing the ROI including the full liver can be seen in Fig. 2.8.

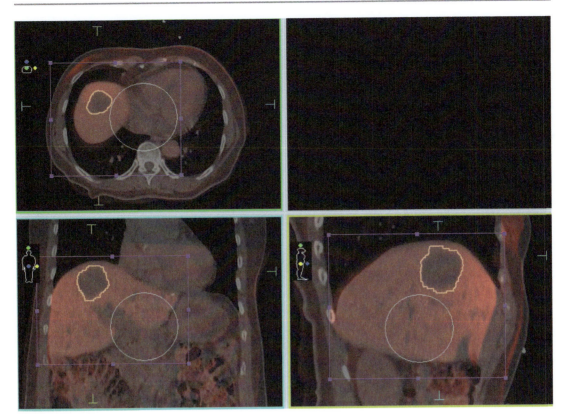

Fig. 2.8 Local intensity-based rigid registration using mutual information for a patient with a liver metastasis from a primary rectal carcinoma, grey overlay images are CT and lava overlay are MRI. ROI used to drive local registration is shown in purple, and the GTV delineated on MRI is shown in brown

2.2.7.5 Spine

It is recommended that the registration be driven locally by a ROI that includes bony anatomy around the spine (including at least two vertebrae superior and inferior to ensure the correct vertebrae are registered) and the posterior lung wall (see Fig. 2.9).

2.2.8 Techniques in the Literature Not Currently Routine in the Clinic

Although rigid registration is not a solved problem, it is relatively standard, and the most image registration research focusses on deformable registration. One approach is structure-based registration using a surface difference minimisation technique to align contours defined on both images. One clinical implementation of this method is the anatomically constrained deformation algorithm (ANACONDA) which supports multimodal deformable image registration (Weistrand and Svensson 2015). Another method of image registration is model based, which requires some a priori knowledge of how tissues within the human body move and deform. One such example using a complex biomechanical model implemented with in-house software was proposed by Brock et al. (2006)

Machine learning (also referred to as deep learning or artificial intelligence in the literature) algorithms could have a big future in image registration (Viergever et al. 2016). These algorithms learn what the properties of tissues on both MRI and CT are from a large database of past cases in order to identify them in new patients and apply a transformation to register these regions.

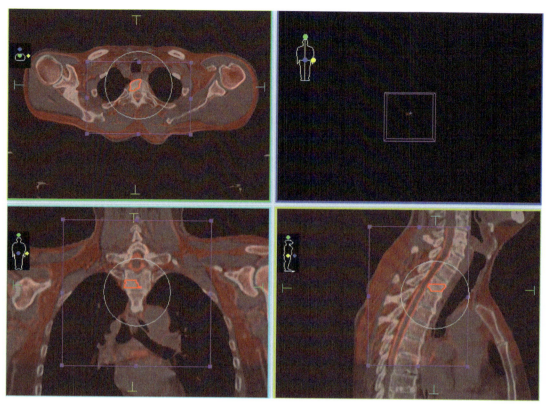

Fig. 2.9 Local intensity-based rigid registration using mutual information for a patient with a T2 spine metastasis, grey overlay images are CT and lava overlay are MRI. ROI used to drive local registration is shown in purple, and the GTV delineated on MRI is shown in red

2.3 Commissioning and Verifying Registration Accuracy per Patient

2.3.1 Goal of Commissioning and Verifying Registration Accuracy per Patient

It was recommended by the AAPM TG53 report that assessing how well multimodal image registration software performs should be split into two parts (Fraass et al. 1998), general commissioning and routine quality control (QC). In this chapter these will be referred to as commissioning, defined as the evaluation of the overall image registration process to ensure accurate image registration can consistently be achieved, and per patient verification, defined as the process of confirming accuracy of image registration for a specific patient (Brock et al. 2017).

Commissioning should be a thorough characterisation of how the software and algorithms work and handle typical patient data. Commissioning can also be performed in phantoms where a ground truth registration is known, unlike in patient registrations. As well as assessing typical image registration accuracy, the commissioning phase must also test the full patent pathway. Once commissioned it is important that the image acquisition parameters remain static as changes to imaging may invalidate commissioning requiring part or all of the process to be repeated.

Commissioning gives the operator information on how accurately algorithms perform on test cases and not on the level of accuracy that can be achieved for individual patients. Therefore it is vital that on an individual patient, tests are undertaken to assess the image registration accuracy for that patient.

In the rest of this chapter, the tools required for assessing image registration quality are introduced and then a system for documenting image registration requests and reporting results is discussed. The AAPM TG132 report (Brock et al. 2017) provides a general approach and recommendations for tests to be performed for both commissioning and per patient verification for all aspects of image registration in radiotherapy. This chapter highlights and discusses the details required to be compliant with these recommendations specifically for MRI to CT image registration. It is important to note that the tests detailed here are recommendations, but the ultimate decision of what tests to use should be made by someone who understands the purpose of the registration in the clinic. It is strongly recommended that once a procedure for commissioning and per patient verification has been developed for your centre, these procedures are formally documented and that roles and responsibilities of all personnel involved are defined (Brock et al. 2017).

2.3.2 Techniques for Assessing Image Registration Quality

2.3.2.1 Qualitative Methods

Qualitative approaches involve visually inspecting registrations to assess how well CT and transformed MRI align. This process is affected by the experience of the operator(s) and therefore is subjective; however this process can be quick and useful in the clinic (Hamdan et al. 2017; Fei et al. 2002). Image registration can have obvious errors easily detected with a visual inspection; however registration error may be subtle, so great care must be taken. Clinical image registration software allows visual inspection to be performed using a variety of tools, such as:

- Overlaying registered MRI and CT.
- Fade or toggle, where the operator can move the visualisation between the two images.
- Displaying contours produced on MRI and/or CT to assess overlap.
- Chequerboard and spyglass, which view both images simultaneously, useful for assessing if edges visible in both images align.
- Displaying points/markers that can be placed in one image and viewed on the other, sometimes referred to as a linked cursor tool.
- Qualitative scoring of registration quality by an experienced operator (Fei et al. 2002).

2.3.2.2 Quantitative Methods

Landmark Matching, Target Registration Error or Euclidean Distances
The simplest quantitative technique is landmark matching, often referred to as target registration error (TRE) or Euclidean distances, which involves measuring the distance between manually identified points on both CT and registered MRI. The maximum and mean distance to agreement can then be quoted. This technique has some value, but it is time-consuming, is subject to inter- and intra-observer error and is suitable only when significant feature points are present (Kim et al. 2015).

Contour-Based Assessment
Another technique for quantitative assessment of registration is contour based. This relies upon performing comparison of contours delineated on both CT and registered MRI. A number of contour comparison metrics (either volumetric or surface based) have been used in the literature including:

- Dice similarity coefficient (DSC) (Fortunati et al. 2014; Hamdan et al. 2017; Sabater et al. 2016; Chuter et al. 2017; Akbarzadeh et al. 2013; Bird et al. 2015).
- Volume differences (or ratio) (Weistrand and Svensson 2015; Akbarzadeh et al. 2013; Tan et al. 2010; Tanaka et al. 2011).
- False positives (the proportion of the volume defined on MRI not covered by the volume defined on CT) (Akbarzadeh et al. 2013).
- False negatives (the proportion of volume defined on CT not covered by the volume defined on MRI) (Akbarzadeh et al. 2013).

- Difference in the centre of mass, also referred to as centre of gravity (Brock et al. 2006; Chuter et al. 2017; Fei et al. 2002).
- Conformity index (Chuter et al. 2017).
- Percentage of surface area differing by a given distance (n mm) (PSAD-n) (Brock et al. 2006).
- Hausdorff surface distance (HSD) (Fortunati et al. 2014; Hamdan et al. 2017; Akbarzadeh et al. 2013).
- Modified Hausdorff surface distance (MHSD) (Fortunati et al. 2014).
- Distance to conformity (or distance to agreement) (Chuter et al. 2017; Jena et al. 2010; Beasley et al. 2016).

An issue using different contour comparison metrics is that a lot of choice is available, and if many are calculated, results from each metric do not agree. For example, Forunati found for H&N patients that MHSD and HSD didn't show the same statistical significance (Fortunati et al. 2014). Therefore results can be biased by which contour comparison metrics are calculated (Beasley et al. 2016). Pragmatically the best solution is to measure a large range of contour comparison metrics and look for trends.

Full Circle or Transitivity

A further technique for quantitative assessment of image registration is the full circle (or transitivity) method developed by van Herk et al. (1998) and further discussed by Bender and Tomé (2009). This technique involves registering a CT image to a first MRI image; the first MRI image is registered to a second MRI image; then finally the second MRI image is registered to the original CT. If all registration steps are accurate, then the product of the three registration matrices should be unity, and any deviation indicates a registration error. The full circle method requires three images which are not always available on a per patient basis, and if an error is detected, it is not possible to identity which registration caused it, so further investigation is required.

The Need for Automated Tools

In the clinic it would be useful to have an automatic tool to assess registration accuracy in order to filter out unacceptable registrations before being used (Fei et al. 2002). This is non-trivial as automated analysis has to be quick and performed in a situation where a ground truth is not known. Nix et al. (2017), Neylon et al. (2017) and Kierkels et al. (2018) have all proposed techniques to automatically assess image registration quantitatively when no ground truth is known.

2.3.3 Techniques Specifically for Assessing Deformable Image Registration Accuracy

In 2010, deformable image registration accuracy was reported to be assessed inconsistently (Brock 2010), and since then methodologies for QA have been suggested (Brock et al. 2017; Kim et al. 2015). Techniques can be broken down into qualitative methods such as a visual assessment of the DVF and quantitative methods such as assessing the Jacobian determinant of the DVF. Both of these techniques will not tell the operator if the deformation applied is correct; however it will let the operator know if the deformation used is not plausible due to unphysical deformations.

2.3.3.1 Visual Assessment of a DVF

Qualitative visual assessment of an applied DVF requires the image registration software used to have tools to allow this; not all commercial software supports this. Some options available in clinical software include displaying the applied DVF as a heat map, warped grid or vector arrows (see examples in Fig. 2.10) or observing the applied DVF in a cine loop. Irrespective of the visualisation method, the operator should identify regions of high deformation and determine if this is plausible (i.e. a region of natural deformation) or not plausible (i.e. a region where deformations are unexpected). If it is not plausible, then the registration in this region must not be used clinically. In a clinical example shown in Fig. 2.11, high regions of deformation are observed outside the patient anteriorly, around the right shoulder, around the posterior of the neck and within the skull. In this case the patient was not in the

2 MRI to CT Image Registration

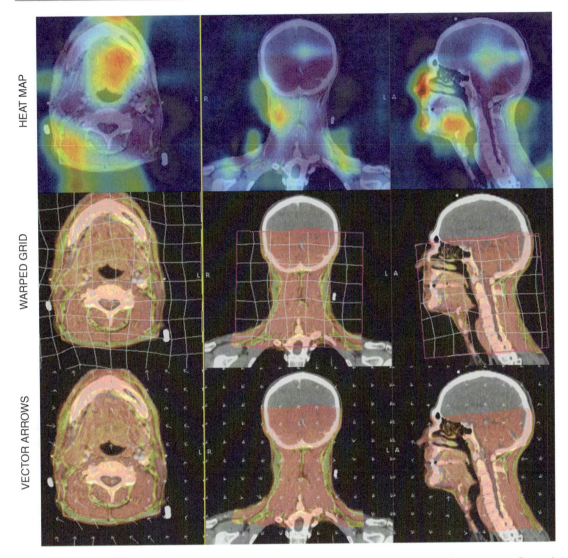

Fig. 2.10 Methods of observing the applied DVF as a heat map (top), warped grids (middle) and vector arrows (bottom) used to visually qualitatively assess deformable image registration accuracy

treatment position for the MRI, and hence the patients' posterior section of the neck and right shoulder was not in the same fixed position, so large amounts of deformation are plausible. The large region of deformation outside the patient anteriorly is due to an MRI wrap artefact which could be removed by using a ROI not including this region to drive registration locally. The region of deformation within the skull is not physically plausible and therefore not acceptable clinically.

2.3.3.2 Jacobian Determinant

The Jacobian determinant of a DVF is a quantitative measure of how much local volume change there is due to the deformation applied. Jacobian determinant values have the following meanings:

- 0–1: Volume compression.
- >1: Volume expansion.
- 1: No volume change.
- ≤0: Regions folded into themselves in a non-physical manner.

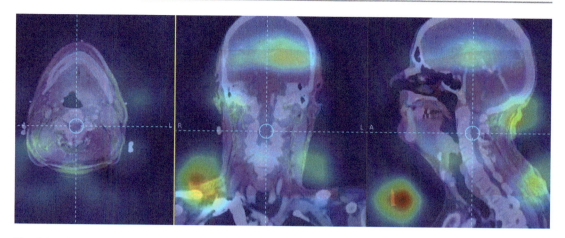

Fig. 2.11 A DVF visualised using a heat map used in a qualitative assessment of deformable registration between a CT acquired in the treatment position and an MRI acquired in a diagnostic position. Large areas of deformation are observed: outside the patient anteriorly; at the right shoulder; at the posterior of the neck; and within the brain

Realistic deformations, e.g. those with a conservation of volume, are characterised by values close to 1 as some small natural expansion and contraction is expected in patients (Fortunati et al. 2014). Regions with Jacobian determinants of ≤0 are indicative of a registration error and should be investigated further.

2.3.4 Phantoms

In the process of commissioning a multimodal image registration algorithm, there is a role for assessing patient data as well as assessing phantom data. Phantom data has the benefits that it can have a known ground truth, unlike patient data, and it can be used to test the performance of the whole image registration process (end to end testing). Phantoms can be either physical or digital, and both types can either be anthropomorphic or geometric. The main problem with using phantoms to assess registration quality is that it is difficult to produce phantoms that accurately mimic natural variations in patients, so they are limited by how closely they represent the clinical situation (Brock et al. 2017).

2.3.4.1 Physical Phantoms

Geometric physical phantoms have limited application in assessing image registration quality as they do not pose the same challenges to an image registration algorithm that a patient does. Anthropomorphic physical phantoms with suitable MRI and CT properties simultaneously are difficult to produce; often MRI properties of such phantoms are suboptimal (Loi et al. 2008).

2.3.4.2 Digital Phantoms

Digital anthropomorphic phantoms can be produced from patient data by selecting MRI and CT images that are well registered. Applying a known function to the MRI image allows the operator to assess if an image registration algorithm can recover the applied function accurately. One of the major issues in using anthropomorphic digital phantoms is that the range of functions that can be applied to the MRI images will have limited clinical relevance; in other words it is very difficult to artificially deform an image in the same way that real tissue deforms in a human (Viergever et al. 2016; Kim et al. 2015).

2.3.5 Image Registration Request and Report

Before discussing the QA tests required for assessing registration, it is important to highlight the importance of communicating both why the registration is needed clinically and the accuracy of the final registration. This communication must be done in such a way that the information can be accessed easily by anyone involved in the patient's care team. AAPM TG132 recommends that this is formalised in two stages, a request and a report (Brock et al. 2017). AAPM TG132 recommends what to include in the request and report; however when registering MRI to CT for the purpose of using MRI for contouring structures, the author of this chapter recommends some modifications as detailed below. The following information should be included in the clinical protocol as it should be similar/the same for all patients in that group:

- Image sets to be registered (if standardised protocols are used in the clinic).
- Local regions of interest (e.g. what structures will be contoured on MRI).
- Method of registration (software and algorithm options).
- Accuracy required; if it varies in different regions, then details should be given.

On an individual patient basis, an image registration request from a clinician should state that the registration follows the desired clinical protocol with any deviations requested detailed. The operator performing the registration should then fill in a report that includes at least the following information: detail any deviations from the clinical protocol; comments on the uncertainties in registration in the regions of importance, highlighting very clearly any regions where registration is too poor to be used clinically; and sample images with annotations if appropriate (Brock et al. 2017).

2.3.6 Commissioning

The recommended tests for commissioning vary dependently on what type of registration is being used. Firstly, rigid registration commissioning tests will be discussed, and then the extra tests required for deformable registration will be discussed. As tests are modified from the AAPM TG132 report, further detail and suggested tolerances can be found in this document (Brock et al. 2017).

2.3.6.1 Rigid Registration Commissioning Tests

End to End with a Physical Phantom

A physical phantom is needed with internal details visible on MRI and CT. The phantom should be scanned on both MRI and CT with a field of view covering the whole phantom in all possible orientations (head first both supine and prone followed by feet first both supine and prone). It is important that when scanning the phantom, it is physically in the same orientation that is inputted on the DICOM tag. Further scans with the phantom rotated by known angles should also be acquired; zero degrees and two other angles between 0° and 45° are sufficient. All images should be imported into the image registration software from both the scanners directly and via PACS. Images including DICOM headers should then be interrogated to ensure the following has transferred correctly:

- Patient orientation.
- Image acquisition parameters such as pixel size, slice thickness and slice spacing.
- Patient demographics.

Image geometry can be assessed, on MRI and CT independently, by measuring distances between the details in the phantom and comparing to known values. Ensuring the imaging system deals with tilted images correctly should be tested by repeating these measurements on the tilted scans.

If image registration in the proposed patient pathway will not be done on the TPS but involves exporting a DICOM object from image registration software to the TPS (the DVF, MRI resampled into the frame of reference of the CT, contours delineated on the MRI or other), then the following DICOM connectivity and integrity tests should be performed. The phantom MRI and CT scans should be registered using the clinical technique and export the DICOM object to be used clinically from the image registration software to the TPS. In the TPS the DICOM object and its header must be assessed for the same parameters discussed previously as well as visualising the DICOM object to ensure transfer has not altered data.

Digital Phantoms

Digital phantoms of MRI and CT scans can be produced in house (using techniques discussed in Sect. 2.3.4), can be purchased or can be downloaded from AAPM TG132 (Brock et al. 2017). The phantoms required have artificially applied offsets, rotations and orientation changes and are degraded with noise. The digital phantoms with known changes should be imported into the image registration software and a registration performed. If the registration software reports the translations/rotations used, then these should be of equal magnitude but in the opposite direction to the applied known values. If the software does not report translations/rotations, then a landmark-based technique, centre of mass of contours produced on both MRI and CT, and/or visual inspection should be used to assess registration accuracy. In either case it is recommended that the registration algorithm should be able to undo the applied function to within a tolerance of less than half of the largest voxel dimension (Brock et al. 2017). Tests should be repeated on images with artificial noise added to characterise algorithm response with suboptimal images.

Clinical Data

Typical MRI and CT datasets for the clinical site(s) being commissioned must be found; it is recommended that at least ten datasets should be used in order to sample a representative variation in patient anatomy. In some cases it will not be possible to acquire the same data that will be used clinically. In this case it is recommended that data from a similar clinical site or from diagnostic imaging should be chosen if available. If the data used during commissioning is not identical to that to be used clinically, then it is recommended that for the first ten clinical patients, the same techniques discussed here are employed to finish these commissioning tests prospectively. For the datasets selected, the proposed clinical registration should be performed, and results should be assessed using a range of suitable quantitative and qualitative methods described in Sects. 2.3.2 and 2.3.3. It is recommended that the qualitative visual assessment is performed in an MDT with all staff groups that will be performing and using the results of registrations clinically. This is a good opportunity for those staff groups to learn about expectations from registration results.

2.3.6.2 Deformable Registration Commissioning Tests

The extra tests recommended for deformable registration are for digital phantoms only. A range of clinically representative deformations should be artificially applied to the MRI digital phantoms. The AAPM TG132 report has a starting point for deformable digital phantoms for prostates; however for other sites more phantoms are required. Once obtained, MRI digital phantoms with known deformations should be registered to the undeformed CT using the technique to be used clinically. If the deformable image registration algorithm works perfectly, then the final registered MRI will be the same as the MRI before the known deformation was applied. A subtraction of the inverse of the applied DVF and the registered DVF (assuming the software you use allows DVFs to be exported) gives the registration error at each voxel. If you use the AAPM TG132 digital phantoms, then the applied DVF is available. The suggested tolerance for this test is for 95% of voxels to be within 2 mm with the maximum error being less than 5 mm.

2.3.7 Verifying Registration Accuracy per Patient

For an individual patient, the accuracy of the registration must be assessed in order for it to be acceptable for the purpose defined in the request, i.e. it must meet required accuracy in the locations to be used for contouring on MRI. The main tool for verifying registration accuracy per patient is a visual inspection using the range of tools shown in Sects. 2.3.2 and 2.3.3. The visual inspection must assess registration accuracy of the organs to be contoured on MRI or directly neighbouring tissue if these are not visible on CT. If this visual assessment finds the boundaries of such regions are not well registered, then the registration should not be used clinically, or if used it should be done so with caution and any uncertainty accounted for in the PTV margin (Brock et al. 2017). As registration errors can be subtle, it is important that visual inspection is carried out carefully and by at least two individual operators separately (often the operator performing the registration and the oncologist using it for contouring).

2.3.7.1 Extra Considerations for Deformable Registration

For deformable image registration, as well as visually assessing the registration, the plausibility of the DVF should be assessed on a per patient basis. This should be performed at least visually but could also include calculating the Jacobian determinant using the tools discussed in Sect. 2.3.3. The aim of this test is to locate regions of large deformation and justify why these have occurred (e.g. due to changes in bowel position for prostate patients). If any region of large deformation cannot be justified (e.g. within the bone or the skull where no deformation is clinically expected), then the registration should not be used in the region of this erroneous deformation. It is important to recognise that these suggested tests assess the plausibility of the deformation applied; and if a deformation is plausible, it does not mean it is correct; this is why visual inspection of the registered images must still be performed.

2.3.7.2 Training Requirements for Operators Who Will Visually Assess Registration Accuracy

It is important that all operators who are going to perform a visual inspection are adequately trained so that consistency in your department is achieved and to ensure safety for all patients. This training should include at least a basic understanding of:

- How CT and MRI images are produced.
- The purpose of the registration (e.g. what regions are important to focus on when performing a registration).
- The accuracy expected from registrations.
- The implications to the treatment if registrations are inaccurate.
- How the registration software works and its limitations.
- The tools available for visually assessing registration results.
- The importance of visualising images properly during an assessment (e.g. optimising window and level settings).

2.3.7.3 The Need for Better Quantitative Tools

Visual inspection may be the best option clinically at the current time, but it is desirable to have a quantitative tool to aid (i.e. not to replace) visual assessment. A quick and simple to use quantitative tool is required as a guide to help with assessing registration on a per patient basis. Although it is well known that this is non-trivial due to a lack of ground truth, a technique similar to the ones discussed by Nix et al. (2017), Seppälä et al. (2015) and Kierkels et al. (2018) would be beneficial in the clinic.

Acknowledgements Dr. Richard Speight is supported by a Cancer Research UK Centres Network Accelerator Award Grant (A21993) to the ART-NET consortium. I would like to thank the editors of this book for the invitation to write this chapter. Ms. Robba Rai (Ingham Institute, Liverpool Cancer Centre, Sydney, Australia) is thanked for useful discussion on prostate fiducial marker registration. I would also like to thank my line manager (Dr. Bashar Al-Qaisieh) and my employer (Leeds Teaching Hospitals, Leeds, UK) for support in writing this chapter.

Finally I would also like to thank all those who read and provided comments and feedback on this chapter, particularly Mrs. Shona Whittam, Mr. David Bird and Dr. David Broadbent (all from Leeds Cancer Centre, Leeds, UK); Associate Professor Ann Henry and Dr. Katherine O'Mahony (University of Leeds, Leeds, UK); Dr. Robert Chuter and Mr. David Lines (both from The Christie NHS Foundation Trust, Manchester, UK); Dr. Jorge Cardoso (Kings Collage London, London, UK); Dr. Jamie McClelland (University College London, London, UK); and Dr. Ben George (CRUK/MRC Institute for Radiation Oncology, University of Oxford, UK).

References

Akbarzadeh A, Gutierrez D, Baskin A, Ay MR, Ahmadian A, Riahi Alam N, Lövblad KO, Zaidi H. Evaluation of whole-body MR to CT deformable image registration. J Appl Clin Med Phys. 2013;14(4):238–53.

Beasley WJ, McWilliam A, Aitkenhead A, Mackay RI, Rowbottom CG. The suitability of common metrics for assessing parotid and larynx autosegmentation accuracy. J Appl Clin Med Phys. 2016;17(2):41–9. https://doi.org/10.1120/jacmp.v17i2.5889.

Bender E, Tomé W. The utilization of consistency metrics for error analysis in deformable image registration. Phys Med Biol. 2009;54(18):55–61. https://doi.org/10.1088/0031-9155/54/18/014.

Bird D, Scarsbrook AF, Sykes J, Ramasamy S, Subesinghe M, Carey B, Wilson DJ, Roberts N, McDermott G, Karakaya E, Bayman E, Sen M, Speight R, Prestwich RDJ. Multimodality imaging with CT, MR and FDG-PET for radiotherapy target volume delineation in oropharyngeal squamous cell. BMC Cancer. 2015;15:844. https://doi.org/10.1186/s12885-015-1867-8.

Bricault I, Ferretti G, Cinquin P. Registration of real and CT-derived virtual bronchoscopic images to assist transbronchial biopsy. IEEE Trans Med Imaging. 1998;17(5):703–14. https://doi.org/10.1109/42.736022.

Brock KK. Results of a multi-institution deformable registration accuracy study (MIDRAS). Int J Radiat Oncol Biol Phys. 2010;76(2):583–96. https://doi.org/10.1016/j.ijrobp.2009.06.031.

Brock KK, Dawson LA. Point: principles of magnetic resonance imaging integration in a computed tomography–based radiotherapy workflow. Semin Radiat Oncol. 2014;24(3):169–74.. https://doi.org/10.1016/j.semradonc.2014.02.006

Brock KK, Dawson LA, Sharpe MB, Moseley DJ, Jaffray DA. feasibility of a novel deformable image registration technique to facilitate classification, targeting, and monitoring of tumor and normal tissue. Int J Radiat Oncol Biol Phys. 2006;64(4):1245–54. https://doi.org/10.1016/j.ijrobp.2005.10.027.

Brock KK, Mutic S, McNutt TR, Li H, Kessler ML. Use of image registration and fusion algorithms and techniques in radiotherapy: report of the AAPM radiation therapy committee task group no. 132. Med Phys. 2017;44(7):e43–76.. https://doi.org/10.1002/mp.12256

Brunt JNH. Computed tomography & magnetic resonance image registration in radiotherapy treatment planning. Clin Oncol. 2010;22:688–97.

Chuter R, Prestwich R, Bird D, Scarsbrook A, Sykes J, Wilson D, Speight R. The use of deformable image registration to integrate diagnostic MRI into the radiotherapy planning pathway for head and neck cancer. Radiother Oncol. 2017;122(2):229–35. https://doi.org/10.1016/j.radonc.2016.07.016.

Devic S. MRI simulation for radiotherapy treatment planning. Med Phys. 2012;39(11):6701–11. https://doi.org/10.1118/1.4758068.

Fei B, Wheaton A, Lee Z, Duerk JL, Wilson DL. Automatic MR volume registration and its evaluation for the pelvis and prostate. Phys Med Biol. 2002;47:823–38.

Ferrant M, Nabavi A, Macq B, Jolesz FA, Kikinis R, Warfield SK. Registration of 3-D intraoperative MR images of the brain using a finite-element biomechanical model. IEEE Trans Med Imaging. 2001;20(12):1384–97. https://doi.org/10.1109/42.974933.

Fortunati V, Verhaart RF, Angeloni F, van der Lugt A, Niessen WJ, Veenland JF, Paulides MM, van Walsum T. Feasibility of multimodal deformable registration for head and neck tumor treatment planning. Int J Radiat Oncol Biol Phys. 2014;90(1):85–93.. https://doi.org/10.1016/j.ijrobp.2014.05.027

Fraass B, Doppke K, Hunt M, Kutcher G, Starkschall G, Stern R, van Dyke J, American Association of Physicists in Medicine Radiation Therapy Committee Task Group 53. Quality assurance for clinical radiotherapy treatment planning. Med Phys. 1998;25(10):1773–829.

Guimond A, Roche A, Ayache N, Meunier J. Three-dimensional multimodal brain warping using the demons algorithm and adaptive intensity corrections. IEEE Trans Med Imaging. 2001;20(1):58–69. https://doi.org/10.1109/42.906425.

Gustafsson C, Sohlin M, Filipsson L. (2016) Method book for the use of MRI in radiotherapy, Version 3, 15/12/2016. http://gentleradiotherapy.se/wp-content/uploads/2016/12/Metodbok_version3_2016-12-15_ENG_final.pdf

Hamdan I, Bert J, Cheze Le Rest C, Tasu JP, Boussion N, Valeri A, Dardenne G, Visvikis D. Fully automatic deformable registration of pretreatment MRI/CT for image-guided prostate radiotherapy planning. Med Phys. 2017;44(12):6447–55. https://doi.org/10.1002/mp.12629.

Hanvey S, Sadozye AH, McJury M, Glegg M, Foster J. The influence of MRI scan position on image registration accuracy, target delineation and calculated dose in prostatic radiotherapy. Br J Radiol. 2012;85:e1256–62.

van Herk M, Bruce A, Kroes APG, Shouman T, Touw A, Lebesque JV. Quantification of organ motion during conformal radiotherapy of the prostate by three dimensional image registration. Int J Radiat Oncol Biol Phys. 1995;33:1311–20.

van Herk M, de Munck JC, Lebesque JV, Muller S, Rasch C, Touw A. Automatic registration of pelvic computed tomography data and magnetic resonance scans including a full circle method for quantitative accuracy evaluation. Med Phys. 1998;25(10):2054–67.

Hill DL, Batchelor PG, Holden M, Hawkes DJ. Medical image registration. Phys Med Biol. 2001;46(3):R1–R45.

Høyer M, Swaminath A, Bydder S, Lock M, Méndez Romero A, Kavanagh B, Goodman KA, Okunieff P, Dawson LA. Radiotherapy for liver metastases: a review of evidence. Int J Radiat Oncol Biol Phys. 2012;82(3):1047–57.

Jacobson TJ, Murphy MJ. Optimized knot placement for B-splines in deformable image registration. Med Phys. 2011;38(8):4579–82. https://doi.org/10.1118/1.3609416.

Jaradat HA, Tomé WA, McNutt TR, Meyerand ME. On the incorporation of multi-modality image registration into the radiotherapy treatment planning process. Technol Cancer Res Treat. 2003;2(1):1–11.

Jena R, Kirkby NF, Burton KE, Hoole AC, Tan LT, Burnet NG. A novel algorithm for the morphometric assessment of radiotherapy treatment planning volumes. Br J Radiol. 2010;83(985):44–51. https://doi.org/10.1259/bjr/27674581.

Khoo VS, Dearnaley DP, Finnigan DJ, Padhani A, Tanner SF, Leach MO. Magnetic resonance imaging (MRI): considerations and applications in radiotherapy treatment planning. Radiother Oncol. 1997;42:1–15.

Kierkels RGJ, den Otter LA, Korevaar EW, Langendijk JA, van der Schaaf A, Knopf AC, Sijtsema NM. An automated, quantitative, and case-specific evaluation of deformable image registration in computed tomography images. Phys Med Biol. 2018;63(4):045026. https://doi.org/10.1088/1361-6560/aa9dc2.

Kim H, Park SB, Monroe JI, Traughber BJ, Zheng Y, Lo SS, Yao M, Mansur D, Ellis R, Machtay M, Sohn JW. Quantitative analysis tools and digital phantoms for deformable image registration quality assurance. Technol Cancer Res Treat. 2015;14(4):428–39. https://doi.org/10.1177/1533034614553891.

Kybic J, Unser M. Fast parametric elastic image registration. IEEE Trans Image Process. 2003;12(11):1427–42. https://doi.org/10.1109/Tip.2003.813139.

Loi G, Dominietto M, Manfredda I, Mones E, Carriero A, Inglese E, Krengli M, Brambilla M. Acceptance test of a commercially available software for automatic image registration of computed tomography (CT), magnetic resonance imaging (MRI) and 99mTc-methoxyisobutylisonitrile (MIBI) single-photon emission computed tomography (SPECT) brain images. J Digit Imaging. 2008;21(3):329–37. https://doi.org/10.1007/s10278-007-9042-7.

Maintz JBA, Viergever MA. A survey of medical image registration. Med Image Anal. 1998;2(1):1–36.

Mutic S, Dempsey JF, Bosch WR, Low DA, Drzymala RE, Chao C, Goddu M, Cutler D, Purdy JA. Multimodality image registration quality assurance for conformal three-dimensional treatment planning. Int J Radiat Oncol Biol Phys. 2001;51(1):255–60.

Neylon J, Min Y, Low DA, Santhanam A. A neural network approach for fast, automated quantification of DIR performance. Med Phys. 2017;44(8):4126–38. https://doi.org/10.1002/mp.12321.

Nix MG, Prestwich RJD, Speight R. Automated, reference-free local error assessment of multimodal deformable image registration for radiotherapy in the head and neck. Radiother Oncol. 2017;125(3):478–84. https://doi.org/10.1016/j.radonc.2017.10.004.

Pennec X, Cachier P, Ayache N. Understanding the "Demon's algorithm": 3D non-rigid registration by gradient descent. Med Image Comput Comput Assist Interv. 1999;1679:597–605. https://doi.org/10.1007/10704282_64.

Rueckert D, Sonoda LI, Hayes C, Hill DLG, Leach MO, Hawkes DJ. Nonrigid registration using free-form deformations: Application to breast MR images. IEEE Trans Med Imaging. 1999;18(8):712–21. https://doi.org/10.1109/42.796284.

Sabater S, Pastor-Juan MR, Berenguer R, Andres I, Sevillano M, Lozano-Setien E, Jimenez-Jimenez E, Rovirosa A, Sanchez-Prieto R, Arenas M. Analysing the integration of MR images acquired in a non-radiotherapy treatment position into the radiotherapy workflow using deformable and rigid registration. Radiother Oncol. 2016;119(1):179–84.. https://doi.org/10.1016/j.radonc.2016.02.032

Seppälä T, Visapää H, Collan J, Kapanen M, Beule A, Kouri M, Tenhunen M, Saarilahti K. Converting from CT- to MRI-only-based target definition in radiotherapy of localized prostate cancer. Strahlenther Onkol. 2015;191:862–8. https://doi.org/10.1007/s00066-015-0868-5.

Tan J, Lim Joon D, Fitt G, Wada M, Lim Joon M, Mercuri A, Marr M, Chao M, Khoo V. The utility of multimodality imaging with CT and MRI in defining rectal tumour volumes for radiotherapy treatment planning: a pilot study. J Med Imaging Radiat Oncol. 2010;54:562–8. https://doi.org/10.1111/j.1754-9485.2010.02212.x.

Tanaka H, Hayashi S, Ohtakara K, Hoshi H, Iida T. Usefulness of CT-MRI fusion in radiotherapy planning for localized prostate cancer. J Radiat Res. 2011;52:782–8. https://doi.org/10.1269/jrr.11053.

Thirion JP. Image matching as a diffusion process: an analogy with Maxwell's demons. Med Image Anal. 1998;2(3):243–60. https://doi.org/10.1016/S1361-8415(98)80022-4.

Torresin A, Grazia Brambilla M, Monti AF, Moscato A, Brockmann MA, Schad L, Attenberger UI, Lohr F. Review of potential improvements using MRI in the radiotherapy workflow. Z Med Phys. 2015;25(3):210–20.. https://doi.org/10.1016/j.zemedi.2014.11.003

Vercauteren T, Pennec X, Perchant A, Ayache N. Diffeomorphic demons: efficient non-parametric image registration. NeuroImage. 2009;45(1):S61–72. https://doi.org/10.1016/j.neuroimage.2008.10.040.

Vercauteren T, Pennec X, Perchant A, Ayache N. Nonparametric diffeomorphic image registration with the demons algorithm. Med Image Comput Comput Assist Interv. 2007;10(2):319–26.

Viergever MA, Maintz JBA, Klein S, Murphy K, Staring M, Pluim JPW. A survey of medical image registration. Med Image Anal. 2016;33:140–4.. https://doi.org/10.1016/j.media.2016.06.030

Weistrand O, Svensson S. The ANACONDA algorithm for deformable image registration in radiotherapy. Med Phys. 2015;42(1):40–53.

Xuan J, Wang Y, Freedman MT, Adali T, Shields P. Nonrigid medical image registration by finite-element deformable sheetcurve models. Int J Biomed Imaging. 2006;2006:73430.. https://doi.org/10.1155/IJBI/2006/73430

Zhang GG, Huang TC, Guerrero T, Lin KP, Stevens C, Starkschall G, Forster K. Use of three-dimensional (3D) optical flow method in mapping 3D anatomic structure and tumor contours across four-dimensional computed tomography data. J Appl Clin Med

Phys. 2008a;9(1):2738. https://doi.org/10.1120/jacmp.v9i1.2738.

Zhang GG, Huang TC, Forster KM, Lin KP, Stevens C, Harris E, Guerrero T. Dose mapping: validation in 4D dosimetry with measurements and application in radiotherapy follow-up evaluation. Comput Methods Prog Biomed. 2008b;90(1):25–37. https://doi.org/10.1016/j.cmpb.2007.11.015.

Zhong HL, Peters T, Siebers JV. FEM-based evaluation of deformable image registration for radiation therapy. Phys Med Biol. 2007;52(16):4721–38. https://doi.org/10.1088/0031-9155/52/16/001.

Quality Assurance

Teo Stanescu and Jihong Wang

3.1 Management of MRI Scanner Performance

3.1.1 Introduction

The quality assurance (QA) of MRI scanners can be a daunting task for the RT physicist given the complexity of the MRI system and the associated procedures required to ensure an optimal and safe integration of the MRI data into the RT workflows. The QA process is required to provide a threshold of confidence that the imaging data acquired in patients is adequate for the clinical objectives of the examinations.

In the QA process, performance metrics and standards are defined to establish action levels and facilitate the routine monitoring of the MRI systems (i.e., hardware and software). For convenience and to minimize logistics, the QA is typically performed by means of phantoms with rather simple and fixed geometries. The QA process implicitly assumes that the phantom-based evaluation is directly correlated with the quality of the imaging done in patients, which exhibit significantly more complex geometries with unpredictable variations from case to case. The assumption that the phantom and patient data are linked together was historically derived from the experience with the x-ray-based imaging devices. For x-ray imaging, the equipment shows a lower level of design complexity and a limited number of degrees of freedom for setting and operating the procedures. In contrast, MRI provides a large number of user-defined and platform-specific parameters to maximizing flexibility in finely tuning the imaging for each case. The MRI scanners also require an extremely stable environment for operation in terms of background magnetic fields, mechanical vibration levels, and spurious radiofrequency (RF) sources (see Chap. 1.2.1). Therefore, MRI QA requires a more detailed understanding of the system design and operation.

A comprehensive QA program is recommended to encompass all key aspects regarding the MR system performance including the scanner and surface coils. ACR, AAPM, and NEMA provide guidelines regarding the type of tests to be performed, evaluation metrics, and incidence of measurements for routine monitoring (AAPM 2010; ACR 2015). The tests and metrics can be

T. Stanescu (✉)
Radiation Medicine Program, Department of Medical Physics, Princess Margaret Cancer Centre, Toronto, ON, Canada

Radiation Oncology, University of Toronto, Toronto, ON, Canada

Techna Institute, University Health Network, Toronto, ON, Canada
e-mail: Teodor.Stanescu@rmp.uhn.on.ca

J. Wang
Division of Radiation Oncology, Department of Radiation Physics, MD Anderson Cancer Center, Houston, TX, USA

adapted to a variety of phantoms: (a) available with the scanner at no extra cost, (b) available to be purchased from a third-party vendor, or (c) manufactured with on-site resources.

3.1.2 Core Performance Tests and QA Program

The most pervasive methodology for quantifying an MR scanner's diagnostic imaging functionality is based on the ACR guidelines (ACR 1998, 2015). A dedicated phantom accompanied by a scanning and analysis procedure was designed to provide a straightforward recipe for quantifying the key vitals of an MR scanner. The ACR guidelines look at several tests such as geometric accuracy, high-contrast spatial resolution, slice thickness accuracy, slice position accuracy, percent intensity uniformity (PIU), percent signal ghosting (PSG), and low-contrast object detectability. ACR also discusses tests related to the magnetic field homogeneity, checks of the RF coils (i.e., PIU, PSG, SNR), and setup and table position accuracy. Depending on relevance and complexity in acquiring or interpreting the data, the QA tests were prescribed different performance frequencies.

For RT applications, it is important to mention that the ACR-type tests represent the minimum requirement for MR scanner QA. RT has more stringent requirements regarding the overall quality of the image data. Spatial accuracy is more demanding in RT than in diagnostic imaging since the image data is used for the delineation of the target, plan simulation, and guidance of the RT treatments. The geometric distortions should not exceed 1–2 mm to limit the propagation of errors in the RT workflow. RT also requires optimal image quality beyond the central axis were the ACR-type tests are performed. Targeted anatomy may lie off-axis, significantly away from the MR isocenter, or large field of views may be desired, for example, in RT workflows relying on MR-only data. RT processes often require dedicated patient setups involving immobilization devices (e.g., compression belts for motion management) or support systems (e.g., flat table tops).

This additional RT equipment needs to be tested to confirm acceptable levels of compatibility with the intended imaging procedures and clinical goals.

To establish a robust QA program for the routine monitoring of an MR scanner, the recommended approach is to acquire test baselines preferably early in the MR scanner lifetime. The baselines should be aligned with the system purchase specifications and the detailed technical and performance outcome of the scanner's acceptance process. The baselines would then be used to set action levels for the monitoring and troubleshooting of the system. Subsequent baselines need to be acquired on an annual basis to track the system performance depreciation over time. When possible it is recommended to synchronize baseline measurements with the service procedures provided by the MR manufacturer. One other factor to be considered refers to regulatory compliance at national, regional, or institutional level. An MRI QA program might not be mandatory but strongly recommended to provide a quantifiable threshold of standardization and accountability.

3.2 Advanced Management of MRI Data Quality for Radiotherapy

Radiation therapy poses a higher demand on the spatial accuracy of the image data that is meant to be utilized for treatment planning and in-room guidance of the patient setup verification and treatment delivery. This is mandated by the RT's need and ability to deliver therapeutic doses of radiation to diseased sites with high accuracy and precision (within 1–2 mm). The MRI's advantage of providing excellent soft-tissue contrast over conventional x-ray-based imaging (i.e., CBCT, CT) is somewhat diminished by its lack of spatial accuracy and intensity inhomogeneities, especially in the case of large field of views.

The image spatial distortions are caused by the imperfections of the hardware as well as by the interaction of the imaged subject with the MRI scanner's magnetic fields. Scanner-related distortions are mainly rooted in the nonlinear performance profile of the imaging gradients and global spatial inhomogeneities of the magnet's main magnetic field. In contrast, the subject or patient-induced spatial distortions are caused by local variations in the content and magnetic properties of adjacent tissues expressed as chemical shift and susceptibility perturbations, respectively. The magnitude of the system-related distortion field (S) can exceed 1 cm when mapped over large imaging volumes (particularly at the periphery) (Wang et al. 2004a; Stanescu et al. 2010; Baldwin et al. 2007), whereas the patient-induced distortion field (P) typically exhibits a level in the range of a few mm and is highly dependent on the imaging parameters (Stanescu et al. 2012). Organ motion adds an extra layer of complexity to S and P, by introducing the temporal component when the fields are assessed in the patient's frame of reference (Stanescu and Jaffray 2016).

The MRI user is presented with image data embedding the composite distortion field (C), which consists of the superposition of the individual S and P fields (Stanescu and Jaffray 2016). The contribution of each source toward the loss of geometric accuracy is often nontrivial, and expert review is needed to identify and mitigate the causes. Fortunately, there is a negligible coupling between S and C, and the distortions can be practically dealt with separately. This means that the system-related and patient-induced geometric distortions can be measured and quantified independent of each other, and corrections can be applied in no particular order. Overall, the spatial distortions need to be assessed and mitigated in the context of individual MRI-based procedure to guarantee the safe integration of MRI data in the radiotherapy workflows.

3.2.1 Scanner-Related Image Spatial Distortions

The scanner-related distortion field (S) is independent of the patient's anatomical specifics and can be quantified by means of a predefined QA process involving a phantom object. The magnitude of S is typically negligible in a small region at the MRI isocenter, and it gradually increases with distance. The management of distortions is provided to some extent by the MRI scanner manufacturers by continuously improving the design, the technologies behind the imaging gradients, and B_0 shimming systems. Furthermore, the manufacturers provide software-based distortion corrections based on theoretical or empirical models (Doran et al. 2005; Janke et al. 2004). Depending on the make and model of the MRI scanner, these corrections can vary widely in terms of spatial coverage and scope (2D or 3D) and can be turned on or off.

The corrections are typically implemented as an image post-processing step and automatically applied to the image sets. Some systems provide the flexibility of applying or removing the image corrections manually and on demand once the image sets are available.

The vendor corrections can be turned on/off by the user depending on the image protocol requirements. For RT purposes, it is strongly recommended to turn the geometric distortion option on, which assumes that the corrections are valid and that some correction is better than none. However, the user should assess this option as part of the MRI scanner commissioning or imaging protocol clinical implementation to ensure that the software corrections do indeed reduce the geometrical errors. It is also important to test and validate that this post-processing option does not introduce additional inaccuracies such as loss of resolution, pixel intensity inhomogeneities, and noise or truncation of the field of view. The DICOM header of the image sets should also be checked to confirm that the scanner's software keeps track of the changes applied to the image data.

The vendor-specific software corrections can be tested by scanning a phantom with a known structure and by switching the 2D/3D correction feature on/off. The two acquisition scenarios should then be compared with the true internal structure of the phantom to assess the extent of local geometric discrepancies by means of:

(a) Rigid registration using standard automatic and manual image registration tools available in any treatment planning system (TPS), in-house, or other any specialized software for image registration. The comparison can be done in relative terms between the MRI scans and by reference to a high-resolution CT scan of the phantom.

(b) Measurements of phantom's known geometric features on the MRI data sets and using as a reference the internal technical specifications of the phantom obtained from the manufacturer—e.g., brochure, CAD drawings.

In spite of significant advancements in improving the quality of the image data by the manufacturers, significant *residual distortions* are still expected, especially for RT applications (Doran et al. 2005; Walker et al. 2014). Therefore, the quantification and mitigation of image distortions for RT application are recommended.

3.2.1.1 Field Homogeneity

Routine testing for the homogeneity and stability of the main magnetic field (i.e., B_0 mapping) is strongly recommended as a prerequisite for high-quality imaging for RT purposes. 3D B_0 mapping techniques are desirable in order to get a comprehensive assessment of the magnetic field. This is beyond the typical ACR test, which is somewhat limited as the approach is based on the measurement of image uniformity for 2D slices. This is only sampling a limited region of the MRI's active imaging field, which is not fully representative for the volume required for RT applications.

The manufacturers typically use a sphere phantom with positive contrast and varying dimensions to measure spatial B_0 nonuniformities as part of their tuning up procedure at the time of MR system installation or routine preventive maintenance. Phantom imaging is often acquired with a GRE double-echo sequence, and magnitude and phase images are reconstructed as separate series. Image analysis is performed on the phase images, which embed the local variations of B_0, and depending on algorithm and the expected level of inhomogeneities, phase unwrapping may be performed for an adequate quantification of the B_0 distribution.

The B_0 mapping data is often reported in parts per million (ppm) via two metrics—i.e., B_{pp} and B_{rms}, representing the peak-to-peak and root-mean-square values of the sampled points in the analysis space. For example, typical upper limits for the baseline specifications are B_{pp} and B_{rms} of 3 ppm and 0.4 ppm, respectively, using a phantom with a 24 cm DSV. The B_0 mapping process is summarized in Fig. 3.1. In case the system performance is outside tolerance, the tuning of the active shim is required to correct the inhomogeneities.

More advanced B_0 techniques rely on imaging sequences involving multiple echoes for a finer quantification of the B_0 map, but this is more common when the acquisition is for correcting patient-specific data rather than dealing with a phantom (Matakos et al. 2014; Reinsberg et al. 2005; Windischberger et al. 2004).

3.2.1.2 Imaging Gradient Nonlinearity

Ideally, the imaging gradients should have a perfect linear profile, providing an accurate spatial relationship between the features depicted as image pixels and the true location and geometry of the imaged subject as shown in Fig. 3.2a. In practice, the linearity is compromised to some degree as the manufacturers aim to achieve a fast gradient rise time by reducing the coils length and number of turns. The deviation from gradient linearity is directly related to loss of spatial accuracy. A sample map of distortions represented as vectors is shown in Fig. 3.2b.

The gradient nonlinearity impact on imaging can be quantified using theoretical and/or experimental methods. MR manufacturers largely prefer to use truncated series of spherical harmonics to characterize the profile of each gradient since they have access to the technical specifications of the imaging system (Doran et al. 2005; Janke et al. 2004). Experimental methods based on a linearity phantom are more popular in the research/clinical community since (a) the direct output of the MR imaging system is quantified including the MR site/install specifics and (b) there are institutional/regulatory requirements for the independent QA validation.

There is no clear consensus on what phantom is best to use for the quantification of gradient

3 Quality Assurance

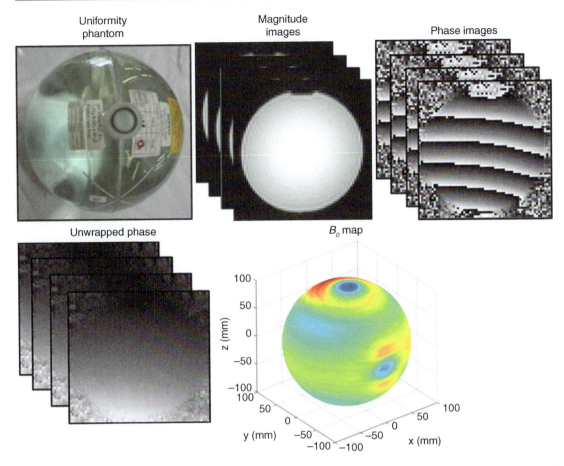

Fig. 3.1 B_0 mapping sample procedure: a spherical uniformity phantom is scanned, and magnitude/phase images are collected. In the case of significant field inhomogeneities, banding regions may be present in the phase images, and phase unwrapping may be necessary to extract and interpret the B_0 values. Spatial maps and statistics are then generated to characterize the level of field homogeneity

nonlinearities. Fortunately, the literature is rich in terms of recommendations and designs with various degrees of success at tackling the issue. The key characteristic is that the phantom needs to have a known and mechanically sound structure. The design relies on multiple aspects driven by the intended application:

(a) *Size of mapping volume*—Small for the head, to be used with a dedicated coil is optional. Large object to be able to map largest anatomical site (e.g., pelvis, chest) in order to acquire body contours needed for adaptive RT planning/dose accumulation.
(b) *Internal structure*—This aspect drives the level of complexity required for the extraction of the distortion field data. Image processing should be kept to a minimum to avoid propagation of errors. The distortion field is commonly extracted point by point given a certain spatial distribution of sampling points or "control points." The definition of a control point is very important—this can be something as simple as the intersection of a 2D/3D grid or a more complex physical feature such as center of mass of a surface located at the intersection of two structures. Another factor is using a single or modular structure with its pros and cons as per consideration (d) below. Using a positive or negative contrast for identifying the control points is a secondary aspect relevant to image data

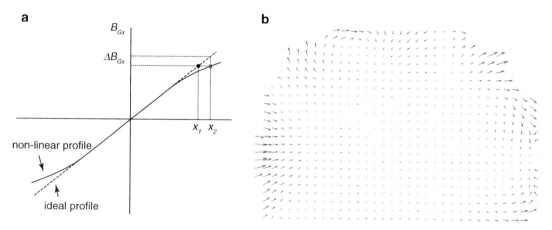

Fig. 3.2 (**a**) AB not specified in the artwork Diagram showing the ideal and realistic profiles of an imaging gradient. The linear difference between x_1 and x_2 represent the geometric error in representing the true location of a feature in the image. The concept can be expanded in two and three dimensions. (**b**) Sample in-plane distortion map showing negligible geometric distortions near the MR isocenter (center of the image). Magnitude of distortions increases with distance toward periphery and can follow different patterns depending on the location of the sampling slice in the imaging volume. The relative magnitude is given here by the length of the vectors, and the FOV is roughly 50 cm × 35 cm

post-processing. The materials used for the construction of the phantom and generation of MR signal are also important. High signal is desired to simplify design and minimize imaging acquisition time. Susceptibility matching between materials is recommended to maximize data quality and simplify acquisition methods—e.g., no need for forward-/reverse-gradient techniques for correction of susceptibility-induced artifacts (Chang and Fitzpatrick 1992). 3D mapping is highly recommended versus 2D. 2D may be still reasonable when used in conjunction with 3D, for spot-checks or routine/daily QA, instead of a large 3D phantom.

(c) *Sampling*—A sufficient number of control points are required to accurately render the distortion field. It is possible to use uniform sampling or adaptive sampling depending on expected behavior of the distortion field—e.g., lower sampling at CAX and denser points toward the periphery. The size of the control points can potentially drive the accuracy and precision in sampling a given VOI, especially in field regions with a higher degree or local variations.

(d) *Manipulation and setup*—The phantom can be designed to sit on a flat table top (more common with the integration or MR in RT) or a setup jig on/off table. Reproducibility of the setup is key. Size, shape, and weight are considerations related to the handling of the phantom, its setup, and ultimately staff safety.

(e) *Cost*—Important factor for maintenance/support and potential adoption of methodology by a larger community.

(f) *Analysis software*—The phantom image data needs to be processed in order to define and extract the distortion field. Once the phantom images are acquired, the MR-defined control points are extracted and rigidly registered to a template, representing the true structure of the phantom/control points. The template can be obtained from the CAD drawings of the phantom by CT scanning the phantom. The first option is desired as the second method may be limited by the intrinsic resolution available in the CT data. From the MR to template registration, the distortion field is computed as the vector deviation between paired points. The field can then be plotted and post-processed to provide a full picture of the impact on overall imaging. It is typical to plot 2D slices or 3D maps and evaluate metrics such as min/max/mean/sd. Plots showing max/mean distortions with distance from MR isocenter are also common and helpful to quickly assess potential impact on RT planning—e.g., contouring, dosimetric computations. The deployment of the analysis software within an organization may be an important factor especially in case of multiple scanners and MR workload. Reporting of the QA results needs to be accessible and relevant to the intended RT application(s).

Gradient nonlinearity and B_0 inhomogeneities effects can be both mapped with a linearity phantom (Stanescu et al. 2010; Walker et al. 2014; Wang et al. 2004b; Tanner et al. 2000). A single scan of the phantom, which is done with a predefined gradient orientation, embeds three effects: gradient, B_0, and susceptibility. By rerunning the same imaging sequence but with the readout gradient direction reversed (when possible), we also reverse the direction of the B_0 and susceptibility effects. By averaging the location of the control points in the two scenarios, we can preserve only the gradient-related distortion field. If the phantom is built with materials matched in terms of susceptibility, then the subtracted field is given by B_0 only.

Given the recent growing interest in the use of MRI in RT, QA device manufacturers started to offer more QA tools for the quantification of system-related distortions. More recent phantom designs aimed to better balance the challenges listed above. Specifically, using harmonic analysis techniques data collected only on the boundary of the phantom, distortion vector field can be reconstructed inside the phantom volume by means of solving a set of second-order partial differential equations. This method can be used for arbitrarily shaped phantom geometries (Stanescu and Jaffray 2018; Tadic et al. 2014). The concept is highlighted in Fig. 3.3.

Regardless of phantom choice and associated image analysis software, the distortion fields have to be assessed and validated for each individual scanner and for specific sequences used for RT. A typical procedure in the literature is to apply the fields and unwarp the images of a phantom with a known structure (i.e., linearity or other) via interpolation techniques. The corrected and raw sets are then compared to evaluate the residual distortions. If the distortion fields are accurate and the interpolation robust then the residual distortion field should be negligible. More commonly, the tolerance is given by the image pixel/voxel resolution of the raw data. Another approach is to rerun the analysis of the linearity phantom on the corrected images and recompute the distortion field. This may be a good approach but can potentially introduce bias.

Since the system-related distortions can be significant, they need to be mitigated in the RT workflow. In certain cases, the image series may need to be corrected by unwarping the raw data with the 3D vector fields derived from the linearity phantom. Extreme care is recommended in the data manipulation especially for the registration process between the reference distortion fields and patient data. The correlation between the DICOM coordinates is nontrivial and scanner (make/model) dependent. Comprehensive validation of the image correction workflow is required.

In summary, the MRI user needs to be aware of the two main avenues for mitigating the MR image distortions: (a) enable vendor corrections per imaging sequence/protocol (this may require extra effort to validate the quality of the overall correction process) and (b) measure distortions with a linearity phantom, assess clinical impact and correct (if needed) geometric distortions above a set threshold.

3.2.2 Patient-Induced Image Spatial Distortions

Anatomical regions may interact differently when exposed to B_0 depending on their magnetic properties characterized by the magnetic susceptibility (χ). Due to significant discontinuities in the χ values at tissue interfaces (e.g., bone-soft tissue, air-soft tissue), the local magnetic field

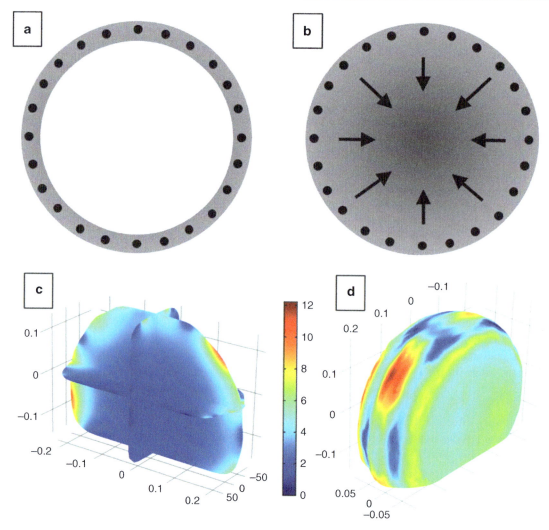

Fig. 3.3 Harmonic analysis applied to 3D distortion fields: (**a**) measurements are done only on the outer boundary of the volume of interest (arbitrary shape); (**b**) distortions are numerically derived for the full inner domain by solving a well-defined boundary value problem; (**c**) and (**d**) show sample maps corresponding to the inside domain and its boundary, respectively, in the case of a large FOV with a non-quadratic shape

may exhibit a level of perturbations which translate into spatial distortions and image intensity artifacts (Ludeke et al. 1985; Schenck 1996). The χ-induced effects are most dominant at the air-soft tissue interfaces and can be extreme when metallic materials are embedded in tissue (e.g., clips, implants, etc.).

The molecular environment specific to each tissue can also introduce small changes in the resonant frequency of neighboring tissues, and this can lead to local anatomical misrepresentations described as chemical shift artifacts. The most common effect is at the water and fat tissues' interface with a perturbation of approximately 3.5 ppm or 220/440 Hz at 1.5/3 T.

The P field, representing the superposition of the χ and chemical shift effects, is typically present along the frequency-encode direction. In particular, chemical shift artifacts can also arise along the phase-encode direction (e.g., EPI) or out of plane in 2DFT imaging.

The magnitude of the χ effects depends mainly on the strength of B_0 and frequency-encoding gradient (G_E) as Δr [mm] = ppm × B_0/G_E.

χ-induced magnetic field maps (in ppm) can be computed via numerical simulations (Stanescu et al. 2012; Bhagwandien et al. 1992) or by measurements via B_0 maps (Jezzard and Balaban 1995; Wang et al. 2013). For a given B_0, the imaging protocols can be optimized to reduce the spatial distortions within a desired threshold using reference plots derived from magnetic field simulations specific to anatomical sites (Stanescu et al. 2012; Stanescu and Jaffray 2016). Alternatively, the B_0 maps in patient can be acquired as part of the imaging protocol—this is needed to make the data relevant to the anatomy/setup of the day. This adds extra imaging time, and image post-processing may be required to subtract the χ effects from the anatomical data intended for the RT workflow. The process can be quite demanding and prone to co-registration errors due to patient motion in case of prolonged imaging times. The above approaches can be tested in a phantom with a simple geometry that provides an interface between two materials (Baldwin et al. 2009). In general, the recommendation is to increase G_E for a given B_0 with the consideration that the SNR will depreciate, and this can impact the quality of the clinical images.

The chemical shift can be computed a priori and reduced within tolerance levels when developing the imaging protocol(s). Given a certain receiver bandwidth (BW) and acquisition matrix size, the BW/pixel can be computed. The water-fat shift is known, and considering the magnitude of B_0, the extent of the chemical shift (in pixels) at 1.5 T is given by 220 Hz × BW/pixel. Similar to the χ effects, a sufficient increase in the BW will reduce the chemical shift artifacts.

In summary, S and P fields are similar in the way that they lead to loss in the linear correlation between the imaged and rendered subject's features but are different in terms of spatial propagation. A QA process is recommended to ensure that a relevant assessment of the overall composite distortion field C is in place.

3.2.3 Lasers

Many of the clinical MRI scanners used for RT planning do not have an external laser system similar to what is typically used for RT patient setup (CT simulation or linac pretreatment verification). One of the reasons is that these systems are available via a diagnostic radiology department. Other RT workflows rely on MR acquisitions guided by patient markings defined at CT in conjunction with the use of MR data as secondary sets for image registration with CT. However, it may be useful to have an external laser system to assess the patient positioning consistency. Such a laser system becomes necessary when MR-only workflows are designed and implemented. Regarding QA, the accuracy of the external laser system and its relationship with the MR's internal laser, in terms of prescribed relative distance and coordinates, need to be checked on a routine basis. A dedicated phantom can be designed to characterize the lasers performance as shown in Fig. 3.4.

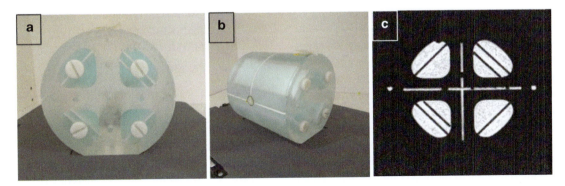

Fig. 3.4 Example of a phantom that can be used for the QA of the laser system: (**a**, **b**) show the design of the phantom, and (**c**) depicts an axial sample image at the center of the phantom (Courtesy of Robba Rai)

3.2.4 Considerations for Radiation Therapy Setups

It is essential to perform MR simulation for RT purpose in the exact treatment position. This requires the use of the same patient immobilization devices—e.g., flat table top, patient constraints support (such as Vac-Lok cradles), site-specific setups (e.g., SBRT half/full baseboards—see Orfit, qFix), etc. Whenever possible, it is recommended to use MR-safe and compatible devices for both MRI and CT acquisition sessions to ensure consistency between RT processes. Depending on resources, these devices may be built-in house if not available commercially. Patient customization may also be needed in certain scenarios—e.g., patient immobilization cradles are made in the CT simulation process immediately prior to the MR simulation to ensure patients are imaged in the same position and with minimal patient anatomy changes. It is also recommended to follow the same motion management schemes (i.e., breath hold, abdominal compression, or free breathing) for the MRI scans as in the CT simulation. All devices required for the patient setup should be part of the end-to-end testing as part of the commissioning process of clinical protocols.

3.3 Strategies for Efficient Management of MRI QA in RT

3.3.1 Rationale

As MR plays an increasing role in RT treatment, simulation, and guidance, the efficient management of MR imaging QA becomes critical. The general principle for MRI QA in RT should be similar to diagnostic imaging. However, additional tests and procedures are needed to ensure that RT-specific characteristics are assessed and mitigated (e.g., 3D geometric distortion, frequency of tests). Additional tests and increased complexity in the interpretation of the data combined with a high patient/data throughput rapidly become a significant challenge for the RT workflow.

3.3.2 Automation of QA

Considering an increased volume of QA—reflected as more tests, higher incidence, and more sophisticated data analysis—it is desirable to automate the QA processes. This aspect becomes especially important when MRI data is acquired and is meant to be readily used for RT planning and in-room guidance. This may be the case for on-demand plan adaptation and treatment delivery. In such scenario, the manual intervention or manipulation of the data should be avoided to expedite the data processing and mitigate for potential human errors. Process automation may be necessary to guarantee process consistency and reliability. Automation may also prove useful for data and system performance standardization across multiple MR scanners.

3.3.3 Example of an Automated Imaging Pipelines for MRI QA

The automation of MRI QA processes requires a robust infrastructure to allow a seamless flow of data. An example of an automated imaging pipeline is shown in Fig. 3.5. The architecture of the pipeline is based on two virtual machines (VMs), which perform specialized tasks and interact with each other. The main functionality of the pipeline is highlighted as follows:

- VM1 hosts a DICOM server and the ability to filter incoming data. VM1 can also trigger specific events based on data classification.
- VM1 hosts the data analysis container, which has a modular structure and can run user-defined applications. Data analysis is performed via serial or parallel processes.
- VM2 hosts a relational database which stores the output generated by VM1, a web server and a web application required for data logging, audit, and online visualization.
- The front end of the web application consists of a user-friendly interface based on dashboards which can display key analytics (e.g., MRI QA metrics—see ACR tests). Access is secured and customized depending on user

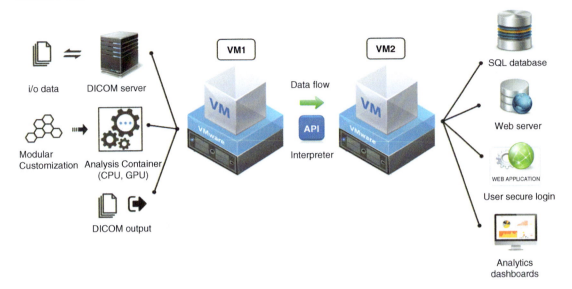

Fig. 3.5 Diagram depicting the architecture of an imaging pipeline developed to enable automation of MRI QA

credentials—e.g., a user can see only one scanner or all scanners available in the database.
- Near real-time feedback is provided to the MR user via email notifications and the online web interface.
- Automated QA includes the use of several phantoms with user-specific analysis.
- Distortion correction is implemented via phantom measurements performed for multiple clinical image acquisition scenarios. A library of 3D vector distortion fields is stored and indexed on VM1. The distortion vector fields are subsequently used to correct image data sets (phantom, patient) on demand.

References

AAPM. AAPM report no. 100: Acceptance testing and quality assurance procedures for magnetic resonance imaging facilities. Alexandria, VA: AAPM; 2010.

ACR. Phantom test guidance for the ACR MRI. Reston, VA: ACR; 1998.

ACR. MRI quality control manual. Reston, VA: ACR; 2015.

Baldwin LN, et al. Characterization, prediction, and correction of geometric distortion in 3 T MR images. Med Phys. 2007;34(2):388–99.

Baldwin LN, Wachowicz K, Fallone BG. A two-step scheme for distortion rectification of magnetic resonance images. Med Phys. 2009;36(9):3917–26.

Bhagwandien R, et al. Numerical analysis of the magnetic field for arbitrary magnetic susceptibility distributions in 2D. Magn Reson Imaging. 1992;10(2):299–313.

Chang H, Fitzpatrick JM. A technique for accurate magnetic resonance imaging in the presence of field inhomogeneities. IEEE Trans Med Imaging. 1992;11(3):319–29.

Doran SJ, et al. A complete distortion correction for MR images: I. Gradient warp correction. Phys Med Biol. 2005;50(7):1343–61.

Janke A, et al. Use of spherical harmonic deconvolution methods to compensate for nonlinear gradient effects on MRI images. Magn Reson Med. 2004;52(1):115–22.

Jezzard P, Balaban RS. Correction for geometric distortion in echo planar images from B0 field variations. Magn Reson Med. 1995;34(1):65–73.

Ludeke KM, Roschmann P, Tischler R. Susceptibility artefacts in NMR imaging. Magn Reson Imaging. 1985;3(4):329–43.

Matakos A, Balter J, Cao Y. Estimation of geometrically undistorted B(0) inhomogeneity maps. Phys Med Biol. 2014;59(17):4945–59.

Reinsberg SA, et al. A complete distortion correction for MR images: II. Rectification of static-field inhomogeneities by similarity-based profile mapping. Phys Med Biol. 2005;50(11):2651–61.

Schenck JF. The role of magnetic susceptibility in magnetic resonance imaging: MRI magnetic compatibility of the first and second kinds. Med Phys. 1996;23(6):815–50.

Stanescu T, Jaffray D. Investigation of the 4D composite MR image distortion field associated with tumor motion for MR-guided radiotherapy. Med Phys. 2016;43(3):1550–62.

Stanescu T, Jaffray D. Technical note: harmonic analysis applied to MR image distortion fields specific to arbitrarily shaped volumes. Med Phys. 2018. https://doi.org/10.1002/mp.13000.

Stanescu T, et al. Investigation of a 3D system distortion correction method for MR images. J Appl Clin Med Phys. 2010;11(1):2961.

Stanescu T, Wachowicz K, Jaffray DA. Characterization of tissue magnetic susceptibility-induced distortions for MRIgRT. Med Phys. 2012;39(12):7185–93.

Tadic T, Jaffray DA, Stanescu T. Harmonic analysis for the characterization and correction of geometric distortion in MRI. Med Phys. 2014;41(11):112303.

Tanner SF, et al. Radiotherapy planning of the pelvis using distortion corrected MR images: the removal of system distortions. Phys Med Biol. 2000;45(8):2117–32.

Walker A, et al. MRI distortion: considerations for MRI based radiotherapy treatment planning. Australas Phys Eng Sci Med. 2014;37(1):103–13.

Wang D, Strugnell W, Cowin G, Doddrell DM, Slaughter R. Geometric distortion in clinical MRI systems part II: correction using a 3D phantom. Magn Reson Imaging. 2004a;22(9):1223–32.

Wang D, et al. Geometric distortion in clinical MRI systems part I: evaluation using a 3D phantom. Magn Reson Imaging. 2004b;22(9):1211–21.

Wang H, Balter J, Cao Y. Patient-induced susceptibility effect on geometric distortion of clinical brain MRI for radiation treatment planning on a 3T scanner. Phys Med Biol. 2013;58(3):465–77.

Windischberger C, et al. Robust field map generation using a triple-echo acquisition. J Magn Reson Imaging. 2004;20(4):730–4.

Clinical Applications of MRI in Radiotherapy Planning

Houda Bahig, Eugene Koay, Maroie Barkati, David C. Fuller, and Cynthia Menard

4.1 Introduction

Owing to the superior soft tissue visualization of MRI compared to computed tomography (CT), the use of MRI in radiotherapy planning has been adopted as part of the standard radiotherapy workflow in several clinical sites. For the majority of sites, MR images used for planning purposes are currently co-registered to the planning CT. CT remains de facto the standard-of-care imaging modality for dose calculation due to its geometric fidelity and electron density information. However, as discussed in Chap. 9, MRI-only planning workflows are actively being developed and are in the early stages of adoption for some clinical sites.

The major advantage of MRI for radiotherapy planning is that of improved tumor and organs at risk (OAR) depiction. In general, it is felt that accurate target volume delineation, combined with the possibilities of functional imaging offered by MRI, has the potential to enhance therapeutic ratios and enhance individualized approaches in radiotherapy planning. At the moment, predominant literature on the use of MRI for radiotherapy planning is focused on head and neck, central nervous system, prostate, gynecological, gastrointestinal, breast, and lung cancer sites. Table 4.1 summarizes the commonly used MRI sequences in each of these tumor sites and their purpose in the clinic. In this chapter, we will provide an overview of the literature supporting the use of planning MRI across these sites.

4.2 Central Nervous System

The role of MRI in radiotherapy planning was first established in brain tumors, and the use of co-registered MRI (planning or diagnostic) is currently considered a requirement for most intracranial tumors. MRI shows marked contrast between white and gray matter in the brain, allowing for improved delineation and reduction of inter-observer variability of the gross tumor volume (GTV), of the surgical cavity in the post-operative setting, and of critical organs at risk (OAR) such as the optic chiasm or brainstem (Scoccianti et al. 2015; Aoyama et al. 2001).

Gliomas present as hypo-intense lesions on T1-weighted MRI sequence. While low-grade gliomas are hyperintense on T2-weighted or fluid attenuation inversion recovery (FLAIR) sequences and show no enhancement post-gadolinium

H. Bahig (✉)
Centre Hospitalier de l'Université de Montréal, Montreal, QC, Canada

The University of Texas MD Anderson Cancer Center, Houston, TX, USA

E. Koay · D. C. Fuller
The University of Texas MD Anderson Cancer Center, Houston, TX, USA

M. Barkati · C. Menard
Centre Hospitalier de l'Université de Montréal, Montreal, QC, Canada

© Springer Nature Switzerland AG 2019
G. Liney, U. van der Heide (eds.), *MRI for Radiotherapy*,
https://doi.org/10.1007/978-3-030-14442-5_4

Table 4.1 Summary of site-specific common MRI sequences and their purpose in the clinic

	Sequences	Purpose
Brain	T1-w + contrast	GTV delineation: high-grade glioma, metastasis, benign pathologies (meningioma; acoustic neuroma)
		3D isotropic (1 mm)—recommended for radiosurgery
	T2-w or FLAIR	GTV delineation: low-grade glioma
		Edema and postoperative changes identification
Spine	T1-w	GTV delineation
	T2-w or STIR	Contrast between spinal cord and cerebrospinal fluid
		Edema visualization
	Consider metal artifact reduction sequences (multi-acquisition variable-resonance image combination or slice-encoding for metal artifact correction (Scoccianti et al. 2015))	Postoperative metallic fixation devices
Head and neck	T1-w fat sat + contrast	GTV and OAR delineation
	T2-w ± fat saturation	Edema identification, salivary glands
	DWI	Detection of metastatic lymph nodes
		Response prediction (investigational)
		Salivary gland function (investigational)
Breast	T1-w ± contrast	Preoperative GTV assessment
		Axillary lymph nodes
	T2-w or STIR	Seroma cavity, internal mammary chain, axillary nodes, and brachial plexus delineation
Lung	T1-w fat-saturation ± contrast (breath hold or respiratory triggered)	GTV and OAR delineation
	T2-w (breath hold or respiratory triggered)	GTV and OAR delineation
	Cine MRI/4D MRI	Motion assessment (investigational)
	DWI	Differentiation of GTV from atelectasis
		Pathological lymph node delineation
Liver and pancreas	T2-w	Duodenal wall delineation
		OAR delineation
	T1-w fat saturation	GTV delineation
		Normal pancreas gland delineation
	T1-w fat saturation + contrast – arterial phase	GTV delineation + lymph nodes
	T1-w fat saturation + contrast – venous phase	GTV and venous structures delineation
	T1-w fat saturation + contrast – delayed venous	Portal vein contouring
	Cine MRI/4D MRI	Motion assessment (investigational)
Cervix	T2-w	Delineation of GTV and OAR
	T1-w fat saturation	Delineation of GTV and OAR
	T2-w HASTE	Brachytherapy—confirmation of applicator positioning
	DWI	GTV delineation (investigational)
		Prediction of treatment response (investigational)
Rectum	T2-w	GTV, rectum and bladder delineation
	T1-w + contrast	GTV delineation
	DWI	GTV delineation (investigational)
Prostate	T2-w	Prostate and tumor delineation
	DWI	GTV delineation
	DCE	GTV delineation (salvage therapy)

GTV gross tumor volume, *w* weighted, *FLAIR* fluid-attenuated inversion recovery, *STIR* short-TI inversion recovery, *DWI* diffusion-weighted imaging, *OAR* organ at risk, *HASTE* half Fourier single-shot turbo spin-echo, *DCE* dynamic contrast enhanced injection, high-grade gliomas usually show irregular enhancement after gadolinium contrast injection in areas of blood-brain barrier breakdown. Vasogenic edema is best visualized on T2-weighted sequences and is often included in the clinical target volume (CTV). In high-grade glioma, both the GTV and CTV contoured on MRI were shown to be significantly larger than those contoured on CT (Fiorentino et al. 2013). In clinical practice, gadolinium-injected 3D T1-weighted as well as axial 2D FLAIR MRI are required in most radiotherapy planning protocols for gliomas (Stall et al. 2010) (Fig. 4.1). For base of skull tumors, the addition of a high-resolution 3D T2-w image should be strongly considered. In general, acquisition parameters should follow the consensus recommendations for a standardized brain tumor imaging protocols in clinical trials (Ellingson et al. 2015).

The recent paradigm shift toward increasing use of stereotactic radiosurgery (SRS) and the recent introduction of hippocampal-sparing whole brain radiotherapy have made MRI an essential component of radiotherapy planning for brain metastasis. For SRS, MRI has superior sensitivity for detection of brain metastasis as well as for detection of leptomeningeal disease (Straathof et al. 1999), two crucial criteria for eligibility to SRS. There is some evidence that the number and size of brain metastasis can change between the time of diagnostic MRI and that of planning MRI (Nagai et al. 2010). This is explained partly by the elapsed time but also by the use of thin-slice MRI for SRS planning. In this context, in addition to increased precision of co-registration with use of a planning MRI (vs. diagnostic MRI), the use of a thin-slice planning MRI has the particular advantage of assessing disease burden and contouring GTV more accurately shortly before treatment start. Hippocampal-sparing whole brain radiotherapy is an experimental approach aiming at reducing neurocognitive toxicity of radiotherapy by preserving neural stem cells located in the hippocampus. Use of MRI is required for proper identification of the gray matter preponderance of the hippocampus, best visualized on a T1-weighted sequence, as detailed in the guidelines of the ongoing RTOG 0933 clinical trial (Gondi et al. 2014).

Diagnostic MRI is the gold standard for diagnosis and characterization of spinal disease. In radiotherapy, diagnostic MRI has long been used

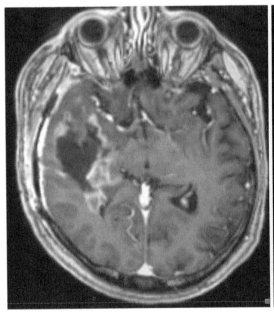
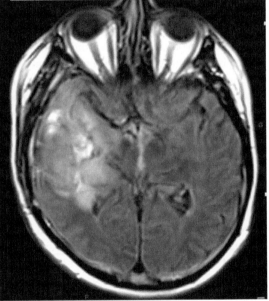

Fig. 4.1 Postoperative glioblastoma. Contrast-enhanced T1-weighted MRI (left) and FLAIR (right) after subtotal resection of glioblastoma at the time of radiotherapy planning. The surgical cavity is surrounded by contrast-enhancing tumor, while FLAIR demonstrates microscopic infiltration of adjacent brain

for assessment of tumoral extension into the spinal canal when there is concern about spinal cord compression. With the emergence of spine stereotactic body radiotherapy (SBRT) as a treatment option for selected spinal tumors, MRI has now evolved to being essential in spinal radiotherapy planning. Spine SBRT consists in delivering ablative radiation doses to the tumor in a short number of fractions while sparing the surrounding critical organs, notably the spinal cord. The extent of epidural disease appreciated on MRI is crucial for determining eligibility to upfront spine SBRT versus consideration for surgical decompression. Importantly, accurate outlining of the GTV and the spinal cord allows for safe dose escalation in close proximity to the spinal cord (Bedford et al. 2012). T1- and T2-weighted MRI sequences are helpful at delimiting spread of bony lesions and at detecting early disease extension in the bone marrow (Mizowaki et al. 2001). Co-registration of these sequences, at the minimum, with the planning CT is required in current spine SBRT guidelines for assessment of soft tissue extension and spinal cord delineation (Ryu et al. 2014; Tseng et al. 2017). In addition, use of gadolinium contrast may be useful for delineating paraspinal disease and for further accentuating bone marrow abnormalities.

Central nervous system functional MRI is a very active area of research, with multiple promising techniques under investigation. Diffusion tensor MRI allows for visualization of axonal (white matter) organization of the brain and has potential for assessing integrity of neural tracts (for tumor delineation), for sparing of white matter fibers such as the optic radiation (Jena et al. 2005), or for predicting cognitive decline (Chapman et al. 2016). MR spectroscopy provides information regarding the presence and concentration of various metabolites and has been used to differentiate radiation necrosis from recurrent tumor (Einstein et al. 2012). Blood-oxygen-level-dependent contrast imaging has been proposed to identify and spare eloquent brain areas (Liu et al. 2000). Like in other clinical sites, DWI and perfusion MRI are being evaluated in both intracranial and spinal tumors for further enhancement of tumor delineation (White et al. 2013) and treatment response prediction (Spratt et al. 2016; Pramanik et al. 2015). Finally, susceptibility-weighted imaging for assessment of microbleeds after radiotherapy is a promising technique for prediction of posttreatment neurovascular toxicity (Belliveau et al. 2017).

4.3 Head and Neck Cancer

The introduction of intensity-modulated radiotherapy (IMRT) as standard of care in head and neck cancer (HNC) has made accurate assessment of tumor volume an essential component of radiotherapy planning. The improved soft tissue contrast of MRI is of particular importance in HNC where discrimination between tumor and surrounding healthy tissues can help avoid unnecessary dose to critical OAR and reduce treatment-related toxicities. Recently published international head and neck radiotherapy consensus guidelines strongly advocate for the use of MRI for delineation of primary tumor in the oral cavity, oropharynx, and nasopharynx, as well as for delineation of several OAR, notably the brainstem, spinal cord, pituitary gland, lacrimal glands, optic structures, parotid glands, and pharyngeal constrictor muscles (Brouwer et al. 2015). Use of MRI in HNC has been associated with reduced inter-observer variability for GTV and OAR contouring, as well as with better definition of tumor extension to surrounding anatomical sites, such as the extrinsic muscles of the tongue (Prestwich et al. 2012). Figure 4.2 shows a case of tonsillar squamous cell cancer where tumor borders are well visualized on contrast-enhanced T1-weighted MRI compared to contrast-enhanced CT. The advantage of MRI in HNC radiotherapy planning is perhaps most evident in base of skull tumors, where MRI enables identification of intracranial extensions, perineural spreads, dural thickening, and subtle skull base bony invasion, all of which are typically poorly visualized on CT imaging and affect both tumor staging and GTV delineation (Zhang et al. 2014; Chung et al. 2004).

Figure 4.3 demonstrates a case of nasopharynx cancer where perineural involvement of the maxillary branch of the trigeminal nerve is well appreciated on contrast-injected T1-weighted

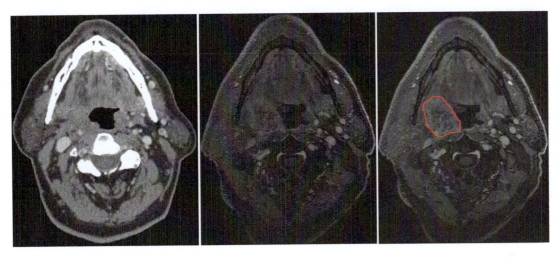

Fig. 4.2 Large squamous cell carcinoma of the right palatine tonsil measuring 3.6 cm × 2.5 cm involving the adjacent right glossopharyngeal sulcus and infiltrating posteriorly the right retropharyngeal space can be visualized on axial contrast-injected CT (left); tumor borders are better appreciated on axial contrast-enhanced T1-weighted MRI (right). Red contour: GTV

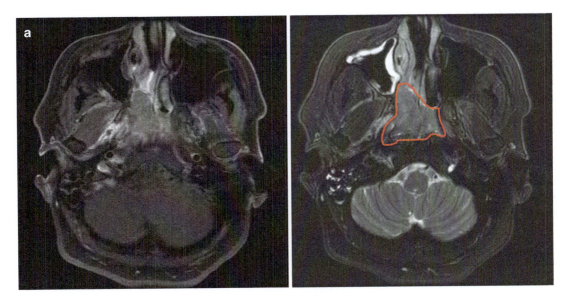

Fig. 4.3 (**a**) Bilateral nasopharyngeal primary tumor is well appreciated on axial contrast-injected T1-weighted (left) and T2-weighted MRI (right). Red contour: GTV. (**b**) Axial and coronal slices showing thickening and enhancement of the maxillary branch (V2) of the trigeminal nerve suspicious for perineural involvement in the right pterygopalatine fossa and right foramen rotundum (arrows)

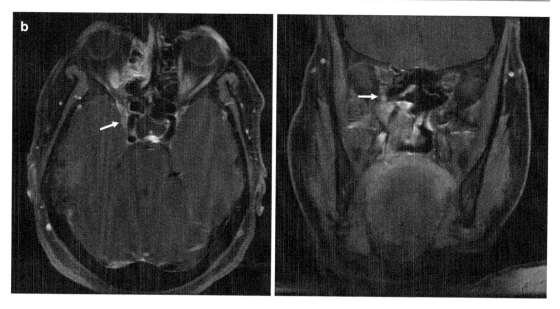

Fig. 4.3 (continued)

MRI. Although bone cortex erosion is often better appreciated on CT, MRI may be superior for detection of skull base invasion (Zhang et al. 2014). Due to image degradation induced by swallowing and respiratory motion, the superiority of MRI over CT for delineation of larynx and hypopharynx tumors remains uncertain. Similarly, the advantage of MRI for delineation of nodal disease is controversial (Sun et al. 2015), but anatomical MRI may have superior sensitivity in the particular context of retropharyngeal lymph nodes (Kato et al. 2014). Lastly, given that poor dentition shares risk factors with HNC, dental artifacts are a common problem in HNC radiotherapy planning. Dental restorations are made of high-attenuation metal, which can cause scatter artifacts and, as a consequence, can severely impair CT-based oral cavity or oropharynx primary tumor delineation (Cooper et al. 2007). With MRI, variations in magnetic field strength at the interface between dental material and soft tissues also cause artifacts, but image quality is usually affected to a lesser extent (Klinke et al. 2012). Functional MRI is an active area of investigation in HNC and includes, among many other applications, use of diffusion-weighted imaging (DWI) for identification of radioresistant disease (Law et al. 2016), detection of lymph node metastases (Perrone et al. 2011), or assessment of baseline and posttreatment salivary gland function (Loimu et al. 2017). Both DWI and dynamic contrast MRI (DCE-MRI) are investigated as noninvasive predictive biomarkers of outcomes (King and Thoeny 2016).

4.4 Thorax

4.4.1 Breast

The use of MRI in breast radiotherapy planning remains experimental, and its role in radiotherapy treatment planning remains controversial. An important pitfall of the integration of MRI in breast radiotherapy planning is that while breast cancer radiation planning is most commonly performed in supine position to maximize beam entry angles, breast MRI in prone position is optimal as it allows to reduce the effects of respiratory motion and geometric inaccuracies. In diagnostic radiology, MRI was shown to have greater sensitivity than mammography for assessment of tumor extension and improved precision for measurement of tumor size as well as for detection of multifocal disease (Chandwani et al. 2014; Sardanelli et al. 2004). These advantages can be attractive in the context of preoperative radiotherapy, such as in the recent strategies of MRI-guided ablative accelerated partial breast irradiation (Charaghvandi et al. 2017; Horton et al. 2015). In the postoperative setting, whole breast irradiation involves inclusion of the entire glandular breast tissue in the CTV. Interestingly, breast MRI in supine position shows higher cranial extension of breast glandular tissue compared to CT in supine position (Giezen et al. 2011). However, given the excellent current outcomes with whole breast irradiation based on CT alone, the necessity to extend the CTV to the most superior regions of MRI-based glandular tissue is unclear and requires further investigation. In addition, there is discordant data on the role of MRI for delineation of the surgical cavity. While some data showed reduced volume of surgical bed delineation and improved inter-observer variability with MRI, other studies suggest no additional information or even discordant information of MRI compared to surgical bed delineation based on CT and surgical clips (Jolicoeur et al. 2011; Giezen et al. 2012; Kirby et al. 2009). Interesting areas of functional imaging involve the use of DWI for GTV and individual lymph node delineation (van Heijst et al. 2016). In addition, the feasibility and clinical value cardiac-gated MRI for imaging of the heart and coronaries, particularly in left radiation planning, is an active area of research.

4.4.2 Lung

Lung MRI has historically been of limited use in both diagnostic radiology and radiotherapy planning due to the issues of respiratory motion and low tissue density of the lungs inducing signal-to-noise ratio reduction and magnetic susceptibility effects. In recent years, technology enhancements have allowed faster acquisition times and improved respiratory gating techniques, which have resulted in better quality of lung MRI (Miller et al. 2014). Literature on use of MRI in lung radiotherapy planning remains scant. Potential benefits of MRI compared to CT may include improvement of evaluation of mediastinal and chest wall invasion, discrimination of tumor from atelectasis and brachial plexus delineation (Cobben et al. 2016). MRI may also have improved sensitivity and accuracy for diagnosis of pathological hilar and mediastinal lymph nodes in non-small cell lung cancer compared to fluorodeoxyglucose positron-emission tomography (Peerlings et al. 2016). Individualized assessment of respiratory motion or selection of appropriate respiratory-gated window through the use of 4D MRI is another pivotal application of MRI in lung radiotherapy (Freedman et al. 2017). While 4D CT is an established technique routinely used in lung radiotherapy planning, a pitfall of 4D CT is that it represents a single breathing cycle which may not be representative of the patient breathing pattern, required regular speed and amplitude of breathing and therefore good cooperation of patients. In the contrary, 4D MRI can capture multiple breathing cycles, over a prolonged period of time, at no radiation cost. It can therefore be more representative of natural breathing motion and be appropriate for uncooperative patients. In addition, the combined evaluation of natural sliding motion of the lungs with soft tissue visualization could help further assess invasion of adjacent structures (Freedman et al. 2017). Dynamic slice-selective 2D acquisition and volumetric 3D acquisition are two potential methods to derive of 4D MRI. The feasibility, geometric distortion, and accuracy of various 4D MRI strategies are currently being assessed by early adopters in lung radiotherapy but also in other sites subject to breathing motion such as the upper abdomen or head and neck region. Functional imaging has a promising role for delineation of involved lymph nodes, discrimination of tumor from atelectasis, prediction of treatment response, as well as assessment of functional lung parenchyma in lung function-sparing strategies (Cobben et al. 2016; Hodge et al. 2010).

4.5 Abdomen and Pelvis

4.5.1 Pancreas and Liver

For both pancreatic and liver tumors, CT remains the standard for radiotherapy planning. However, as highlighted by the recently published multi-institutional MRI-based contouring guidelines for pancreatic tumors and adjacent organs at risks (Heerkens et al. 2017), the role of MRI is rapidly growing. While dose escalation has been hypothesized to improve the current dismal outcomes of pancreatic cancer, the presence of dose-limiting adjacent organs at risk (duodenum, stomach, and jejunum) in close vicinity prevents safe dose escalation (Crane and Koay 2016). Better assessment of local tumor extension and improved discrimination of GTV from adjacent structures with MRI compared to CT has the potential to allow dose escalation strategies (Saisho and Yamaguchi 2004; Koay et al. 2017). In pancreas, commonly used MRI sequences include a T2-weighted sequence for optimal duodenal wall delineation, a fat-suppressed T1-weighted sequence for discrimination of normal pancreas, and a post-contrast late arterial phase fat-suppressed T1-weighted sequence for tumor and lymph node delineation (Koay et al. 2018). In the liver, radiotherapy planning of both primary and metastatic tumors is challenging due to the minimal contrast between the tumor and surrounding normal liver. Typical helpful MRI sequences include T1- and T2-weighted sequences. Figure 4.4 shows a well-demarcated large hepatocellular carcinoma on T2-weighted MRI. In addition, post-contrast fat-suppressed T1-weighted sequence and multiphase CT are frequently used for target delineation. While the early arterial phase enhancement and venous phase washout best characterize hepatocellular carcinomas, the venous phase is optimal for most metastatic liver lesions (Choi and Lee 2010; Fowler et al. 2011). Liver GTV derived from MRI was shown to be 180–250% larger than that derived from CT (Pech et al. 2008). Respiratory motion affecting the upper abdominal organs is another difficulty of liver and pancreas radiotherapy planning. While 4D CT is generally used for motion assessment, 4D MRI is gaining an increasing role. The advantage of 4D MRI is that of assessment of motion over several respiratory cycles, at no ionizing radiation cost. This can translate into use of personalized planning target volumes based on individual assessment of respiratory motion or selection of appropriate respiratory-gated window (Brock and Dawson 2010; Stemkens et al. 2015). A promising future application of 4D MRI is that of real-time tumor tracking for further reduction of PTV margin, which could be made possible with the recent development of MR-linac technology and may further facilitate dose escalation strategies (Lagendijk et al. 2014).

4.5.2 Rectum

MRI is considered the gold standard for rectal imaging, and it is routine clinical practice to use co-registered MRI for target volume delineation

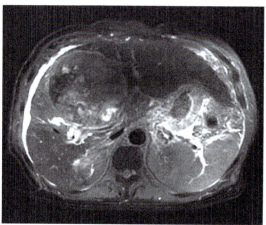 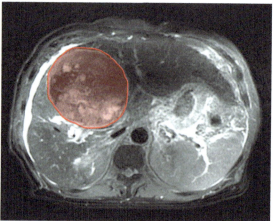

Fig. 4.4 Axial T2-weighted image showing large heterogeneous mass, biopsy-proven hepatocellular carcinoma, involving liver segments II/III and IV (red)

in radiotherapy planning. Use of multi-planar imaging helps to better appreciate anatomy and is useful to determine cranio-caudal extension of the GTV. In general, rectal tumors show mild hyperintensity on T2-weighted sequences, enhance on post-gadolinium injection, and show restricted diffusion on DWI. Depth of invasion through the rectal wall as well as extension to surrounding structures is also better appreciated on MRI (Gwynne et al. 2012). Perhaps the most important benefit of MRI in rectal cancer treatment planning is that GTV derived from MRI is generally smaller and, in low rectal tumor, often further from the anal sphincter compared to CT-based delineation, allowing for relative sparing of the anal sphincter/pelvic floor (Tan et al. 2010). Reduction of GTV dimensions in cranio-caudal direction also reduces CTV, leading to a reduction in dose to organs at risk including the bladder, bowel, ovary, uterus, testes, penile bulb, and anal sphincter (Tan et al. 2010). In addition to reducing toxicities, this could facilitate dose escalation strategies (Tan et al. 2010). To reduce variations in rectal and bladder filling between planning CT and MRI, patient preparation including use of muscle relaxant and identical bladder filling protocols is recommended. Like in other clinical sites, use of functional MRI including both diffusion and DCE-MRI generally remains investigational, and active research is ongoing to determine their role for tumor delineation, treatment response prediction, and detection of regional lymph node metastasis (Lambrecht et al. 2012; Pham et al. 2017).

4.5.3 Prostate

The prostate is another organ site where the role of MRI in radiotherapy planning has been extensively studied. Multiparametric MRI, including T2-weighted, high-*b*-value DWI, and DCE sequences, is now an established protocol for detection of intraprostatic lesions and disease staging, as per PI-RADS v2 guidelines (Weinreb et al. 2016). While CT has traditionally been used to contour the prostate gland, boundaries of the prostate gland are well depicted on T2-weighted MRI, where the high signal intensity of the prostate can help locate the prostatic apex and discriminate adjacent structures (i.e., levator ani muscle, rectum, distal urethral sphincter, and urogenital diaphragm) (Villeirs and De Meerleer 2007; Milosevic et al. 1998). This generally leads to smaller CTV compared to those obtained with CT and therefore offers the advantage of OAR and potentially reduction of toxicities (Sander et al. 2014). In fact, MRI-aided CTV delineation was shown to reduce radiation dose to the rectum, penile bulb, and neurovascular bundle (Steenbakkers et al. 2003; Cassidy et al. 2016) but has not yet demonstrated convincing evidence of impact on toxicity outcomes. MRI was also shown to reduce inter-observer variability in prostate delineation (Villeirs et al. 2005) as well as to better assess tumor extension, both extraprostatic (extracapsular or seminal vesicle extension) (Chang et al. 2014) and intraprostatic (dominant lesion location, discrimination between the peripheral and central zones) (De Meerleer et al. 2005). While standard practice is to treat the entire prostate to a homogeneous dose, focal treatment or dose escalation strategies to dominant lesion visible on MRI becomes possible, with the aim of improving the therapeutic window between tumor control and toxicity (Tanderup et al. 2014; Aluwini et al. 2013). The benefit of focal dose escalation to intraprostatic disease defined on multiparametric MRI is currently being assessed in randomized controlled trials (Lips et al. 2011). Importantly, the role of MRI in planning also extends to the post-prostatectomy setting; the potential for MRI to detect foci of local relapse in biochemical recurrences post-prostatectomy could facilitate targeted salvage radiotherapy strategies (Dirix et al. 2017). In general, imaging protocols should follow the recently published consensus recommendations from the MRinRT symposium (Menard et al. 2018; Salembier et al. 2018).

4.5.3.1 Prostate Brachytherapy

While prostate brachytherapy workflow has historically involved use of transrectal ultrasound or CT, superior visualization of the dominant intraprostatic lesions, prostate apex, neurovascular bundle, and urinary sphincter achieved with MRI has made the latter an attractive modality for brachytherapy planning. MRI can in fact play a key role in every step of prostate brachytherapy workflow, including (1) prostate delineation and real-time MR guidance at time of implantation for both high-dose rate (HDR) and low-dose rate (LDR) brachytherapy, (2) dose optimization in HDR brachytherapy, and (3) post-implant dosimetry assessment for quality assurance in LDR brachytherapy (Tanderup et al. 2014). Needle guidance can be performed either under real-time MRI (Menard et al. 2004) or more commonly with fusion of diagnostic MRI to transrectal ultrasound (TRUS). Treatment planning can also be performed directly on MR images (Menard et al. 2018) or fused TRUS/MRI (Frank et al. 2017). For the MRI-only workflow, use of safe MRI-compatible applicators, for example, plastic- and titanium-based, to avoid tissue injuries, is a crucial consideration. Applicators and brachytherapy sources appear as areas of signal void and titanium-based applicators are associated with significant susceptibility artifacts. Conversely when using a TRUS-MRI workflow, accuracies in image registration through the course of the intervention are paramount (Poulin et al. 2018). Finally, post-implant MRI for quality assurance after LDR brachytherapy is highly encouraged as it provides precise quantification of dose to main intraprostatic lesions as well as to the CTV and OAR. Functional information derived from multiparametric MRI could improve identification of intraprostatic GTV (Fig. 4.5), which is of particular interest for focal brachytherapy and is an area of active research (Bauman et al. 2013).

4.5.4 Cervix

Standard treatment for cervical cancer typically involves a combination of external beam radiotherapy and brachytherapy. Conventional radiotherapy involves a three-dimensional conformal radiotherapy of the pelvis, followed by intracavitary brachytherapy. In the last few years, IMRT has been increasingly used as a means to reduce normal tissue toxicity. Guidelines from the Gynecologic IMRT Consortium group strongly recommend the use of MRI for delineation of target volume and OAR for cervical cancer external beam radiation planning (Lim et al. 2011). The most significant benefit of MRI in cervical cancer

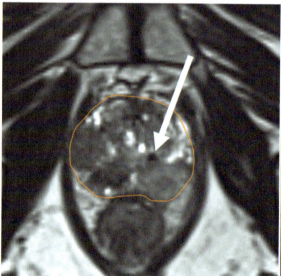

Fig. 4.5 High-resolution 3D T2-weighted image (left) 4 days after placement of fiducial markers in a patient with prostate cancer (arrow). Calculated high-b-value diffusion image (right) showing bright tumor in right lateral peripheral zone of the prostate (arrow). Hemorrhage artifact is evident in the posterior peripheral zone bilaterally

is that of optimal visualization of the cervical tumor in multi-planar imaging, allowing for precise volumetric definition of the GTV. Like in other clinical sites, MRI-based tumor and organ at risk delineation has been shown to reduce inter-observer variability (Lim et al. 2011) and to improve assessment of tumor extension, particularly for estimation of tumor size, parametrial extension, uterine body extension, and adjacent soft tissue extensions (bladder, rectum) (Bipat et al. 2003; Park et al. 2005). Cervical tumors appear as high signal intensity lesions on T2-weighted MRI and can be discriminated from the surrounding low signal intensity normal cervical stroma (Fig. 4.6). In the context of IMRT planning, an important consideration is that of pelvic organs inter- and intra-fraction mobility, which should be taken into account at time of planning. To reduce variations in rectal and bladder filling between planning CT and MRI, patient preparation including use of muscle relaxant and identical bladder filling protocols is recommended. Fast 4D MRI is a useful tool to determine internal motion margin of the target volume and OAR that are subject to changes in bladder filling, rectal filling, and other internal motion, at no radiation cost (Kerkhof et al. 2009). Some promising uses of DWI include cancer staging (detection of extrauterine disease and metastatic lymph nodes) and outcome prediction (Ho et al. 2017; Gong et al. 2017).

4.5.4.1 Cervix Brachytherapy

Conventional 2D brachytherapy can be associated with under- or overdosing of target volume owing to individual variations of residual disease size and patient's anatomy (Tanderup et al. 2010). Conversely, use of MRI-based 3D imaging at the time of brachytherapy allows for tailored brachytherapy based on residual tumor volume (Tanderup et al. 2010), optimal dosimetric coverage of target volumes, dose volume adaptation, and sparing the nearby radiosensitive organs such as the rectum, sigmoid, bowel, and bladder (Dolezel et al. 2011). The Gynaecological GEC-ESTRO Working Group for cervix cancer advocates for acquisition of pelvic MRI before external beam radiotherapy start and at time of brachytherapy (Dimopoulos et al. 2012). A multi-planar T2-weighted sequence, preferably with the applicator in place and oriented according to the applicator, is used for delineation of residual GTV, high-risk CTV, and intermediate-risk CTV (Fig. 4.7). Delineation of the residual GTV based on MRI was previously shown to be systematically smaller than CT-based delineation (Viswanathan et al. 2007). When feasible, real-time MR guidance for optimal positioning of the applicator while visualizing the

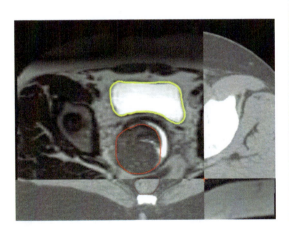

Fig. 4.6 Axial T2-weighted MRI and CT scan co-registered for external beam radiotherapy planning for cervix cancer. Red contour: GTV; yellow contour: bladder; brown contour: rectum

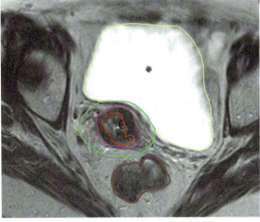

Fig. 4.7 Axial T2-weighted MRI for cervix brachytherapy. Red, GTV at time of brachytherapy; magenta, high-risk CTV; green, intermediate-risk CTV; yellow, bladder; brown, rectum

tumor can be used in institutions that have access to a dedicated MRI in their radiation oncology department. Improvements in local control, overall survival, and toxicities with MRI-guided brachytherapy compared to the conventional 2D approach have been reported in mono-institutional studies (Lindegaard et al. 2013). In addition, multi-institutional assessment of outcomes from MRI-guided treatment is currently of prospective trials lead by the EMBRACE collaborative group (Potter et al. 2018; Jastaniyah et al. 2016). The role of functional imaging, in particular DW-MRI, is also investigated for delineation of GTV in brachytherapy setting, as well as noninvasive biomarker to predict treatment outcomes (Dyk et al. 2014).

4.6 Conclusion

The use of MRI has become an integral part of radiotherapy planning across multiple clinical sites including head and neck, brain, cervix, and prostate. With the help of ongoing technology enhancements, the role of MRI in radiotherapy is now also rapidly making its way in clinical sites previously felt less suitable for MRI due to geometric distortions and magnetic susceptibility effects. The development of MR-linac systems and the advent of MR-only workflows will further accelerate the use of MRI in radiotherapy planning and will set the stage for a new era of daily MRI-based radiation planning. In addition, the use of functional MRI for prediction of tumor response and spatiotemporal mapping of radioresistant tumor regions may become a crucial tool for the promising avenues of radiotherapy adaptation and dose painting. To date, MRI remains a complementary imaging modality used along with planning CT for safe delineation of target volumes and organs at risk. Robust evidence demonstrating the clinical benefits of anatomical and functional MRI in radiotherapy planning is needed in order to justify the increased workload and costs associated with its widespread implementation.

References

Aluwini S, van Rooij P, Hoogeman M, Kirkels W, Kolkman-Deurloo IK, Bangma C. Stereotactic body radiotherapy with a focal boost to the MRI-visible tumor as monotherapy for low- and intermediate-risk prostate cancer: early results. Radiat Oncol. 2013;8:84.

Aoyama H, Shirato H, Nishioka T, Hashimoto S, Tsuchiya K, Kagei K, et al. Magnetic resonance imaging system for three-dimensional conformal radiotherapy and its impact on gross tumor volume delineation of central nervous system tumors. Int J Radiat Oncol Biol Phys. 2001;50(3):821–7.

Bauman G, Haider M, Van der Heide UA, Menard C. Boosting imaging defined dominant prostatic tumors: a systematic review. Radiother Oncol. 2013;107(3):274–81.

Bedford JL, Convery HM, Hansen VN, Saran FH. Paraspinal volumetric modulated arc therapy. Br J Radiol. 2012;85(1016):1128–33.

Belliveau JG, Bauman GS, Tay KY, Ho D, Menon RS. Initial investigation into microbleeds and white matter signal changes following radiotherapy for low-grade and benign brain tumors using ultra-high-field MRI techniques. AJNR Am J Neuroradiol. 2017;38(12):2251–6.

Bipat S, Glas AS, van der Velden J, Zwinderman AH, Bossuyt PM, Stoker J. Computed tomography and magnetic resonance imaging in staging of uterine cervical carcinoma: a systematic review. Gynecol Oncol. 2003;91(1):59–66.

Brock KK, Dawson LA. Adaptive management of liver cancer radiotherapy. Semin Radiat Oncol. 2010;20(2):107–15.

Brouwer CL, Steenbakkers RJ, Bourhis J, Budach W, Grau C, Gregoire V, et al. CT-based delineation of organs at risk in the head and neck region: DAHANCA, EORTC, GORTEC, HKNPCSG, NCIC CTG, NCRI, NRG Oncology and TROG consensus guidelines. Radiother Oncol. 2015;117(1):83–90.

Cassidy RJ, Yang X, Liu T, Thomas M, Nour SG, Jani AB. Neurovascular bundle-sparing radiotherapy for prostate cancer using MRI-CT registration: a dosimetric feasibility study. Med Dosim. 2016;41(4):339–43.

Chandwani S, George PA, Azu M, Bandera EV, Ambrosone CB, Rhoads GG, et al. Role of preoperative magnetic resonance imaging in the surgical management of early-stage breast cancer. Ann Surg Oncol. 2014;21(11):3473–80.

Chang JH, Lim Joon D, Nguyen BT, Hiew CY, Esler S, Angus D, et al. MRI scans significantly change target coverage decisions in radical radiotherapy for prostate cancer. J Med Imaging Radiat Oncol. 2014;58(2):237–43.

Chapman CH, Zhu T, Nazem-Zadeh M, Tao Y, Buchtel HA, Tsien CI, et al. Diffusion tensor imaging predicts cognitive function change following partial brain radiotherapy for low-grade and benign tumors. Radiother Oncol. 2016;120(2):234–40.

Charaghvandi RK, van Asselen B, Philippens ME, Verkooijen HM, van Gils CH, van Diest PJ, et al. Redefining radiotherapy for early-stage breast cancer with single dose ablative treatment: a study protocol. BMC Cancer. 2017;17(1):181.

Choi BI, Lee JM. Advancement in HCC imaging: diagnosis, staging and treatment efficacy assessments: imaging diagnosis and staging of hepatocellular carcinoma. J Hepatobiliary Pancreat Sci. 2010;17(4):369–73.

Chung NN, Ting LL, Hsu WC, Lui LT, Wang PM. Impact of magnetic resonance imaging versus CT on nasopharyngeal carcinoma: primary tumor target delineation for radiotherapy. Head Neck. 2004;26(3):241–6.

Cobben DC, de Boer HC, Tijssen RH, Rutten EG, van Vulpen M, Peerlings J, et al. Emerging role of MRI for radiation treatment planning in lung cancer. Technol Cancer Res Treat. 2016;15(6):47–60.

Cooper JS, Mukherji SK, Toledano AY, Beldon C, Schmalfuss IM, Amdur R, et al. An evaluation of the variability of tumor-shape definition derived by experienced observers from CT images of supraglottic carcinomas (ACRIN protocol 6658). Int J Radiat Oncol Biol Phys. 2007;67(4):972–5.

Crane CH, Koay EJ. Solutions that enable ablative radiotherapy for large liver tumors: Fractionated dose painting, simultaneous integrated protection, motion management, and computed tomography image guidance. Cancer. 2016;122(13):1974–86.

De Meerleer G, Villeirs G, Bral S, Paelinck L, De Gersem W, Dekuyper P, et al. The magnetic resonance detected intraprostatic lesion in prostate cancer: planning and delivery of intensity-modulated radiotherapy. Radiother Oncol. 2005;75(3):325–33.

Dimopoulos JC, Petrow P, Tanderup K, Petric P, Berger D, Kirisits C, et al. Recommendations from Gynaecological (GYN) GEC-ESTRO Working Group (IV): Basic principles and parameters for MR imaging within the frame of image based adaptive cervix cancer brachytherapy. Radiother Oncol. 2012;103(1):113–22.

Dirix P, van Walle L, Deckers F, Van Mieghem F, Buelens G, Meijnders P, et al. Proposal for magnetic resonance imaging-guided salvage radiotherapy for prostate cancer. Acta Oncol (Stockh). 2017;56(1):27–32.

Dolezel M, Odrazka K, Vanasek J, Kohlova T, Kroulik T, Kudelka K, et al. MRI-based pre-planning in patients with cervical cancer treated with three-dimensional brachytherapy. Br J Radiol. 2011;84(1005):850–6.

Dyk P, Jiang N, Sun B, DeWees TA, Fowler KJ, Narra V, et al. Cervical gross tumor volume dose predicts local control using magnetic resonance imaging/diffusion-weighted imaging-guided high-dose-rate and positron emission tomography/computed tomography-guided intensity modulated radiation therapy. Int J Radiat Oncol Biol Phys. 2014;90(4):794–801.

Einstein DB, Wessels B, Bangert B, Fu P, Nelson AD, Cohen M, et al. Phase II trial of radiosurgery to magnetic resonance spectroscopy-defined high-risk tumor volumes in patients with glioblastoma multiforme. Int J Radiat Oncol Biol Phys. 2012;84(3):668–74.

Ellingson BM, Bendszus M, Boxerman J, Barboriak D, Erickson BJ, Smits M, et al. Consensus recommendations for a standardized brain tumor imaging protocol in clinical trials. Neuro-Oncology. 2015;17(9):1188–98.

Fiorentino A, Caivano R, Pedicini P, Fusco V. Clinical target volume definition for glioblastoma radiotherapy planning: magnetic resonance imaging and computed tomography. Clin Transl Oncol. 2013;15(9):754–8.

Fowler KJ, Brown JJ, Narra VR. Magnetic resonance imaging of focal liver lesions: approach to imaging diagnosis. Hepatology. 2011;54(6):2227–37.

Frank SJ, Mourtada F, Crook J, Menard C. Use of magnetic resonance imaging in low-dose-rate and high-dose-rate prostate brachytherapy from diagnosis to treatment assessment: defining the knowledge gaps, technical challenges, and barriers to implementation. Brachytherapy. 2017;16(4):672–8.

Freedman JN, Collins DJ, Bainbridge H, Rank CM, Nill S, Kachelriess M, et al. T2-Weighted 4D magnetic resonance imaging for application in magnetic resonance-guided radiotherapy treatment planning. Investig Radiol. 2017;52(10):563–73.

Giezen M, Kouwenhoven E, Scholten AN, Coerkamp EG, Heijenbrok M, Jansen WP, et al. Magnetic resonance imaging- versus computed tomography-based target volume delineation of the glandular breast tissue (clinical target volume breast) in breast-conserving therapy: an exploratory study. Int J Radiat Oncol Biol Phys. 2011;81(3):804–11.

Giezen M, Kouwenhoven E, Scholten AN, Coerkamp EG, Heijenbrok M, Jansen WP, et al. MRI- versus CT-based volume delineation of lumpectomy cavity in supine position in breast-conserving therapy: an exploratory study. Int J Radiat Oncol Biol Phys. 2012;82(4):1332–40.

Gondi V, Pugh SL, Tome WA, Caine C, Corn B, Kanner A, et al. Preservation of memory with conformal avoidance of the hippocampal neural stem-cell compartment during whole-brain radiotherapy for brain metastases (RTOG 0933): a phase II multi-institutional trial. J Clin Oncol. 2014;32(34):3810–6.

Gong Y, Wang Q, Dong L, Jia Y, Hua C, Mi F, et al. Different imaging techniques for the detection of pelvic lymph nodes metastasis from gynecological malignancies: a systematic review and meta-analysis. Oncotarget. 2017;8(8):14107–25.

Gwynne S, Mukherjee S, Webster R, Spezi E, Staffurth J, Coles B, et al. Imaging for target volume delineation in rectal cancer radiotherapy—a systematic review. Clin Oncol. 2012;24(1):52–63.

Heerkens HD, Hall WA, Li XA, Knechtges P, Dalah E, Paulson ES, et al. Recommendations for MRI-based contouring of gross tumor volume and organs at risk for radiation therapy of pancreatic cancer. Pract Radiat Oncol. 2017;7(2):126–36.

van Heijst TC, van Asselen B, Pijnappel RM, Cloos-van Balen M, Lagendijk JJ, van den Bongard D, et al. MRI sequences for the detection of individual lymph nodes in regional breast radiotherapy planning. Br J Radiol. 2016;89(1063):20160072.

Ho JC, Allen PK, Bhosale PR, Rauch GM, Fuller CD, Mohamed AS, et al. Diffusion-weighted magnetic resonance imaging as a predictor of outcome in cervical cancer after chemoradiation. Int J Radiat Oncol Biol Phys. 2017;97(3):546–53.

Hodge CW, Tome WA, Fain SB, Bentzen SM, Mehta MP. On the use of hyperpolarized helium MRI for conformal avoidance lung radiotherapy. Med Dosim. 2010;35(4):297–303.

Horton JK, Blitzblau RC, Yoo S, Geradts J, Chang Z, Baker JA, et al. Preoperative single-fraction partial breast radiation therapy: a novel phase 1, dose-escalation protocol with radiation response biomarkers. Int J Radiat Oncol Biol Phys. 2015;92(4):846–55.

Jastaniyah N, Yoshida K, Tanderup K, Lindegaard JC, Sturdza A, Kirisits C, et al. A volumetric analysis of GTVD and CTVHR as defined by the GEC ESTRO recommendations in FIGO stage IIB and IIIB cervical cancer patients treated with IGABT in a prospective multicentric trial (EMBRACE). Radiother Oncol. 2016;120(3):404–11.

Jena R, Price SJ, Baker C, Jefferies SJ, Pickard JD, Gillard JH, et al. Diffusion tensor imaging: possible implications for radiotherapy treatment planning of patients with high-grade glioma. Clin Oncol. 2005;17(8):581–90.

Jolicoeur M, Racine ML, Trop I, Hathout L, Nguyen D, Derashodian T, et al. Localization of the surgical bed using supine magnetic resonance and computed tomography scan fusion for planification of breast interstitial brachytherapy. Radiother Oncol. 2011;100(3):480–4.

Kato H, Kanematsu M, Watanabe H, Mizuta K, Aoki M. Metastatic retropharyngeal lymph nodes: comparison of CT and MR imaging for diagnostic accuracy. Eur J Radiol. 2014;83(7):1157–62.

Kerkhof EM, van der Put RW, Raaymakers BW, van der Heide UA, Jurgenliemk-Schulz IM, Lagendijk JJ. Intrafraction motion in patients with cervical cancer: the benefit of soft tissue registration using MRI. Radiother Oncol. 2009;93(1):115–21.

King AD, Thoeny HC. Functional MRI for the prediction of treatment response in head and neck squamous cell carcinoma: potential and limitations. Cancer Imaging. 2016;16(1):23.

Kirby AM, Yarnold JR, Evans PM, Morgan VA, Schmidt MA, Scurr ED, et al. Tumor bed delineation for partial breast and breast boost radiotherapy planned in the prone position: what does MRI add to X-ray CT localization of titanium clips placed in the excision cavity wall? Int J Radiat Oncol Biol Phys. 2009;74(4):1276–82.

Klinke T, Daboul A, Maron J, Gredes T, Puls R, Jaghsi A, et al. Artifacts in magnetic resonance imaging and computed tomography caused by dental materials. PLoS One. 2012;7(2):e31766.

Koay EJ, Hall W, Park PC, Erickson B, Herman JM. The role of imaging in the clinical practice of radiation oncology for pancreatic cancer. Abdom Radiol (NY). 2018;43(2):393–403.

Lagendijk JJ, Raaymakers BW, Van den Berg CA, Moerland MA, Philippens ME, van Vulpen M. MR guidance in radiotherapy. Phys Med Biol. 2014;59(21):R349–69.

Lambrecht M, Vandecaveye V, De Keyzer F, Roels S, Penninckx F, Van Cutsem E, et al. Value of diffusion-weighted magnetic resonance imaging for prediction and early assessment of response to neoadjuvant radiochemotherapy in rectal cancer: preliminary results. Int J Radiat Oncol Biol Phys. 2012;82(2):863–70.

Law BK, King AD, Bhatia KS, Ahuja AT, Kam MK, Ma BB, et al. Diffusion-weighted imaging of nasopharyngeal carcinoma: can pretreatment DWI predict local failure based on long-term outcome? AJNR Am J Neuroradiol. 2016;37(9):1706–12.

Lim K, Small W Jr, Portelance L, Creutzberg C, Jurgenliemk-Schulz IM, Mundt A, et al. Consensus guidelines for delineation of clinical target volume for intensity-modulated pelvic radiotherapy for the definitive treatment of cervix cancer. Int J Radiat Oncol Biol Phys. 2011;79(2):348–55.

Lindegaard JC, Fokdal LU, Nielsen SK, Juul-Christensen J, Tanderup K. MRI-guided adaptive radiotherapy in locally advanced cervical cancer from a Nordic perspective. Acta Oncol (Stockh). 2013;52(7):1510–9.

Lips IM, van der Heide UA, Haustermans K, van Lin EN, Pos F, Franken SP, et al. Single blind randomized phase III trial to investigate the benefit of a focal lesion ablative microboost in prostate cancer (FLAME-trial): study protocol for a randomized controlled trial. Trials. 2011;12:255.

Liu WC, Schulder M, Narra V, Kalnin AJ, Cathcart C, Jacobs A, et al. Functional magnetic resonance imaging aided radiation treatment planning. Med Phys. 2000;27(7):1563–72.

Loimu V, Seppala T, Kapanen M, Tuomikoski L, Nurmi H, Makitie A, et al. Diffusion-weighted magnetic resonance imaging for evaluation of salivary gland function in head and neck cancer patients treated with intensity-modulated radiotherapy. Radiother Oncol. 2017;122(2):178–84.

Menard C, Susil RC, Choyke P, Gustafson GS, Kammerer W, Ning H, et al. MRI-guided HDR prostate brachytherapy in standard 1.5T scanner. Int J Radiat Oncol Biol Phys. 2004;59(5):1414–23.

Menard C, Paulson E, Nyholm T, McLaughlin P, Liney G, Dirix P, et al. Role of prostate MR imaging in radiation oncology. Radiol Clin N Am. 2018;56(2):319–25.

Miller GW, Mugler JP III, Sa RC, Altes TA, Prisk GK, Hopkins SR. Advances in functional and structural imaging of the human lung using proton MRI. NMR Biomed. 2014;27(12):1542–56.

Milosevic M, Voruganti S, Blend R, Alasti H, Warde P, McLean M, et al. Magnetic resonance imaging (MRI) for localization of the prostatic apex: comparison to computed tomography (CT) and urethrography. Radiother Oncol. 1998;47(3):277–84.

Mizowaki T, Araki N, Nagata Y, Negoro Y, Aoki T, Hiraoka M. The use of a permanent magnetic resonance imaging system for radiotherapy treatment planning of bone metastases. Int J Radiat Oncol Biol Phys. 2001;49(2):605–11.

Nagai A, Shibamoto Y, Mori Y, Hashizume C, Hagiwara M, Kobayashi T. Increases in the number of brain metastases detected at frame-fixed, thin-slice MRI for gamma knife surgery planning. Neuro-Oncology. 2010;12(11):1187–92.

Park W, Park YJ, Huh SJ, Kim BG, Bae DS, Lee J, et al. The usefulness of MRI and PET imaging for the detection of parametrial involvement and lymph node metastasis in patients with cervical cancer. Jpn J Clin Oncol. 2005;35(5):260–4.

Pech M, Mohnike K, Wieners G, Bialek E, Dudeck O, Seidensticker M, et al. Radiotherapy of liver metastases. Comparison of target volumes and dose-volume histograms employing CT- or MRI-based treatment planning. Strahlenther Onkol. 2008;184(5):256–61.

Peerlings J, Troost EG, Nelemans PJ, Cobben DC, de Boer JC, Hoffmann AL, et al. The diagnostic value of MR imaging in determining the lymph node status of patients with non-small cell lung cancer: a meta-analysis. Radiology. 2016;281(1):86–98.

Perrone A, Guerrisi P, Izzo L, D'Angeli I, Sassi S, Mele LL, et al. Diffusion-weighted MRI in cervical lymph nodes: differentiation between benign and malignant lesions. Eur J Radiol. 2011;77(2):281–6.

Pham TT, Liney G, Wong K, Rai R, Lee M, Moses D, et al. Study protocol: multi-parametric magnetic resonance imaging for therapeutic response prediction in rectal cancer. BMC Cancer. 2017;17(1):465.

Potter R, Tanderup K, Kirisits C, de Leeuw A, Kirchheiner K, Nout R, et al. The EMBRACE II study: the outcome and prospect of two decades of evolution within the GEC-ESTRO GYN working group and the EMBRACE studies. Clin Transl Radiat Oncol. 2018;9:48–60.

Poulin E, Boudam K, Pinter C, Kadoury S, Lasso A, Fichtinger G, et al. Validation of MRI to TRUS registration for high-dose-rate prostate brachytherapy. Brachytherapy. 2018;17(2):283–90.

Pramanik PP, Parmar HA, Mammoser AG, Junck LR, Kim MM, Tsien CI, et al. Hypercellularity components of glioblastoma identified by high b-value diffusion-weighted imaging. Int J Radiat Oncol Biol Phys. 2015;92(4):811–9.

Prestwich RJ, Sykes J, Carey B, Sen M, Dyker KE, Scarsbrook AF. Improving target definition for head and neck radiotherapy: a place for magnetic resonance imaging and 18-fluoride fluorodeoxyglucose positron emission tomography? Clin Oncol. 2012;24(8):577–89.

Ryu S, Pugh SL, Gerszten PC, Yin FF, Timmerman RD, Hitchcock YJ, et al. RTOG 0631 phase 2/3 study of image guided stereotactic radiosurgery for localized (1–3) spine metastases: phase 2 results. Pract Radiat Oncol. 2014;4(2):76–81.

Saisho H, Yamaguchi T. Diagnostic imaging for pancreatic cancer: computed tomography, magnetic resonance imaging, and positron emission tomography. Pancreas. 2004;28(3):273–8.

Salembier C, Villeirs G, De Bari B, Hoskin P, Pieters BR, Van Vulpen M, et al. ESTRO ACROP consensus guideline on CT- and MRI-based target volume delineation for primary radiation therapy of localized prostate cancer. Radiother Oncol. 2018;127(1):49–61.

Sander L, Langkilde NC, Holmberg M, Carl J. MRI target delineation may reduce long-term toxicity after prostate radiotherapy. Acta Oncol (Stockh). 2014;53(6):809–14.

Sardanelli F, Giuseppetti GM, Panizza P, Bazzocchi M, Fausto A, Simonetti G, et al. Sensitivity of MRI versus mammography for detecting foci of multifocal, multicentric breast cancer in fatty and dense breasts using the whole-breast pathologic examination as a gold standard. AJR Am J Roentgenol. 2004;183(4):1149–57.

Scoccianti S, Detti B, Gadda D, Greto D, Furfaro I, Meacci F, et al. Organs at risk in the brain and their dose-constraints in adults and in children: a radiation oncologist's guide for delineation in everyday practice. Radiother Oncol. 2015;114(2):230–8.

Spratt DE, Arevalo-Perez J, Leeman JE, Gerber NK, Folkert M, Taunk NK, et al. Early magnetic resonance imaging biomarkers to predict local control after high dose stereotactic body radiotherapy for patients with sarcoma spine metastases. Spine J. 2016;16(3):291–8.

Stall B, Zach L, Ning H, Ondos J, Arora B, Shankavaram U, et al. Comparison of T2 and FLAIR imaging for target delineation in high grade gliomas. Radiat Oncol. 2010;5:5.

Steenbakkers RJ, Deurloo KE, Nowak PJ, Lebesque JV, van Herk M, Rasch CR. Reduction of dose delivered to the rectum and bulb of the penis using MRI delineation for radiotherapy of the prostate. Int J Radiat Oncol Biol Phys. 2003;57(5):1269–79.

Stemkens B, Tijssen RH, de Senneville BD, Heerkens HD, van Vulpen M, Lagendijk JJ, et al. Optimizing 4-dimensional magnetic resonance imaging data sampling for respiratory motion analysis of pancreatic tumors. Int J Radiat Oncol Biol Phys. 2015;91(3):571–8.

Straathof CS, de Bruin HG, Dippel DW, Vecht CJ. The diagnostic accuracy of magnetic resonance imaging and cerebrospinal fluid cytology in leptomeningeal metastasis. J Neurol. 1999;246(9):810–4.

Sun J, Li B, Li CJ, Li Y, Su F, Gao QH, et al. Computed tomography versus magnetic resonance imaging for diagnosing cervical lymph node metastasis of head and neck cancer: a systematic review and meta-analysis. OncoTargets Ther. 2015;8:1291–313.

Tan J, Lim Joon D, Fitt G, Wada M, Lim Joon M, Mercuri A, et al. The utility of multimodality imaging with CT and MRI in defining rectal tumour volumes for radiotherapy treatment planning: a pilot study. J Med Imaging Radiat Oncol. 2010;54(6):562–8.

Tanderup K, Nielsen SK, Nyvang GB, Pedersen EM, Rohl L, Aagaard T, et al. From point A to the sculpted pear: MR image guidance significantly improves tumour dose and sparing of organs at risk in brachytherapy of cervical cancer. Radiother Oncol. 2010;94(2):173–80.

Tanderup K, Viswanathan AN, Kirisits C, Frank SJ. Magnetic resonance image guided brachytherapy. Semin Radiat Oncol. 2014;24(3):181–91.

Tseng CL, Eppinga W, Charest-Morin R, Soliman H, Myrehaug S, Maralani PJ, et al. Spine stereotactic body radiotherapy: indications, outcomes, and points of caution. Global Spine J. 2017;7(2):179–97.

Villeirs GM, De Meerleer GO. Magnetic resonance imaging (MRI) anatomy of the prostate and application of MRI in radiotherapy planning. Eur J Radiol. 2007;63(3):361–8.

Villeirs GM, Van Vaerenbergh K, Vakaet L, Bral S, Claus F, De Neve WJ, et al. Interobserver delineation variation using CT versus combined CT + MRI in intensity-modulated radiotherapy for prostate cancer. Strahlenther Onkol. 2005;181(7):424–30.

Viswanathan AN, Dimopoulos J, Kirisits C, Berger D, Potter R. Computed tomography versus magnetic resonance imaging-based contouring in cervical cancer brachytherapy: results of a prospective trial and preliminary guidelines for standardized contours. Int J Radiat Oncol Biol Phys. 2007;68(2):491–8.

Weinreb JC, Barentsz JO, Choyke PL, Cornud F, Haider MA, Macura KJ, et al. PI-RADS prostate imaging – reporting and data system: 2015, version 2. Eur Urol. 2016;69(1):16–40.

White NS, McDonald CR, Farid N, Kuperman JM, Kesari S, Dale AM. Improved conspicuity and delineation of high-grade primary and metastatic brain tumors using "restriction spectrum imaging": quantitative comparison with high B-value DWI and ADC. AJNR Am J Neuroradiol. 2013;34(5):958–64, s1.

Zhang SX, Han PH, Zhang GQ, Wang RH, Ge YB, Ren ZG, et al. Comparison of SPECT/CT, MRI and CT in diagnosis of skull base bone invasion in nasopharyngeal carcinoma. Biomed Mater Eng. 2014;24(1):1117–24.

Part II

MRI During Treatment

Functional MR Imaging

Marielle Philippens and Roberto García-Álvarez

5.1 General Introduction

In recent years, anatomical T1- and T2-weighted MR imaging has become one of the standard tools, besides CT and PET, to define the target volume. In addition, functional MR imaging is used to better define the target volume based on physiologic features of the tissue. Functional imaging can also be used to predict outcome, to assess outcome during treatment and to diagnose recurrences. Besides, function or organization of organs at risk can be explored and incorporated in radiotherapy treatment planning. The distinctive properties of tumors are described by Hanahan and Weinberg as sustained proliferation, evasion of growth suppressors, resistance to cell death, replicative immortality, induction of angiogenesis, invasion, metastasis and changed metabolism induced by deficient DNA repair (Hanahan and Weinberg 2000, 2011). This results in tumor cells with leaky vessels, high cell density and changed metabolites. Tumors differ in vascularization due to angiogenesis, cell density caused by high proliferation, and metabolism due to high proliferation and less cell differentiation.

Four different techniques will be described in this chapter: diffusion-weighted MRI, dynamic contrast MRI, fMRI, and MR spectroscopy. The first technique mostly reflects the microanatomical organization of a tissue, while DCE-MRI reflects vascular function and capillary organization. BOLD fMRI of the brain reflects brain activity and can therefore be used to avoid functional brain structures. Applications and future perspectives of diffusion-weighted MRI, DCE-MRI, and MR spectroscopy are described in Chaps. 4, 6, and 12.

The application of BOLD fMRI is still relatively limited. Therefore, several studies are summarized in this chapter. The concept of incorporating functional areas into the planning of radiotherapy was first introduced in 1997 by Hamilton et al. (1997). He demonstrated the feasibility of treatment plans that spare functional brain while identical dose to target volumes was provided. In later years, this dose reduction to functional OAR was demonstrated using mapping the motor, visual acoustic and somatosensory areas for treatment planning of radiosurgery (Liu et al. 2000; Torresin et al. 2015). The combination of DWI tractography with fMRI can further reduce the dose to functional areas, as was demonstrated in a cohort of brain patients undergoing stereotactic radiosurgery and high-grade glioma patients (Pantelis et al. 2010; Wang et al. 2015). Fiber tracts and fMRI activation areas, were incorporated as organs at risk during the treatment planning process. Pantelis et al. (2010) concluded that these fOAR could receive twice the dose if they were not

M. Philippens (✉)
Department of Radiotherapy, University Medical Center Utrecht, Utrecht, The Netherlands
e-mail: m.philippens@umcutrecht.nl

R. García-Álvarez
Ingham Institute, Liverpool Hospital,
Sydney, NSW, Australia

© Springer Nature Switzerland AG 2019
G. Liney, U. van der Heide (eds.), *MRI for Radiotherapy*,
https://doi.org/10.1007/978-3-030-14442-5_5

taken into account Besides the identification of fOAR in the brain, Garcia-Alvarez et al. (2006) introduced a margin concept based on repeatability of fMRI to account for spatial uncertainty for functional organs at risk (fOAR). They derived margins of 2.9 mm and 2.2 mm for the left and right primary motor cortices, respectively. This chapter will mainly focus on the biophysics background and technical aspects, such as image acquisition techniques and data analysis.

5.2 Diffusion-Weighted MR Imaging

Diffusion-weighted MR imaging (DWI) is an increasingly widely applied technique in oncology. Until now, DWI has been the only noninvasive technique for in vivo measurement of the tissue microstructure. Dense structures such as tumors, lymph nodes, or brain tissue show a high signal intensity on DWI. Moreover, as the diffusion properties of white matter are anisotropic, the connectivity in the anatomical networks in the brain can be explored. The diffusion contrast is based on the restriction or hindrance of motion of water molecules due to physical barriers in tissue, such as membranes, large molecules, or organelles. The resulting signal intensity reflects the underlying microstructure of the tissue.

5.2.1 DWI Biophysical Principles

In a phantom without restrictive barriers, the displacement of a water molecule due to diffusion is driven by the kinetic energy of the system and dependent on temperature and the friction of the system related to viscosity and particle shape. The larger the displacement, the larger the diffusion coefficient is. In tissues, generally diffusion restriction or hindrance and thus of displacement of water molecules is related to the microstructure of the tissue. In dense tissues, small displacements will result in a low diffusion coefficient. As the coefficient is not only dependent on temperature and viscosity, it is referred to as apparent diffusion coefficient (ADC). In standard clinical diffusion-weighted MRI, the diffusion time is around 50 ms and the diffusion coefficient of water at 37 °C is around 3×10^{-9} m^2/s. This will give a mean displacement of 17 μm if free diffusion is possible, which is an ideal scale for probing the microanatomy (Le Bihan et al. 2006).

The diffusion restriction in tissues can be isotropic, i.e., in most tumors, or anisotropic. Anisotropic diffusion is studied mainly in white matter tracks in central nervous system (Basser et al. 1994) and in peripheral nerves (Takahara et al. 2011).

5.2.2 DWI Acquisition Techniques

The acquisition of diffusion-weighted imaging consists of two main parts. The first consists of the diffusion weighting and the second of the signal acquisition. Additionally, fat suppression is important in DWI, to prevent large chemical shift artifacts and to ensure the distinction of tumors from fat with an intrinsic low ADC.

5.2.2.1 Diffusion Weighting

Originally, Stejskal and Tanner introduced B0 field gradients in a nuclear magnetic resonance experiment for motion probing long before MR imaging was introduced (Stejskal and Tanner 1965). A pair of balanced diffusion-sensitizing gradients was introduced around a 180° refocusing pulse to probe diffusional motion. This first gradient induces dephasing, while the second gradient will rephase the magnetization unless motion has taken place during the diffusion time. This loss of coherence will attenuate the acquired signal. As the base of the DWI is a spin echo, the contrast in the diffusion-weighted scan is T2 with diffusion weighting due to the duration of the diffusion gradients. In highly diffusion-weighted scans, the attenuation due to motion probing will exceed the T2 weighting (Fig. 5.1). If the diffusion weighting is not high enough, high signal intensities due to long T2 values can still be more prominent than the signal decay due to diffusion weighting. This is referred to as T2 shine through.

Originally the technique was referred to as pulsed-field gradient-nuclear magnetic resonance (PFG-NMR). It introduces an exponential signal decay resulting from diffusion motion described

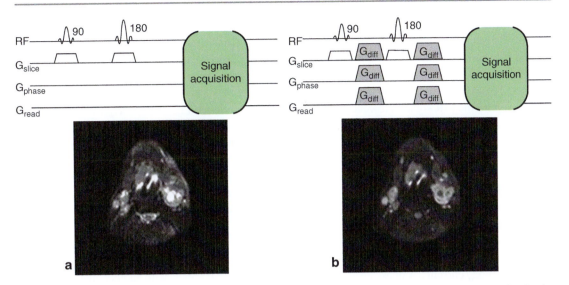

Fig. 5.1 Diffusion-weighted sequence with corresponding DW images. On the left side the image and sequence with $b = 0$ mm²/s (**a**) and on the right side with $b = 800$ mm²/s is shown (**b**). The diffusion weighting results in a relative signal intensity preservation in the tumor and the lymph nodes, while the signal intensity in the necrotic core of the tumor decreases largely

in the Stejskal-Tanner formula, which is still used in clinical DWI.

$$S_{diff} = S_0 e^{-bD} \quad (5.1)$$

where b for rectangular gradient shape is described as

$$b = \gamma^2 G^2 \delta^2 \left(-\frac{\delta}{3} \right) \quad (5.2)$$

In Eq. (5.1) the signal intensity (S) is described as function of the signal intensity identical to the diffusion-weighted sequence but without diffusion weighting (S_0), the diffusion weighting, the so-called b-value (b), and the (apparent) diffusion coefficient (D). The b-value which describes the translational diffusion is dependent on the gradient strength (G), the gradient duration (δ), the diffusion time (Δ), and the shape of the diffusion gradient (Sinnaeve 2012). In clinical practice, generally only the b-value is mentioned. However, differences in diffusion time, Δ, and in gradient shape can lead to different ADC values if the diffusion time is not long enough to sample the microanatomy and experience full motion restriction (Callaghan 1991). To measure the ADC, a series of experiments is needed. Generally, only the gradient strength is varied between the different measurements, while diffusion time and gradient duration are kept constant. In addition, three orthogonal gradient directions are measured consecutively to approach average directionality, or if the directionality of the diffusion motion is of interest as in tractography of the brain, six or more gradient directions are used.

The strong gradients induce eddy currents that affect the ADC values and the geometric accuracy of EPI-based DWI. Eddy currents can be induced in any conductive part of the magnet and increase with the strength and the slew rate of the gradient pulse. To reduce this effect, double refocus techniques can be used to null the cumulative eddy currents (Reese et al. 2003).

The ADC will also be affected by the nonlinearity of the gradients (Malyarenko et al. 2014). This can lead to underestimation of ADC off-center regions.

5.2.2.2 Signal Acquisition

The strong motion probing gradients necessary for diffusion probing will also sensitize the measurement to bulk or subvoxel motion. As this motion is not random, it will lead to substantial phase offset of the acquired magnetization. Phase offsets will be different for every shot leading to severe motion artifacts and signal loss which results in an overestimation of the ADC (Le Bihan et al. 2006). This is generally solved by using a single-shot readout. Echo planar imaging is a very efficient acquisition scheme. It is very fast, has a high SNR, and is not SAR demanding. Besides EPI also single-shot fast spin echo (FSE) or turbo spine echo (TSE) can be used to acquire the MR signal. However, both single-shot acquisitions will restrict the image resolution as transverse relaxation will attenuate the signal during readout. Generally EPI is used to acquire the MR signal but both EPI and FSE have their own drawbacks.

For EPI (see Chap. 1), the first challenge is that the accuracy of the spatial encoding is very sensitive to inhomogeneities in the main magnetic field (B0 field), induced by the susceptibility of the patient or by eddy currents. A phase error will build up during the "zig-zag" traversal of k-space. Therefore, the bandwidth in this direction will be small leading to geometric distortions in the phase-encode direction (Schakel et al. 2013). If the distortions are not too large, these geometric distortions can be retrospectively unwarped using a B0 field map or reversed gradient method which uses opposing phase-encode directions (Chap. 3) (Jezzard and Balaban 1995). As the distortions are nonlinear, signal pileup can take place, which cannot be resolved (Jones and Cercignani 2010).

B0 displacements can to some extent be reduced using methods to homogenize the B0 field, referred to as B0 shimming, or increase the bandwidth in the phase-encoding direction using acceleration methods, such as SENSE or GRAPPA (Chap. 1.3.2.6). This will reduce the displacements by the acceleration factor, which is typically a factor 2–3.

Distortions due to eddy current will be dependent on the direction of the diffusion gradient resulting in a shear, shift, or scaling (Jezzard et al. 1998). Furthermore, the displacements will scale up with the b-value. Commonly, retrospective correction of these distortions is performed using a deformable registration between the distorted images with higher b-values and the non-diffusion-weighted images ($b = 0$ s/mm^2) (Rohde et al. 2004).

Similar to the large displacements due to B0 inhomogeneities, fat will show large displacements due to chemical shift. On 3 T, the water-fat shift is ~430 Hz. As the bandwidth per pixel is typically around 40 Hz, this results in a displacement of fat of ~10 pixels, which gives a fat shift of 2.5 cm. Therefore, fat suppression is needed in DWI. Generally, spectral saturation is used (SPIR, SPAIR) or short tau inversion recovery (STIR), which is not sensitive to B0 distortions (Chap. 1.3.1.2).

Fast spin echo is another acquisition technique using refocusing pulses instead of gradients to create an echo (Hennig et al. 1986). Although FSE is more time consuming than EPI and leads to higher energy absorption, the advantage is that the geometric fidelity is comparable to conventional anatomical MR images (Schakel et al. 2017). To avoid differences in phase shifts due to bulk or microscopic motion during diffusion preparation, generally each slice is acquired in a single shot. However, the use of FSE comes with another challenge as the combination of diffusion-sensitizing gradients and a spin-echo train is not trivial. An FSE is prone to errors if the Carr-Purcell-Meiboom-Gill (CPMG) conditions are not met. In DWI, two of the CPMG conditions are violated as (1) phase offsets exist and (2) refocusing pulses not equal to 180° are used. This will result in a rapid decline of the echo amplitude (Schick 1997). To create stable echo trains under these circumstances, several approaches have been proposed. This included phase cycling of the refocusing pulse (Le Roux 2002), removal of the component with phase offset (Alsop 1997), and the echo parity selection method (Norris 2007). Here, an imbalanced readout gradient was applied to separate echo families which have experienced odd or even number of refocusing pulses. This comes with the expense of half the SNR for the latter two methods. Schick has proposed a method where both echo parities are acquired and added as magnitude images after reconstruction (Schick 1997). To achieve reasonable acquisition times for clinical applications in DW-FSE, acceleration is needed.

5.2.3 DWI Data Analysis

In particular for response prediction, assessment, and monitoring, robust and reproducible ADC values are important. The simplest analysis is a mono-exponential fit of the signal intensity to derive the ADC value (Eq. (5.1)) (Fig. 5.2).

However, in practice, the diffusion decay curve deviates from mono-exponential behavior.

5 Functional MR Imaging

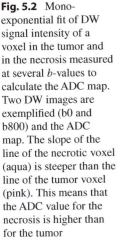

Fig. 5.2 Mono-exponential fit of DW signal intensity of a voxel in the tumor and in the necrosis measured at several *b*-values to calculate the ADC map. Two DW images are exemplified (b0 and b800) and the ADC map. The slope of the line of the necrotic voxel (aqua) is steeper than the line of the tumor voxel (pink). This means that the ADC value for the necrosis is higher than for the tumor

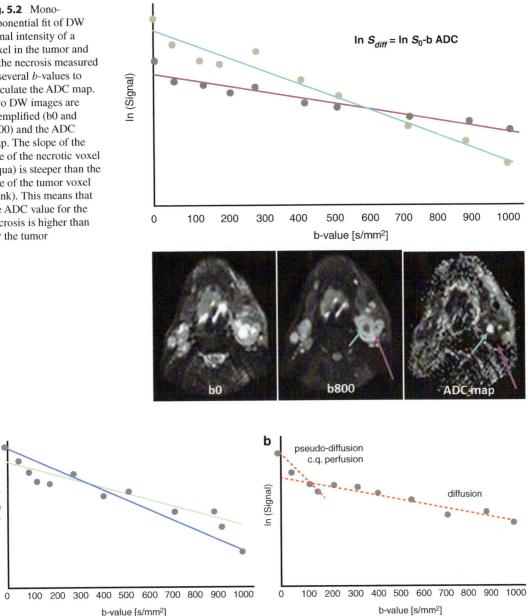

Fig. 5.3 The effect of non-mono-exponential decay on the ADC calculated. The effect of the choice of *b*-values on the ADC is shown (**a**) and an IVIM fit is depicted in **b**

The diffusion attenuation curve shows a steeper decay at low *b*-values, than at higher *b*-values (Le Bihan 2017). This indicates that the ADC calculated using a mono-exponential model is sensitive to the choice of *b*-values (Fig. 5.3a).

The steeper decay at low *b*-values was also observed in the early days of diffusion-weighted MRI, and intravoxel incoherent motion (IVIM) was introduced to show that at low *b*-values, the signal attenuation in brain was based on a fast and a slow diffusion component (Fig. 5.3b). This fast component was assigned to microcirculation, which is around ten times faster than diffusion of free water and referred to as pseudo-diffusion, which is considered to be related to perfusion (Koh et al. 2011a; Lebihan et al. 1986). In the last years, IVIM has experienced a revival in oncology for diagnostic purposes and response evaluation (Iima and Le Bihan 2016). The signal can be described as

$$S = S_0 \left(f_{IVIM} e^{-b(D_{IVIM}+D)} + (1 - f_{IVIM}) e^{-bD} \right) \quad (5.3)$$

with S being the signal intensity, S_0 the signal intensity at $b = 0$ mm²/s, f_{IVIM}, D_{ivim} the pseudo-diffusion due to microcirculation, and D the ADC in tissue. However, there are several other methods to solve the challenges of fitting the IVIM data (Le Bihan 2017).

Another issue is the non-Gaussian behavior of water undergoing hindered diffusion will also lead to a non-mono-exponential diffusion signal decay curve. To account for non-Gaussian behavior, several models have been proposed of which the Kurtosis model is the most popular (Jensen et al. 2005). Here, the deviation at high b-values of non-exponential behavior is accounted for by a quadratic function of the ADC at $b = 0$ s/mm² (ADC_0) and the kurtosis parameter (K) that describes deviation from mono-exponential behavior.

$$S = S_0 e^{-b ADC_0 + (b ADC_0)^2 K/6} \quad (5.4)$$

Additionally, noise handling is important for a correct estimation of the ADC, IVIM, and Kurtosis parameters. As magnitude signal is used in MRI, noise has a non-Gaussian nature and will lead to a so-called noise floor at high b-values where the signal to noise ratio is low, which mimics non-mono-exponential behavior of the diffusion decay curve (Gudbjartsson and Patz 1995; Henkelman 1985). Therefore, particularly estimation of IVIM and Kurtosis parameters has to be interpreted with great caution taking into account both the signal acquisition and fitting procedure.

5.3 Dynamic Contrast Enhanced MRI

5.3.1 DCE-MRI Biophysical Principles

One of the features of malignant tumors is increased angiogenesis, which generally leads to a chaotically structured vasculature with a high permeability. In clinical CT and MRI protocols, imaging after contrast administration is standard, because most malignant lesions demonstrate an increased extravasation of the small-molecular-weight contrast agents in malignant tumors. This enhancement pattern is a fairly late snapshot during contrast distribution. Temporospatial distribution patterns of the contrast agent have shown to be important in staging, segmentation (Chap. 4), and response evaluation in oncology (Chap. 6). Both CT and MRI are used for perfusion measurement. The technique was proposed in the mid-1980s, and to describe perfusion and extravasation of the contrast agent, a high temporal resolution is needed, particularly when pharmacokinetic modeling is used to describe the perfusion and permeability parameters. In CT, the amount of contrast is directly related to the in HU, while in MRI, the contrast concentration is not linear with the signal intensity. Actually, the gadolinium contrast agents increase the R_1 (=1/T_1) or R_2 (=1/T_2) relaxation rate of water near the contrast. The disadvantage of CT is the ionizing radiation used for the dynamic scanning limiting the power used (mAs) and the number of scans. Moreover, the field of view in the feet-head direction is limited by the size of the detector. Therefore, DCE-MRI is more widely used to trace the dynamic distribution of contrast agent. The quantification of contrast agent in MRI can be analyzed in three different ways: (1) qualitatively following the contrast distribution, (2) model-free distribution analysis, and (3) full pharmacokinetic analysis.

Although most contrast agents show both T_2 and T_1 relaxations and also have a susceptibility effect (T_2^*), we will focus on the T1 effect in this chapter as this is mostly used in oncology. Moreover, only small molecule gadolinium-based contrast agents are covered.

The effect of contrast agent on the T1 relaxation times can be described by the Solomon-Bloembergen equation (Gowland et al. 1992), which shows that the effective relaxation rate R_1 (=1/T_1) is the sum of the relaxation rate of the protons with and without contrast agent (Eqs. (5.5) and (5.6)).

$$\frac{1}{T_1} = \frac{1}{T_{10}} + \frac{1}{T_{1,c}} \quad (5.5)$$

5 Functional MR Imaging

$$\frac{1}{T_1} = \frac{1}{T_{10}} + r_1 \left[c_{\text{contrast agent}} \right] \quad (5.6)$$

Here, $T_{1,0}$ and $T_{1,c}$ are the T1 relaxation time of the tissue with contrast agent concentration 0 and c, respectively, $r1$ is the relaxivity constant of the contrast agent, and $[c_{\text{contrast agent}}]$ is the concentration of the contrast agent. The relaxivity is field strength dependent and is determined by the chemical structure of the contrast agent.

5.3.2 DCE-MRI Acquisition Techniques

5.3.2.1 T1 Measurement of Contrast Agent Concentration

To describe the vascularity based on contrast agent distribution, a fast dynamic sequence is needed that is sensitive to T1 changes and with minimal T2* effects. To capture the first pass of the contrast agent, temporal resolution of 5 s is required. Mostly a spoiled gradient echo sequence (SPGR) is used. This sequence goes with different names: FLASH, SPGR, and T1-FFE. T1 contrast despite the short TR values is preserved because the transverse magnetization is destroyed by either gradient spoiling of the transverse magnetization or by using rf phase cycling of 117° (Zur et al. 1991). The signal intensity is depending on the flip angle (α), which is typically smaller than 25° and a repetition time (TR) mostly smaller than 10 ms (Chap. 1). The echo time (TE) is short to be able to neglect the T2* effect during the time series. The signal intensity as function of T1 can be described by

$$S = g\rho \frac{\sin(\alpha)\left(1 - \exp\left(-\frac{TR}{T_1}\right)\right)}{1 - \cos(\alpha)\exp\left(-\frac{TR}{T_1}\right)} \exp\left(-\frac{TE}{T_2^*}\right)$$

(5.7)

Here, the parameters g and ρ account for the system and reconstruction settings (g) and the proton density (ρ), respectively. The image contrast depends on flip angle (α) and TR and is dependent on T1 relaxation time. MRI signal intensity is not an absolute value due to variability of patients, sequence, MR system, receive coils, and reconstruction settings. For absolute contrast distribution determination and to model perfusion and permeability, the measured signal intensity has to be transferred into concentration of the contrast agent. Therefore, T1 maps are needed to measure T_{10}, which allows to calculate the concentration of contrast agent. The relationship between signal intensity and T1 can be approached as a linear relationship between S and $1/T1$ and rearranged as (Rosen et al. 1990):

$$\frac{S_{\text{Gd}} - S_0}{S_0} = r_1 T_{10} \left[c_{\text{contrast agent}} \right] \quad (5.8)$$

This demonstrates that the relative increase in signal intensity after contrast agent administration is not only related to the concentration of contrast agent but also to the native T1 of the tissue (Fig. 5.4).

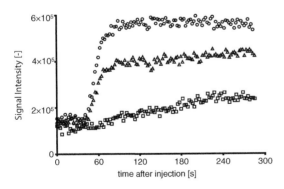 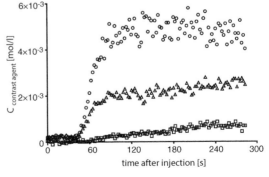

Fig. 5.4 The signal intensity (left) and the concentration (right) of three voxels is shown in a prostate. The voxels were selected in normal periperal zone (squares), tumor (triangles), and benign hyperplasia (rhombus). The non-linear relation between signal intensity (left) and contrast agent concentration (right) is clearly visible

As absolute T1 values are required to solve Eq. (5.9), T1 measurements have to be performed. The most accurate method is the inversion recovery method, but this will be very time consuming (Bydder and Young 1985). Another method is to acquire two images with different repetition times (TR), but this will also require long acquisition times. Therefore, mostly the variable flip angle method is used, exploiting a SPGR with different flip angles (Homer and Beevers 1985). Rearrangement of Eq. (5.8) shows that a plot of $y = S_\alpha/\sin(\alpha)$ versus $x = S_\alpha/\tan(\alpha)$ will give a linear relation with a slope of $e^{-TR/T1}$. In principle, two flip angles in a suitable range depending on the T1 of interest might be sufficient for the T1 calculation. However, more flip angles will give a more accurate estimation of T1 relaxation time and might be preferable if the T1 is unknown. In a 2D acquisition, the excitation slice profile can reduce the accuracy of the flip angle and by that the quantification of the concentration. Therefore, a 3D SPGR is preferred.

5.3.2.2 Measuring Contrast Agent Distribution

Similar to the T1 quantification, generally 3D SPGR with a flip angle optimized for T1 and TR is used for the contrast distribution (Brooks et al. 1999). For a specific tissue, the flip angle giving the highest signal intensity can be chosen, the Ernst angle, which is dependent on T1 and TR, but this might not be the flip angle for the best contrast. The temporal resolution is determined by the model of choice. For pharmacokinetic modeling, the spatial resolution needs to be higher than 6 and ideally 12 dynamics per minute (5–10 s/dynamic), while for qualitative dynamic imaging, up to 1 min per dynamic is used (Shukla-Dave et al. 2018). A high temporal resolution restricts the spatial resolution.

5.3.2.3 Acquisition of Arterial Input Function

For full pharmacokinetic modeling, also an arterial or vessel input function (AIF) is used. One of the choices to be made is if an individually measured or a population-averaged AIF is used. Optimally, the measured vessel should be an artery feeding the tumor. However, in practice, this might not be possible. Accurate characterization of the AIF needs very high temporal resolution, around 1 s. In practice, a vessel is chosen that is within the field of view and is large enough to select. Further, as the change in T1 of blood can decrease considerably after a bolus injection, the sequence has to be sensitive for a wide range of T1 values. This is a trade-off for sensitivity for the much smaller changes in T1 of the tumor and tissues of interest. Further, to establish steady state in the incoming blood, a saturation band is needed. Another approach is the use of a phase base AIF (Akbudak and Conturo 1996; Akbudak et al. 1997). The advantage is that the phase of the system is linearly related to the concentration contrast agent. The drawback is that phase drifts due to machine instabilities are commonly present and have to be corrected for, which is not trivial (Simonis et al. 2016). To overcome the requirements of spatial and temporal resolution and T1 range, often a population-averaged AIF has been used, which is retrieved from literature or measured in a number of patients or volunteers.

5.3.3 DCE-MRI Data Analysis

The analysis of tracer kinetics enables characterization of tumor microvasculature for diagnosis, delineation, and response evaluation. Several approaches have been proposed ranging from simple qualitative methods based on the shape of the uptake curve to challenging model fits.

The basics of all tracer kinetic models are that the response of the tissue is related to the dose injected (linear) and that the response function does not change over time (stationary), a linear stationary model. The simplest input of the system is a delta function, but in practice the input is a bolus of contrast agent injected in a couple of seconds, dispersed and delayed in the vascular system, which is depicted in the review of Koh et al. (2011b). Therefore, the kinetics of the contrast concentration in the tissue $c_t(t)$ is defined as a convolution of the tissue response function ($R(t)$) and the arterial input function ($c_a(t)$). Tissue and arterial tracer kinetics can be measured to

5 Functional MR Imaging

resolve the tissue response function and the plasma flow (F_p) (Brix et al. 2010). The tissue response function describes how contrast agent entering from the vasculature disperses in the system.

$$c_t(t) = F_p \times R(t) \otimes c_a(t) \quad (5.9)$$

5.3.3.1 Qualitative Methods

The simplest evaluation of DCE-MRI is visual assessment, which is widely used by radiologists in daily clinical. Here, contrast arrival, wash-in, and wash-out are visually evaluated. Different parts of the dynamic curve reflect different stages of the contrast distribution. The first stage is the time to arrival and the second the upslope to the peak which is, respectively, related to the blood flow and total blood flow and volume. The third phase, the early washout, is determined by the leakage of the contrast agent into the extracellular extravascular space (EES), which reflects both the permeability and the microvascular surface area. The later washout face is mostly related to the EES (Fig. 5.5).

5.3.3.2 Model Free Analysis

An example of model-free analysis is the fairly simple quantitative measurement of the initial area under the curve (IAUC) (Fig. 5.5). Both time of injection and time of arrival in the tissue of the contrast agent are used.

$$\mathrm{IAUC} = \int_t^0 \left[c_{\text{contrast agent}} \right](t')\,dt' \quad (5.10)$$

Generally an integration over 60–100 s is used. Other measures to describe the uptake curve are time of arrival, time to peak, uptake slope, and washout slope. Normalizing of the IAUC to the integral over the AIF will give an indication of the total distribution volume (Padhani and Leach 2005). All these measurements can be performed using signal intensity or contrast agent concentration. However, if signal intensity is used, the absolute values are arbitrary and therefore meaningless.

Another model-free approach is a deconvolution of Eq. (5.10) using the measured $c_a(t)$ and $c_t(t)$, either algebraically or using a Fourier transform (Ostergaard et al. 1996a, b; Wirestam et al. 2000). As deconvolution enhances noise, regularization of the deconvolution is required (Koh and Hou 2002; Liu et al. 1999). The results will be a curve of $F_p \times R(t)$ and needs further interpretation to deduce physiological implications.

5.3.3.3 Pharmacokinetic Modeling

Pharmacokinetic modeling of contrast agents is a research field on its own, and several reviews and book chapters have been published (Brix et al. 2010; Jackson et al. 2006; Koh et al. 2011b; Sourbron and Buckley 2013). In these models, the response function ($F_p \times R(t)$) is described using a tissue model to quantify the changed

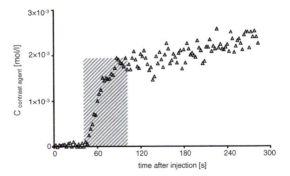

Fig. 5.5 Dynamic contrast curves of a prostate cancer patient showing differences in time-to-peak, upslope (wash-in), and wash-out for normal prostatic peripheral zone (blue), tumor (red), and benign hyperplasia (green) (left). The AUC for 60 s from the time to arrival (shaded area on the right)

endothelial permeability and perfusion of tumors. For kinetic modeling three steps are required: (1) conversion of the signal intensity to concentration of contrast agent, which is described above, (2) choice of an appropriate tissue model, and (3) parameter fitting of the model.

Two different approaches for the tissue models have been taken: compartmental models (Kety and Schmidt 1945) and plug-flow models (Miles and Griffiths 2003). In the compartmental models, the contrast agent in the vascular system is assumed to be mixed, which means that the concentration is spatially uniform. In contrast, the plug-flow approximation a contrast agent travels with a single uniform velocity in a tube. This assumes a parallel organized capillary bed, while the compartmental model might be more applicable for chaotic organized capillary beds.

Although reality might be complex, a simple diffusive model is used with exchange driven by differences in concentration of contrast agent in compartments and the permeability of membranes in between. The distribution of contrast agent after injection is described as the exchange of contrast agent between the different compartments, which comprise of the intravascular plasma compartment (v_p) and the extravascular extracellular compartment (EES or v_e). The plasma volume fraction (v_p) of the blood is the blood volume (v_b) minus the hematocrit (Hct).

$$v_p = v_b(1 - \text{Hct}) \quad (5.11)$$

In compartmental models, the tissue models assume the contrast agent to be distributed over several compartments with exchange of the contrast agent between the compartments (Fig. 5.6).

A conventional two-compartment model can be described as mass balance between of contrast agent between the plasm compartment and the extracellular extravascular compartment. Here, $c_e(t)$ and $c_p(t)$ denote the concentrations of contrast agent in v_e and v_p.

$$v_p \frac{dc_p(t)}{dt} = -\text{PS}[c_p(t) - c_e(t)] - F_p c_p(t) + c_0(t)\delta(t) \quad (5.12)$$

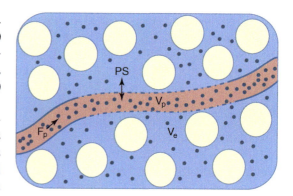

Fig. 5.6 Schematic illustration of a tissue as used for pharmacokinetic models. The plasma volume (v_p), the extravascular extracellular space (v_e), and the permeability surface area product (PS) are indicated. The contrast agent is depicted as black dots, while the yellow circles represent cells, which are not permeable for contrast agent. The dashed line indicates the permeable endothelium of the microvasculature

$$v_e \frac{dc_e(t)}{dt} = \text{PS}[c_p(t) - c_e(t)] \quad (5.13)$$

As both vasculature and tissue are present in a voxel, distribution curves are a superposition of the contrast agent in the microvasculature and interstitium. In the early 1990s, Tofts, Brix, Larsson, and colleagues (Brix et al. 1991; Larsson et al. 1990; Tofts and Kermode 1991) proposed independently comparable models, the generalized kinetic models which are currently mostly referred to as Tofts models. These models are in analogy with tracer kinetic model of Kety and Schmidt (1945). They do not include blood flow, as the acquisition speed was not high enough to measure the first pass of the contrast agent.

The exchange between the compartments is defined as the rate constants, K^{trans} and k_{ep}. Exchange rate K^{trans} describes the kinetics from the vascular to the EES. Depending on the vascular conditions, K^{trans} can be either blood flow (F_p)- or permeability (PS)-limited or a mixture of both. The efflux rate constant is represented by $k_{\text{ep}} = K^{\text{trans}}/v_e$. The derivation of the model is described clearly in Koh et al. (2011b).

$$\frac{dc_t(t)}{dt} = K^{\text{trans}} c_p(t) - k_{\text{ep}} c_t(t) \quad (5.14)$$

This can be solved as

$$c_t(t) = K^{trans} c_p(t) \otimes e^{-k_{ep}t} \quad (5.15)$$

where $c_t(t)$ is measured in the tissue of interest, $c_p(t)$ is given or measured from the arterial input function, and K^{trans} and k_{ep} can be solved.

The extended generalized kinetic models included the vascular component in addition to the extravascular extracellular component (Brix et al. 2004; Henderson et al. 2000; Pradel et al. 2003). As Eq. (5.16) only describes the tissue compartment, the tissue concentration will be extended with v_p, and the tissue concentration will become

$$c_t(t) = v_p c_p(t) + K^{trans} c_p(t) \otimes e^{-k_{ep}t} \quad (5.16)$$

This is known as the extended Tofts model.

A simplified version of this model is the Patlak model, where the efflux from the interstitium is neglected to enable linearization as denoted in Eqs. (5.17)–(5.19).

$$x(t) = \frac{\int_0^t c_p(u)\,du}{c_p(t)} \quad (5.17)$$

$$y(t) = \frac{c_t(t)}{c_p(t)} \quad (5.18)$$

$$y(t) = v_p + K^{trans} x(t) \quad (5.19)$$

The plug-flow models or distributed parameter models basically assume a cylindrical vascular space with a tracer-concentration gradient along both the intravascular space and EES. Therefore, mass balance equations have to account for both changes in time and space along the cylindrical axis. St. Lawrence and Lee simplified the model in the AATH model, the adiabatic approximation to the tissue homogeneity model, by assuming that the exchange between the v_p and v_e only occurs at the venous outlet of the capillary which is described by the first-pass extraction fraction (E) (St Lawrence and Lee 1998a, b). In practice, this means that plug flow exists during the vascular phase. In the interstitium phase, a tissue homogeneity model is used which assumes a well-mixed compartment neglecting the vascular space. The solution of the mass balance of the AATH model is the impulse residue function ($R_{AATH}(t)$), which is split into two physiological phases, the vascular and the interstitium phase for a two-compartmental model, where t_p denotes v_p/F_p

$$R_{AATH}(t) = \begin{cases} 1 & 0 < t \le t_p \\ E\exp\left[-\frac{EF_p}{v_e}(t - t_p)\right] & t > t_p \end{cases} \quad (5.20)$$

with

$$E = 1 - \exp\left(\frac{PS}{F_p}\right) \quad (5.21)$$

The relation between the different models, the assumptions made, and the interpretations of the model parameters are depicted and listed in the review of Sourbron and Buckley (2013).

In summary, the optimal model for a given measurement is dependent both on the tissue properties as on the scan parameters. Tissue properties, such as the level of vascularization, the permeability, and the blood flow, are important in relation to the scan parameters including temporal resolution of the scan series, injection rate of the contrast bolus, and noise level of the scans.

5.4 BOLD fMRI

One of the most used clinical applications which makes used of the BOLD endogenous contrast is the functional magnetic resonance imaging, also referred to as BOLD fMRI technique. In a simple fMRI experiment, a large number of the so-called blood-oxygen-level-dependent (BOLD)-sensitive images are collected during condition A (e.g., patient lying at rest in scanner bed) and during neural stimulation condition B (patient performing a task). Localized changes of nuclear magnetic relaxation times (T2 and T2*), blood flow and blood volume between conditions A and B produce small signal changes in the image. By performing statistical analysis on a pixel-by-pixel basis, the location of brains' response to a specific stimulus can be depicted.

5.4.1 Neuronal Activation and the BOLD Contrast

A neuron can be defined as an excitable cell specialized for the transmission of electrical signals over long distances. The neurons receive input signal from sensory cells or other neurons and send output signals to muscles or other neurons. Neurons connect with each other via specialized junctions called synapses. Metabolic changes in neurons are energy requiring, where more of this energy is used at or around synapses. Because most brain energy production depends on oxidation processes, there is an increase in local oxygen demand with increased synaptic activity. As a consequence, neuronal activity is accompanied by increased local blood flow. This phenomenon was first observed in 1890 by the English novel laureate Sir Charles Scott Sherrington who demonstrated that stimulation of the brain induces a local increase in blood flow. This increase in blood flow is accompanied by a small increase in local blood volume and a local oxygen consumption. These physiological changes provide the basics of BOLD contrast imaging techniques in the brain.

In general, blood can be considered to be a concentrated solution of hemoglobin (~12 g per 100 cm^3), which is an oxygen-carrying protein. Oxygenated hemoglobin is diamagnetic, while deoxygenated hemoglobin is paramagnetic. Consequently, variations in hemoglobin oxygenation induce changes in the local magnetic field causing changes on the T2*- and T2-weighted images.

In 1990, Ogawa et al. (1990) obtained the first BOLD contrast image. Ogawa observed numerous dark lines of various sizes in the brains of live mice and rats at high field (7.0 T). These lines represented blood vessels depicted because of the increase in deoxyhemoglobin content in red cells. Blood deoxygenation increases the magnetic susceptibility in local vessels which induces a decrease in water tissue T2* relaxation time. Prior to Ogawa's experiment, Thulborn et al. demonstrated that the rate of T2 relaxation decay of blood changed exponentially with the amount of deoxygenated hemoglobin. These two pieces of work suggest that changes in T2 and T2* relaxation times have a direct effect on the BOLD contrast.

The changes in BOLD signal over time are known as the BOLD response. The typical BOLD response morphology is illustrated in Fig. 5.7.

A BOLD response can be subdivided into three different stages. The first one takes place immediately after the triggering of neural electrical activity. This consists of a short period of time ranging from half to one second with the MR signal decreasing by approximately 0.5% below baseline. The so-called initial dip is followed by a rapid increase of the MR signal by typically 2–3% at 1.5 T. This corresponds to the positive BOLD signal, and it is the one measured by the majority of fMRI studies. This second period normally peaks at 5–8 s after initiation of the stimulus at the so-called overshoot. The initial dip is thought to arise from immediate oxygen consumption, which

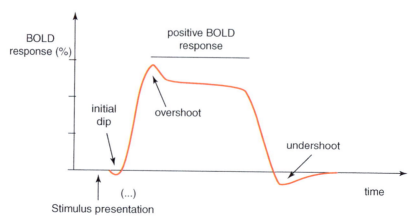

Fig. 5.7 Schematic representation of the BOLD response

is followed by a disproportionate increase in oxygen supply (Yacoub and Hu 1999).

Finally, toward the end of the stimulus, the MR signal decreases back to the baseline, which is frequently accompanied by an undershoot period. Throughout this final stage, the signal remains below baseline for several seconds.

5.4.2 Image Acquisition

Although BOLD contrast can be achieved via spin echo (SE), the most commonly used pulse sequence, mainly due to its superior SNR, is gradient echo (GE)-based (Chap. 1.6.5). In the typical fMRI examination, a whole volume or phase (a collection of contiguous slices covering the desired anatomy) is acquired in the duration of one TR period.

5.4.3 BOLD fMRI Concepts and Study Design Strategies

fMRI can be used to map those regions of the brain associated with cognitive, emotional, and behavioral functions such as sensation, movement, language, and memory. As described earlier, during an fMRI acquisition, the patient performs a task while rapid BOLD-sensitive images covering the whole brain are acquired. This whole brain collection of images (Fig. 5.8) is denoted as volume, phase, pass, or sample and is typically collected every 1–3 s. Volumes are consecutively acquired through the duration of the fMRI study, which ranges from a couple up to several minutes.

There are few fMRI study designs utilizing BOLD contrast to map brain activity either at rest or during a controlled task. The most frequently used techniques based on the chosen stimulus presentation paradigm are block design, event-related, mixed, and resting state (Amaro and Barker 2006). The latter is used to map the various neuronal networks that occur when the subject is at rest. In either block design or event-related, neuronal activity is triggered by presenting a series of tasks which are carried out by the subject while lying in the scanner.

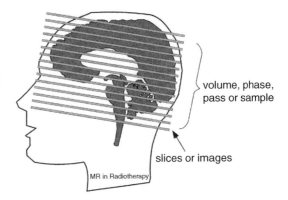

Fig. 5.8 Collection of 2D BOLD images known as volume, phase, pass, or sample in the field of fMRI usually collected in one repetition time (TR)

In block-design paradigms, the objective is to maintain cognitive engagement by presenting sequential stimuli within blocked conditions. A block can be defined as a time period of about 15–30 s and is alternated with periods of rest-denominated control blocks. A general block design is illustrated in Fig. 5.9. For example, a task during a conventional language paradigm (AFSNR Paradigms Task Force 2017) consists of presenting letters every couple of seconds. Subject is then instructed to silently generate as many words as possible that begin with projected words. During control periods, subject is instructed to either rest or engage in a different task. Ideally, control conditions are carefully chosen to only vary in the studied brain function. The pair control and task constitutes a cycle, which is repeated to allow enough data to be accumulated.

A typical block-design paradigm consists of:

- Four to six cycles with equal number of tasks and controls.
- Task and control duration: 15–30 s each.
- Number of volumes: about 40–60 volumes per cycle.
- Total scan duration: 4–6 min allowing for approximately 10–15 s of dummy scans.

Event-related paradigms enable detection of short variations in hemodynamic response function (HRF) from individual stimuli, which are introduced as brain regions can exhibit a different HRF to the same stimulus (Buxton et al. 2004).

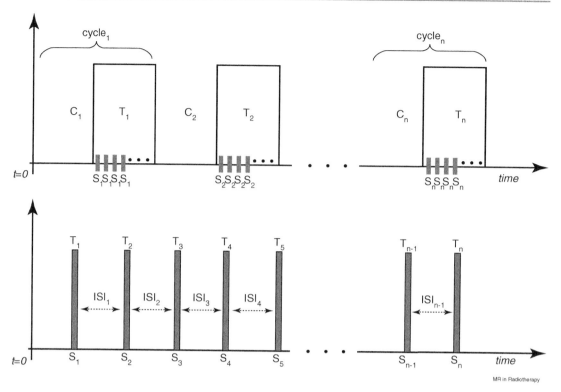

Fig. 5.9 Block-design paradigm (upper) and event-related paradigm (lower). Ti (Task) represents a time period during which sequential stimuli, represented with letter Si, of the same condition are presented. Ci represents a control period and ISIi an interstimulus interval

In event-related paradigms, every stimulus is presented individually during a very short period of time, typically 1–2 s.

In an event-related paradigm (Fig. 5.9), the concept of task is reduced to a single stimulus. The time between stimulus presentations, ISI (interstimulus interval), can vary across the acquisition reducing subject ability of prediction and maintaining attention levels across the acquisition (D'Esposito et al. 1999).

Experiments where ISI (typically 4 s) is chosen to be shorter than the HRF of the previous stimulus are classified as rapid event-related paradigms. Rapid event-related paradigms are very flexible, allowing variability of ISI and the randomization of presented stimuli. In general, ISI duration, its variability and stimuli randomization should be chosen carefully to warrant the success of the experiment.

Finally, resting-state fMRI (RS-fMRI) is a relatively recent technique and is very different than block or event-related, as it does not depend on any stimulus presentation. RS-fMRI relies on synchronized spontaneous BOLD fluctuation at low frequencies (between 0.01 and 0.1 Hz) between spatially differentiated areas of the brain at rest and was first introduced by Biswal (2012) and Biswal et al. (1995). These functionally linked brain regions are defined as resting-state networks. Various groups have identified networks such as the default mode, somatosensory, visual, attention, and language networks (Rosazza and Minati 2011).

During a typical resting-state experiment, the subject is instructed to close eyes and to think of nothing, without falling asleep. Scan duration ranges between 3 and 11 min.

5.4.4 BOLD fMRI Data Analysis

Pre-processing of fMRI data typically consists of slice-timing correction, three-dimensional rigid-body (Lee et al. 2013) motion correction, Gaussian temporal and spatial data smoothing, linear trend removal, and filtering in the frequency domain. After data pre-processing, statistical analysis takes place. As described earlier, the basic objective is to localize regions of the brain associated with a series of stimuli presentations. In the case of RS-fMRI, the aim is the depiction of the various neuronal networks.

In this context, the general linear model (GLM) (Smith and Matthews 2003) has become the most popular statistical method to analyze fMRI data. The GLM assumes that both HRF and stimulus are known. For more complex data analysis where there is no prior assumption of the HRF, other statistical analysis methods are utilized. This is, for example, the case in RS-fMRI studies. These statistical methods are seed-based analysis, independent component analysis (ICA), and graph analysis among others (Lee et al. 2013).

5.4.5 BOLD fMRI Distortion Artifacts and Challenges

Fast imaging techniques based on EPI are vulnerable to a variety of artifacts. The three main artifacts associated with EPI are the Nyquist ghosting, chemical shift derived from fat, and spatial distortion. The first one occurs because of hardware imperfections during the fast switching between the positive and negative components of the frequency encoding gradient. The other two are a consequence of small bandwidths in the phase direction and eddy currents induced by the rapid oscillating gradients.

When using fMRI data in radiotherapy, a special attention needs to be given to distortion. Details on the origin and correction of distortions are described in Chap.1.7.

5.4.6 Discussion

In general, there is not a perfect BOLD fMRI technique. It all depends on the intended clinical or research application. Block-design technique offers some advantages over event-related. This includes a better statistical power and larger BOLD signal change in relation to baseline (Petersen and Dubis 2012). Nonetheless, event-related fMRI is less sensitive to head motion artifacts; it also permits randomization of stimulus presentation. In general, event-related works better for maintaining subject attention. RS-fMRI has become a robust technique for the study of population differences of the various neuronal networks. However, it lacks statistical power in single-subject analysis.

In the context of BOLD fMRI in radiotherapy, the most used study approach is based on block-design fMRI. It is mainly due to its superior BOLD signal and statistical power.

5.5 Magnetic Resonance Spectroscopy (MRS)

MRS, also known as nuclear magnetic resonance (NMR) spectroscopy, was initially developed for the study of non-biological samples for the analysis of molecular interactions and chemical compounds identification.

This section intends to briefly cover the fundamental principles of in vivo clinical H^1 MRS. Typical studies in this field are based on the comparison of spectra from abnormal and normal tissue used for classification of abnormalities or monitoring of therapeutic treatments. The key feature of this technique is the capability to collect the MR signal of a specific volume of tissue. The localization techniques for MRS are very similar to those used in MRI, but due to the comparatively smaller concentration of H^1 metabolites, the MR spectra are obtained from a larger volume of tissue (typically ~8 cm^3). One of the main differences between MRI and MRS is that the former uses frequency encoding for spatial localization, whereas in MRS frequency is the desired measurement.

5.5.1 Spectra Formation

From a classical mechanics point of view, an RF pulse is an oscillating magnetic field (B_1) produced by a transmitter coil which generates transverse magnetization and decays with time in the form of a free induction decay (FID). After Fourier transformation of the FID, a function of frequency is obtained, which represents the spectrum (see Fig. 5.10).

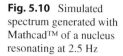
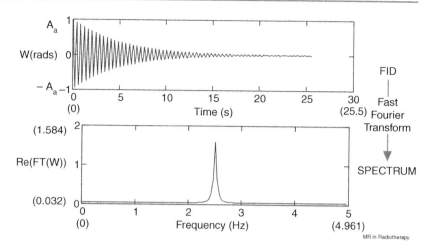

Fig. 5.10 Simulated spectrum generated with Mathcad™ of a nucleus resonating at 2.5 Hz

In Fig. 5.10, the upper graph shows how the waveform, ω (rads), of a hypothetical nucleus resonating at a frequency of 2.5 Hz, varies with respect to time. The lower graph represents the spectrum obtained after plotting the real part of the Fourier transform of the nucleus waveform, $RE(FT(\omega))$, with respect to angular frequency (ω). The peak reveals the existence of a nucleus or group of nuclei resonating at 2.5 Hz, while the area under the peak would corresponds to the relative concentration of nuclei detected.

Basic pre-processing operations of MRS consist of seven main steps: spectral and spatial filtering or apidization, spectral zero-filling, spectral FFT (fast Fourier transform), water reference, baseline correction, and zero-order auto-phase correction. Details of the correction steps are described in the review of van der Graaf (2010). The filtering steps are a trade-off between SNR, resolution, and voxel bleeding.

5.5.2 MRS Data Acquisition and Localization Method

Spatial selectivity in clinical MRS is accomplished using magnetic field gradients. Most localization techniques are based on the same slice selection and phase-encoding technique used in conventional MRI. Typical clinical methods for H^1 brain spectroscopy include stimulated echo acquisition mode (STEAM) and point-resolved spectroscopy (PRESS). However, the preferred technique mainly due to its higher SNR is the PRESS pulse sequence. The multivoxel version of the PRESS pulse sequence (Fig. 5.11) is commonly known as chemical shift imaging (CSI) or magnetic resonance spectroscopic imaging (MRSI).

This sequence consists of a 90° pulse followed by two 180° pulses. Each pulse is accompanied by various slice selection (SS) gradients and crusher gradients (CG) in the three orthogonal planes (G_x, G_y, and G_z). The crusher areas are compensated to include the slice refocus (after the 90° SS gradient) and phase-encoding gradients. This combination of pulses and slice selection gradients results in the excitation of a single voxel of tissue in the desired location. In 3D MRSI, data is collected from an array of voxels (or grid) which are spatially localized by the phase-encoding gradients in the three orthogonal planes. The size of the voxels is determined by the field of view divided by the number of phase-encoding steps in each direction. Prior to the volume excitation, it is necessary to use chemical shift selective (CHESS) saturation followed by very selective suppression (VSS) pulses to suppress the large water signal and reduce voxel contamination (Tran et al. 2000). Most commercial PRESS implementations include six default VSS pulses, each suppressing signal from around the edges of the excitation volume.

Fig. 5.11 A conventional PRESS pulse sequence diagram

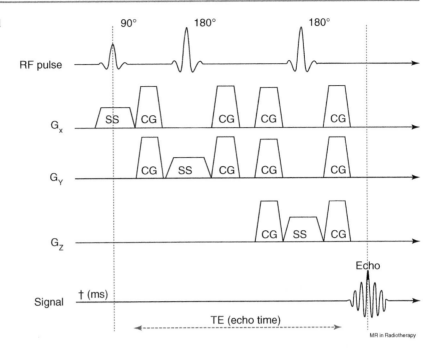

5.5.3 Chemical Shift and Parts per Million (ppm) Scale

The chemical shift concept is derived from the separation of resonance frequencies of different nuclei at a local magnetic field strength. Interactions between nuclei and their local chemical environment are responsible for shifts of the central resonance frequency. This is also known as a "chemical shift," where the degree of shift is related to the chemical species studied. Chemical shift often permits numerous chemical species to be distinctively identified. A weaker, and more complex, frequency shift may result from nuclear interactions in closer proximity. This effect is called spin-spin coupling or J-coupling.

Since a wide range of scanners of various field strengths are used to generate spectra, the horizontal axis of the spectrum is commonly depicted in parts per million (ppm). This is a dimensionless frequency scale independent of field strength. This can be defined as follows:

$$\delta(\text{ppm}) = \frac{f_i - f_{\text{ref}}}{f_{\text{ref}}}$$

where f_i is the frequency of interest and f_{ref} the frequency of the reference compound. In H^1 MRS the reference compound is tetramethylsilane (TMS), which is assigned a value of 0 ppm. Due to TMS having a highly shielded structure, it is to the right of most organic molecules measured with MRS.

5.5.4 MRS Data Analysis and Quantification (Peak Measurement)

The three main characteristics of a spectral peak are its integrated area, P_a, frequency δ(ppm), and linewidth, $\Delta f_{1/2}$. The peak frequency (f), measured in Hz, is proportional to the gyromagnetic ratio, γ, and the local magnetic field experienced by the nucleus (see Larmor equation definition (McRobbie et al. 2006)). The integrated area of each peak, P_a, is proportional to the number of nuclei resonating at that particular frequency. The linewidth ($\Delta f_{1/2}$ in Hz) determines the shape of the spectral absorption peak, and it is defined as the full width at half-peak amplitude. $\Delta f_{1/2}$ is inversely proportional to the total transverse relaxation time (T2*) as follows:

$$f_{1/2} = \frac{1}{2\pi T_2^*}$$

where $\Delta f_{1/2}$ represents the frequency difference or bandwidth at half-peak amplitude. From this equation for smaller T_2^* values, greater $\Delta f_{1/2}$ are obtained. Hence nuclei which demonstrate rapid signal decay (short $T2^*$) are represented by broader lines in the spectrum. Conversely, for greater T_2^* values, sharper spectral peaks are generated.

Spectral peaks with a broad linewidth can cause difficulties in spectral analysis, because of the reduced spectral resolution and diminished peak SNR. Line broadening can be corrected by improving local B0 inhomogeneities. This process is called shimming and can be applied linearly or in a polynomial fashion; the latter is referred to as high-order shimming.

Metabolite quantification is mostly measured in MR spectroscopy measuring the area or the amplitude of each peak, which is proportional to its concentration. However, obtaining reproducible values remains problematic. In the field of MRS radiology, most clinical practice uses peak ratios instead of absolute peak concentration (McKnight et al. 2001).

Figure 5.12 shows in vitro H^1-MRS spectrum obtained at a 1.5 T scanner from a $2 \times 2 \times 2$ cm^3 voxel place at the center of an 18 cm MRS sphere phantom (General Electric), using a quadrature head coil and a PRESS pulse sequence with a TE = 35 ms. This MRS phantom is filled with a homogeneous aqueous solution used to mimic the metabolic properties of a healthy human brain except of the lactate peak (Lac).

Detected peaks and corresponding resonance frequency (in ppm) are summarized in Table 5.1

5.5.5 MRSI Artifacts and Challenges

There are various factors determining the quality of MRSI. Primarily it is affected by the difficulty of achieving a good shim and water suppression over a large volume of interest (VOI) which may include areas of change in magnetic susceptibility such as air to tissue interfaces found in the nasal sinuses. Also, the point spread function (PSF) frequently referred to as voxel bleed is worse in MRSI. The contamination of each voxel within the VOI is contaminated with signal from the neighboring voxels due to finite sampling of data in k-space.

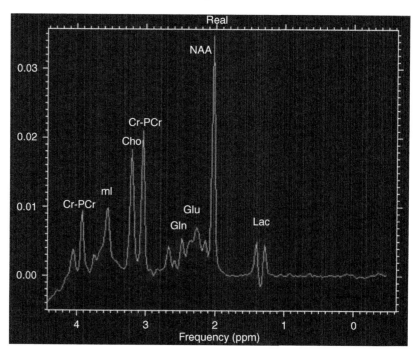

Fig. 5.12 ^{1}H-spectrum obtained from a MRS sphere phantom mimicking human brain metabolites

Table 5.1 Detected metabolite peaks and corresponding resonance frequencies in ppm

Metabolites	Resonance frequency, δ (ppm)
Lactate (Lac) – doublet	1.33
N-acetylaspartate (NAA)	2.02
Glutamate (Glu)	2.10
Glutamine (Gln)	2.50
Creatine/phosphocreatine(Cr/PCr)	3.03
Choline (Cho)	3.22
Myoinositol (mI)	3.60

There is another artifact, also present in normal imaging, known as a chemical shift error. This consists of a spatial displacement of the various chemical species during the slice selection due to the shifted resonance frequency of these species. In spectroscopic imaging this results in a poor definition of the VOI edges. The excitation profile of the VOI can be improved by over prescribing the VOI, which consists of an increase of the VOI size followed by a truncation to its original size by the use of VSS pulses. For example, the spatial mismatch or volume offset between NAA and Cho with respect to the central frequency on a 3.0 T scanner, of a single-voxel spectrum acquired with a bandwidth of 5.0 kHz and a VOI of $10 \times 10 \times 10$ mm^3, for NAA and Cho with respect to the central frequency is 0.3 and 0.2 mm, respectively.

References

AFSNR Paradigms Task Force AFSNR BOLD paradigms. Secondary AFSNR BOLD paradigms. 2017.

Akbudak E, Conturo TE. Arterial input functions from MR phase imaging. Magn Reson Med. 1996;36(6):809–15. https://doi.org/10.1002/mrm.1910360602.

Akbudak E, Norberg RE, Conturo TE. Contrast-agent phase effects: an experimental system for analysis of susceptibility, concentration, and bolus input function kinetics. Magn Reson Med. 1997;38(6):990–1002. https://doi.org/10.1002/mrm.1910380619.

Alsop DC. Phase insensitive preparation of single-shot RARE: application to diffusion imaging in humans. Magn Reson Med. 1997;38(4):527–33. https://doi.org/10.1002/mrm.1910380404.

Amaro E, Barker GJ. Study design in fMRI: basic principles. Brain Cogn. 2006;60(3):220–32. https://doi.org/10.1016/j.bandc.2005.11.009.

Basser PJ, Mattiello J, LeBihan D. MR diffusion tensor spectroscopy and imaging. Biophys J. 1994;66(1):259–67. https://doi.org/10.1016/S0006-3495(94)80775-1.

Biswal BB. Resting state fMRI: a personal history. NeuroImage. 2012;62(2):938–44. https://doi.org/10.1016/j.neuroimage.2012.01.090.

Biswal B, Yetkin FZ, Haughton VM, Hyde JS. Functional connectivity in the motor cortex of resting human brain using echo-planar MRI. Magn Reson Med. 1995;34(4):537–41. https://doi.org/10.1002/mrm.1910340409.

Brix G, Semmler W, Port R, Schad LR, Layer G, Lorenz WJ. Pharmacokinetic parameters in CNS GD-DTPA enhanced MR imaging. J Comput Assist Tomogr. 1991;15(4):621–8. https://doi.org/10.1097/00004728-199107000-00018.

Brix G, Kiessling F, Lucht R, et al. Microcirculation and microvasculature in breast tumors: pharmacokinetic analysis of dynamic MR image series. Magn Reson Med. 2004;52(2):420–9. https://doi.org/10.1002/mrm.20161.

Brix G, Griebel J, Kiessling F, Wenz F. Tracer kinetic modelling of tumour angiogenesis based on dynamic contrast-enhanced CT and MRI measurements. Eur J Nucl Med Mol Imaging. 2010;37:S30–51. https://doi.org/10.1007/s00259-010-1448-7.

Brooks JCW, Roberts N, Kemp GJ, Martin PA, Whitehouse GH. Magnetic resonance imaging-based compartmentation and its application to measuring metabolite concentrations in the frontal lobe. Magn Reson Med. 1999;41(5):883–8.

Buxton RB, Uludag K, Dubowitz DJ, Liu TT. Modeling the hemodynamic response to brain activation. NeuroImage. 2004;23:S220–33. https://doi.org/10.1016/j.neuroimage.2004.07.013.

Bydder GM, Young IR. MR imaging – clinical use of the inversion recovery sequence. J Comput Assist Tomogr. 1985;9(4):659–75. https://doi.org/10.1097/00004728-198507010-00002.

Callaghan PT. Principles of nuclear magnetic resonance microscopy. Oxford: Oxford University Press; 1991.

van der Graaf M. In vivo magnetic resonance spectroscopy: basic methodology and clinical applications. Eur Biophys J. 2010;39(4):527–40. https://doi.org/10.1007/s00249-009-0517-y.

D'Esposito M, Zarahn E, Aguirre GK. Event-related functional MRI: implications for cognitive psychology. Psychol Bull. 1999;125(1):155–64. https://doi.org/10.1037/0033-2909.125.1.155.

Garcia-Alvarez R, Liney G, Manton D, Beavis A, Turnbull L. Spectro image registration and metabolite-mapping software (SIRAMAS), a new open source research tool. 13th Annual meeting ISMRM. Miami. 2005.

Garcia-Alvarez R, Liney GP, Beavis AW. Repeatability of functional MRI for conformal avoidance radiotherapy planning. J Magn Reson Imaging. 2006;23(2):108–14. https://doi.org/10.1002/jmri.20493.

Gowland P, Mansfield P, Bullock P, Stehling M, Worthington B, Firth J. Dynamic studies of gadolinium uptake in brain-tumors using inversion-recovery echo-planar imaging. Magn Reson Med. 1992;26(2):241–58. https://doi.org/10.1002/mrm.1910260206.

Gudbjartsson H, Patz S. The rician distribution of noisy MRI data. Magn Reson Med. 1995;34(6):910–4. https://doi.org/10.1002/mrm.1910340618.

Hamilton RJ, Sweeney PJ, Pelizzari CA, et al. Functional imaging in treatment planning of brain lesions. Int J Radiat Oncol Biol Phys. 1997;37(1):181–8. https://doi.org/10.1016/s0360-3016(96)00475-0.

Hanahan D, Weinberg RA. The hallmarks of cancer. Cell. 2000;100(1):57–70. https://doi.org/10.1016/s0092-8674(00)81683-9.

Hanahan D, Weinberg RA. Hallmarks of cancer: the next generation. Cell. 2011;144(5):646–74. https://doi.org/10.1016/j.cell.2011.02.013.

Henderson E, Sykes J, Drost D, Weinmann HJ, Rutt BK, Lee TY. Simultaneous MRI measurement of blood flow, blood volume, and capillary permeability in mammary tumors using two different contrast agents. J Magn Reson Imaging. 2000;12(6):991–1003. https://doi.org/10.1002/1522-2586(200012)12:6<991::aid-jmri26>3.3.co;2-t.

Henkelman RM. Measurement of signal intensities in the presence of noise in MR images. Med Phys. 1985;12(2):232–3. https://doi.org/10.1118/1.595711.

Hennig J, Nauerth A, Friedburg H. Rare imaging – a fast imaging method for clinical MR. Magn Reson Med. 1986;3(6):823–33. https://doi.org/10.1002/mrm.1910030602.

Homer J, Beevers MS. Driven-equilibrium single-pulse observation of t1 relaxation – a reevaluation of a rapid new method for determining NMR spin-lattice relaxation-times. J Magn Reson. 1985;63(2):287–97. https://doi.org/10.1016/0022-2364(85)90318-x.

Iima M, Le Bihan D. Clinical intravoxel incoherent motion and diffusion MR imaging: past, present, and future. Radiology. 2016;278(1):13–32. https://doi.org/10.1148/radiol.2015150244.

A Jackson, DL Buckley, GJM Parker (2006) Tracer kinetic modelling for T1-weighted CE-MRI in dynamic contrast-enhanced magnetic resonance imaging in oncology. AL Baert, K Sartor. Dynamic contrast-enhanced magnetic resonance imaging in oncology: Springer, New York, NY.

Jensen JH, Helpern JA, Ramani A, Lu HZ, Kaczynski K. Diffusional kurtosis imaging: the quantification of non-Gaussian water diffusion by means of magnetic resonance imaging. Magn Reson Med. 2005;53(6):1432–40. https://doi.org/10.1002/mrm.20508.

Jezzard P, Balaban RS. Correction for geometric distortion in echo-planar images from B-0 field variations. Magn Reson Med. 1995;34(1):65–73. https://doi.org/10.1002/mrm.1910340111.

Jezzard P, Barnett AS, Pierpaoli C. Characterization of and correction for eddy current artifacts in echo planar diffusion imaging. Magn Reson Med. 1998;39(5):801–12. https://doi.org/10.1002/mrm.1910390518.

Jones DK, Cercignani M. Twenty-five pitfalls in the analysis of diffusion MRI data. NMR Biomed. 2010;23(7):803–20. https://doi.org/10.1002/nbm.1543.

Kety SS, Schmidt CF. The determination of cerebral blood flow in man by the use of nitrous oxide in low concentrations. Am J Physiol. 1945;143(1):53–66.

Koh TS, Hou Z. A numerical method for estimating blood flow by dynamic functional imaging. Med Eng Phys. 2002;24(2):151–8. https://doi.org/10.1016/s1350-4533(01)00105-9.

Koh D-M, Collins DJ, Orton MR. Intravoxel incoherent motion in body diffusion-weighted MRI: reality and challenges. Am J Roentgenol. 2011a;196(6):1351–61. https://doi.org/10.2214/ajr.10.5515.

Koh TS, Bisdas S, Koh DM, Thng CH. Fundamentals of tracer kinetics for dynamic contrast-enhanced MRI. J Magn Reson Imaging. 2011b;34(6):1262–76. https://doi.org/10.1002/jmri.22795.

Larsson HBW, Stubgaard M, Frederiksen JL, Jensen M, Henriksen O, Paulson OB. Quantitation of blood-brain-barrier defect by magnetic-resonance-imaging and gadolinium-DTPA in patients with multiple-sclerosis and brain-tumors. Magn Reson Med. 1990;16(1):117–31. https://doi.org/10.1002/mrm.1910160111.

Le Bihan D. What can we see with IVIM MRI? NeuroImage. 2017. https://doi.org/10.1016/j.neuroimage.2017.12.062.

Le Bihan D, Poupon C, Amadon A, Lethimonnier F. Artifacts and pitfalls in diffusion MRI. J Magn Reson Imaging. 2006;24(3):478–88. https://doi.org/10.1002/jmri.20683.

Le Roux P. Non-CPMG fast spin echo with full signal. J Magn Reson. 2002;155(2):278–92. https://doi.org/10.1006/jmre.2002.2523.

Lebihan D, Breton E, Lallemand D, Grenier P, Cabanis E, Lavaljeantet M. MR imaging of intravoxel incoherent motions – application to diffusion and perfusion in neurologic disorders. Radiology. 1986;161(2):401–7. https://doi.org/10.1148/radiology.161.2.3763909.

Lee MH, Smyser CD, Shimony JS. Resting-state fMRI: a review of methods and clinical applications. Am J Neuroradiol. 2013;34(10):1866–72. https://doi.org/10.3174/ajnr.A3263.

Liu HL, Pu YL, Liu YJ, et al. Cerebral blood flow measurement by dynamic contrast MRI using singular value decomposition with an adaptive threshold. Magn Reson Med. 1999;42(1):167–72. https://doi.org/10.1002/(sici)1522-2594(199907)42:1<167::aid-mrm22>3.3.co;2-h.

Liu WC, Schulder M, Narra V, et al. Functional magnetic resonance imaging aided radiation treatment planning. Med Phys. 2000;27(7):1563–72. https://doi.org/10.1118/1.599022.

Malyarenko DI, Ross BD, Chenevert TL. Analysis and correction of gradient nonlinearity bias in apparent diffusion coefficient measurements. Magn Reson Med. 2014;71(3):1312–23. https://doi.org/10.1002/mrm.24773.

McKnight TR, Noworolski SM, Vigneron DB, Nelson SJ. An automated technique for the quantitative assessment of 3D-MRSI data from patients with glioma. J

Magn Reson Imaging. 2001;13(2):167–77. https://doi.org/10.1002/1522-2586(200102)13:2<167::aid-jmri1026>3.3.co.

McRobbie DW, Moore EA, Prince MR, Grave MJ. MRI from picture to proton. Cambridge: Cambridge University Press; 2006.

Miles KA, Griffiths MR. Perfusion CT: a worthwhile enhancement? Br J Radiol. 2003;76(904):220–31. https://doi.org/10.1259/bjr/13564625.

Nelson SJ, Graves E, Pirzkall A, et al. In vivo molecular imaging for planning radiation therapy of gliomas: an application of 1H MRSI. J Magn Reson Imaging. 2002;16(4):464–76. https://doi.org/10.1002/jmri.10183.

Norris DG. Selective parity RARE imaging. Magn Reson Med. 2007;58(4):643–9. https://doi.org/10.1002/mrm.21339.

Ogawa S, Lee TM, Kay AR, Tank DW. Brain magnetic-resonance-imaging with contrast dependent on blood oxygenation. Proc Natl Acad Sci U S A. 1990;87(24):9868–72. https://doi.org/10.1073/pnas.87.24.9868.

Ostergaard L, Sorensen AG, Kwong KK, Weisskoff RM, Gyldensted C, Rosen BR. High resolution measurement of cerebral blood flow using intravascular tracer bolus passages. 2. Experimental comparison and preliminary results. Magn Reson Med. 1996a;36(5):726–36. https://doi.org/10.1002/mrm.1910360511.

Ostergaard L, Weisskoff RM, Chesler DA, Gyldensted C, Rosen BR. High resolution measurement of cerebral blood flow using intravascular tracer bolus passages. 1. Mathematical approach and statistical analysis. Magn Reson Med. 1996b;36(5):715–25. https://doi.org/10.1002/mrm.1910360510.

Padhani AR, Leach MO. Antivascular cancer treatments: functional assessments by dynamic contrast-enhanced magnetic resonance imaging. Abdom Imaging. 2005;30(3):324–41. https://doi.org/10.1007/s00261-004-0265-5.

Pantelis E, Papadakis N, Verigos K, et al. Integration of functional mri and white matter tractography in stereotactic radiosurgery clinical practice. Int J Radiat Oncol Biol Phys. 2010;78(1):257–67. https://doi.org/10.1016/j.ijrobp.2009.10.064.

Petersen SE, Dubis JW. The mixed block/event-related design. NeuroImage. 2012;62(2):1177–84. https://doi.org/10.1016/j.neuroimage.2011.09.084.

Pirzkall A, McKnight TR, Graves EE, et al. MR-spectroscopy guided target delineation for high-grade gliomas. Int J Radiat Oncol Biol Phys. 2001;50(4):915–28. https://doi.org/10.1016/s0360-3016(01)01548-6.

Pirzkall A, Nelson SJ, McKnight TR, et al. Metabolic imaging of low-grade gliomas with three-dimensional magnetic resonance spectroscopy. Int J Radiat Oncol Biol Phys. 2002;53(5):1254–64. https://doi.org/10.1016/s0360-3016(02)02869-9.

Pradel C, Siauve N, Bruneteau G, et al. Reduced capillary perfusion and permeability in human tumour xenografts treated with the VEGF signalling inhibitor ZD4190: an in vivo assessment using dynamic MR imaging and macromolecular contrast media. Magn Reson Imaging. 2003;21(8):845–51. https://doi.org/10.1016/s0730-725x(03)00186-3.

Reese TG, Heid O, Weisskoff RM, Wedeen VJ. Reduction of eddy-current-induced distortion in diffusion MRI using a twice-refocused spin echo. Magn Reson Med. 2003;49(1):177–82. https://doi.org/10.1002/mrm.10308.

Rohde GK, Barnett AS, Basser PJ, Marenco S, Pierpaoli C. Comprehensive approach for correction of motion and distortion in diffusion-weighted MRI. Magn Reson Med. 2004;51(1):103–14. https://doi.org/10.1002/mrm.10677.

Rosazza C, Minati L. Resting-state brain networks: literature review and clinical applications. Neurol Sci. 2011;32(5):773–85. https://doi.org/10.1007/s10072-011-0636-y.

Rosen BR, Belliveau JW, Vevea JM, Brady TJ. Perfusion imaging with NMR contrast agents. Magn Reson Med. 1990;14(2):249–65. https://doi.org/10.1002/mrm.1910140211.

Schakel T, Hoogduin JM, Terhaard CHJ, Philippens MEP. Diffusion weighted MRI in head-and-neck cancer: geometrical accuracy. Radiother Oncol. 2013;109(3):394–7. https://doi.org/10.1016/j.radonc.2013.10.004.

Schakel T, Hoogduin JM, Terhaard CHJ, Philippens MEP. Technical note: diffusion-weighted MRI with minimal distortion in head-and-neck radiotherapy using a turbo spin echo acquisition method. Med Phys. 2017;44(8):4188–93. https://doi.org/10.1002/mp.12363.

Schick F. SPLICE: sub-second diffusion-sensitive MR imaging using a modified fast spin-echo acquisition made. Magn Reson Med. 1997;38(4):638–44. https://doi.org/10.1002/mrm.1910380418.

Shukla-Dave A, Obuchowski NA, Chenevert TL, et al. Quantitative imaging biomarkers alliance (QIBA) recommendations for improved precision of DWI and DCE-MRI derived biomarkers in multicenter oncology trials. J Magn Reson Imaging. 2018. https://doi.org/10.1002/jmri.26518.

Simonis FFJ, Sbrizzi A, Beld E, Lagendijk JJW, van den Berg CAT. Improving the arterial input function in dynamic contrast enhanced MRI by fitting the signal in the complex plane. Magn Reson Med. 2016;76(4):1236–45. https://doi.org/10.1002/mrm.26023.

Sinnaeve D. The Stejskal-Tanner equation generalized for any gradient shape-an overview of most pulse sequences measuring free diffusion. Concepts Magn Reson A. 2012;40A(2):39–65. https://doi.org/10.1002/cmr.a.21223.

Smith SM, Matthews PM, editors. Functional MRI an introduction to methods. An introduction to methods. Oxford: Oxford University Press; 2003.

Sourbron SP, Buckley DL. Classic models for dynamic contrast-enhanced MRI. NMR Biomed. 2013;26(8):1004–27. https://doi.org/10.1002/nbm.2940.

St Lawrence KS, Lee TY. An adiabatic approximation to the tissue homogeneity model for water exchange in the brain: I. Theoretical derivation. J Cereb Blood Flow Metab. 1998a;18(12):1365–77.

St Lawrence KS, Lee TY. An adiabatic approximation to the tissue homogeneity model for water exchange in the brain: II. Experimental validation. J Cereb Blood Flow Metab. 1998b;18(12):1378–85.

Stejskal EO, Tanner JE. Spin diffusion measurements: spin echoes in the presence of a time-dependent field gradient. J Chem Phys. 1965;42(1):288. https://doi.org/10.1063/1.1695690.

Takahara T, Kwee TC, Hendrikse J, et al. Subtraction of unidirectionally encoded images for suppression of heavily isotropic objects (SUSHI) for selective visualization of peripheral nerves. Neuroradiology. 2011;53(2):109–16. https://doi.org/10.1007/s00234-010-0713-6.

Tofts PS, Kermode AG. Measurement of the blood-brain-barrier permeability and leakage space using dynamic MR imaging. 1. Fundamental-concepts. Magn Reson Med. 1991;17(2):357–67. https://doi.org/10.1002/mrm.1910170208.

Torresin A, Brambilla MG, Monti AF, et al. Review of potential improvements using MRI in the radiotherapy workflow. Zeitschr Med Phys. 2015;25(3):210–20. https://doi.org/10.1016/j.zemedi.2014.11.003.

Tran TKC, Vigneron DB, Sailasuta N, et al. Very selective suppression pulses for clinical MRSI studies of brain and prostate cancer. Magn Reson Med. 2000;43(1):23–33. https://doi.org/10.1002/(sici)1522-2594(200001)43:1<23::aid-mrm4>3.0.co;2-e.

Wang ML, Ma H, Wang XD, et al. Integration of BOLD-fMRI and DTI into radiation treatment planning for high-grade gliomas located near the primary motor cortexes and corticospinal tracts. Radiat Oncol. 2015;10. doi: https://doi.org/10.1186/s13014-015-0364-1.

Wirestam R, Andersson L, Ostergaard L, et al. Assessment of regional cerebral blood flow by dynamic susceptibility contrast MRI using different deconvolution techniques. Magn Reson Med. 2000;43(5):691–700. https://doi.org/10.1002/(sici)1522-2594(200005)43:5<691::aid-mrm11>3.0.co;2-b.

Yacoub E, Hu X. Detection of the early negative response in fMRI at 1.5 tesla. Magn Reson Med. 1999;41(6):1088–92. https://doi.org/10.1002/(sici)1522-2594(199906)41:6<1088::aid-mrm3>3.0.co;2-q.

Zur Y, Wood ML, Neuringer LJ. Spoiling of transverse magnetization in steady-state sequences. Magn Reson Med. 1991;21(2):251–63. https://doi.org/10.1002/mrm.1910210210.

Response Assessment

Ines Joye and Piet Dirix

6.1 Introduction

Truly personalized "precision" medicine is only possible through some sort of early response prediction and/or assessment. Especially in the case of radiotherapy (RT), which is still generally delivered over multiple fractions, it is crucial to differentiate between "responders" and "nonresponders" at the earliest opportunity to allow for treatment (de-)intensification or indeed "salvage" surgery or other alternatives. While technology-driven improvement of RT conformity is reaching its zenith, major gains can still be expected from the increased understanding of the "biological" side of radiation treatment, e.g., biomarker-guided prescription, combined treatment modalities, and adaptation of treatment during its course (Baumann et al. 2016). Clearly, to translate recent insights in tumor biology into routine radiotherapy practice, noninvasive ways to probe the tumor and its microenvironment are critical. Realistically, this leaves (repeated) imaging and/or liquid biopsies as the only potential drivers of personalized radiotherapy.

Computed tomography (CT) is now routinely used in many phases of cancer management, including screening, diagnosis, staging, treatment planning, response evaluation, and subsequent follow-up. It has an established value in the assessment of structural features of cancer, but CT is unable to depict functional or molecular details of solid tumors. Functional imaging techniques such as positron-emission tomography (PET) and magnetic resonance imaging (MRI) reflect physiological processes such as metabolism, proliferation, diffusion, and perfusion. Hence, these modalities are able to depict changes in tissue microstructure before morphological changes become apparent.

Unfortunately, PET, with whichever tracer, is usually hampered by the inflammation that is almost immediately caused by radiotherapy as well as its limited spatial resolution and is therefore only of limited use during RT. MRI on the other hand has the unique capability of providing anatomical and functional information with excellent spatial resolution in a single imaging session. Moreover, some of its functional quantitative imaging can easily distinguish between inflammation and viable tumor, even during RT. Additionally, the lack of ionizing radiation exposure and its wide availability make MRI the ideal candidate for repeated imaging, i.e., before, during, and after radiation therapy.

The volume and variety of imaging data challenges the traditional qualitative expert

I. Joye (✉) · P. Dirix
Department of Radiation Oncology, Iridium Cancer Network, Antwerpen, Wilrijk, Belgium

Molecular Imaging, Pathology, Radiotherapy & Oncology (MIPRO), University of Antwerp, Antwerpen, Belgium
e-mail: Piet.Dirix@gza.be

© Springer Nature Switzerland AG 2019
G. Liney, U. van der Heide (eds.), *MRI for Radiotherapy*,
https://doi.org/10.1007/978-3-030-14442-5_6

observer-based analysis. This is where the field of "radiomics" comes into play: by applying automated methods, quantitative imaging features are extracted and applied within clinical decision support systems to improve diagnostic, prognostic, and predictive accuracy (Lambin et al. 2012). The extraction of large amounts of image features is now emerging as a biomarker for screening, staging, survival, pathological response, and tumor recurrence (Lambin et al. 2017; Wu et al. 2018). The integration of these automated and comprehensive imaging analytics with pre- and peri-therapeutic markers derived from advances in molecular pathology (e.g., tumor genomics, circulating tumor cell assays) is creating an exciting future in which radiation oncology is becoming increasingly precise and personalized (Jaffray et al. 2018).

This chapter focuses on which role MRI currently has prior to, during, and after radiotherapy for a variety of tumor types and on how MRI can guide physicians in clinical decision-making.

6.2 Response Prediction on Initial MRI

As highly conformal radiotherapy permits lowering the dose to the organs at risk outside the target volume, the maximum dose becomes restricted by the presence of dose-limiting structures within the target volume, such as cartilage, connective tissue, nerves, and bone. It was therefore suggested that, rather than requiring dose uniformity within the PTV, traditionally the mainstay of conformal RT planning, dose escalation on areas of increased radioresistance within the tumor should be attempted in an effort to improve locoregional control (Galvin and De Neve 2007). Consequently, the concept of "dose-painting" on a biological target volume (BTV) was introduced (Ling et al. 2000). Clearly, this can only be successfully implemented by detailed imaging of the tumor and its microenvironment. Also, patient selection for other types of treatment intensification, or indeed de-intensification, through the concomitant prescription (or not) of systemic treatments, hinges on the ability to estimate the behavior of the tumor beforehand.

6.2.1 Head and Neck Cancer

In head and neck cancer, MRI can be used to estimate areas of more radioresistant disease within the tumor. For example, apparent diffusion coefficient (ADC) values on diffusion-weighted imaging (DWI) were significantly correlated with T-classification (Hatakenaka et al. 2011). Kim et al. (2009) performed DWI before, 1 week during, and approximately 2 weeks after concomitant chemoradiotherapy (CRT) in 33 head and neck cancer patients and correlated ADC measurements with clinical and in some cases pathological outcome data. They found that patients who responded favorably had significantly lower pre-treatment ADC values than partial or non-responders. In a larger database of 161 head and neck cancer patients treated with primary radiotherapy, Lambrecht et al. (2014) showed that pre-treatment ADC derived from high b-values (ADC_{high}) was a prognostic factor for disease recurrence (adjusted hazard ratio, 1.14 per 10^{-4} mm^2 s^{-1}; 95% CI 1.04–1.25).

However, the underlying biology of pre-treatment ADC, an obvious prerequisite for DWI-based dose-painting, is not yet fully understood. Important work in that respect was performed by the Utrecht group. Driessen et al. (2014) showed that ADC was significantly correlated with cellularity, stromal component, and nuclear-cytoplasmic ratio. The positive correlation of ADC and stromal component suggested that the poor prognostic value of high pre-treatment ADC might partly be attributed to the tumor-stroma component, a known predictor of local failure. Recently, the same group showed that high pre-treatment ADC is correlated with low T-cell influx, suggesting that the higher stromal component seen in these tumors has an immunosuppressive effect (Swartz et al. 2018). This suggests that pre-treatment DWI could play a role in selecting future combinations of CRT with immunotherapy.

Also in head and neck cancer, a pivotal trial on pre-treatment dynamic contrast-enhanced (DCE) MRI in patients undergoing CRT or surgery showed that the intra-tumoral distribution of K^{trans} was the strongest predictor of outcome (Shukla-Dave et al. 2012). Similarly, Kim et al. (2010) showed that pre-treatment K^{trans} was significantly higher in patients with complete response compared to patients with only partial response at 6 months after concomitant CRT. Clearly, if DWI and/or DCE-MRI have the ability to identify poor responders and can indicate the regions within the tumor that will be the focal point of locoregional failure, they provide both the motive and the opportunity to "paint" a higher dose on these areas in an effort to improve locoregional control (Dirix et al. 2009; Bauman et al. 2013).

6.2.2 Central Nervous System

For high-grade gliomas, MRI is firmly established as the superior imaging modality for diagnostic purposes. In diffusion tensor (DTI) MRI, diffusion gradients are applied in several different directions, and the dominant direction of diffusion within each voxel is determined, in addition to its magnitude, and is quantified as fractional anisotropy (FA). It was suggested that migrating cancer cells follow the paths of least resistance as determined from DTI and that anisotropic margins, based on DTI in each individual patient, could be used to reduce unnecessary irradiation of normal brain tissue and at the same time improve disease control (Krishnan et al. 2008).

6.2.3 Prostate

In prostate cancer, multiparametric MRI (mpMRI) allows to detect the site(s) of major cancer burden against a background of normal prostate tissue or low-grade, clinically irrelevant disease (Weinreb et al. 2016). Consequently, if mpMRI is performed as a triage test before prostate biopsies in men with high-serum prostate-specific antigen (PSA) levels, biopsies can be avoided in 25–30% of patients with clinically insignificant prostate cancer, while MRI-targeted biopsies generally allow to detect clinically significant cancer in 10–20% more patients (Ahmed et al. 2017; Kasivisvanathan et al. 2018). Interestingly, there is increasing evidence that these MRI-detected sites of major cancer burden, so-called index lesion(s), are also the site(s) of local recurrence(s) after radiotherapy (Joseph et al. 2009; Fuchsjager et al. 2010; Chopra et al. 2012; Arrayeh et al. 2012). Therefore, a more personalized, dose-painted approach of whole-gland irradiation with simultaneous boost on the index lesion(s) was advocated (Bauman et al. 2013). Several trials were initiated, the largest of which (the FLAME trial, NCT01168479) recently completed accrual (Monninkhof et al. 2018).

6.2.4 Gastrointestinal

6.2.4.1 Rectum

Rectal cancer studies generally show either no relation between initial ADC and tumor response or suggest that a lower pre-treatment ADC is associated with a better tumor response to preoperative CRT (Sun et al. 2010; Lambrecht et al. 2012; Barbaro et al. 2012; Cai et al. 2013; Intven et al. 2013). The negative correlation between initial ADC and tumor response is hypothesized to be attributed to the presence of necrotic areas (characterized by a high ADC), in which tumor cells are exposed to a more acidic and hypoxic environment, diminishing the effectiveness of radiotherapy and chemotherapeutic agents (Harrison and Blackwell 2004). However, the opposite finding that a lower ADC is associated with less response to CRT might be explained by a higher tumor cellularity and thus a larger tumor burden. In any case, radiological-pathological correlative studies on this issue are currently lacking, and explanations regarding initial ADC and treatment response in rectal cancer remain hypothetical.

6.2.4.2 Esophagus

Research on the predictive role of DWI performed prior to CRT in esophageal cancer has led to contradictory results: while one study on esophageal squamous cell carcinoma reported that a higher initial ADC was associated with a better response to CRT, other studies were inconclusive or contrarily found a higher initial ADC in non-responders (Aoyagi et al. 2011; De Cobelli et al. 2013; Van Rossum et al. 2015). Beside a potential role in response prediction, initial ADC may be indicative for tumor characteristics such as histology (adenocarcinoma vs. squamous cell carcinoma) and clinical T-stage (Van Rossum et al. 2015).

6.3 MRI During RT and Early After for Treatment Individualization

It has been suggested that DWI as well as DCE-MRI can identify physiological changes within the first weeks of treatment that are correlated with long-term clinical outcome. This would obviously allow to adapt the treatment at a very early opportunity and allow to maximize the changes of salvage treatments in non-responders as well as organ sparing in excellent responders.

6.3.1 Head and Neck Cancer

In head and neck cancer, the aforementioned study by the group from the University of Pennsylvania found that normalized ADC values after the first week of treatment had the highest accuracy for separating complete responders versus partial or non-responders to CRT (Kim et al. 2009). Perhaps, this increase in ADC correlates to the histologic presence of apoptosis, necrosis, and/or fibrosis and thus loss of tumoral structural integrity. In a similar study by the Leuven group, DWI was performed before treatment as well as 2 and 4 weeks into CRT (Vandecaveye et al. 2010). The absence of an ADC increase corresponded to lesions that would not disappear or would recur after treatment. In a follow-up study, Vandecaveye et al. found that the difference in ADC (ΔADC) between baseline and a new scan 3 weeks after CRT showed a positive predictive value of 89% and a negative predictive value of 100% for response (Vandecaveye et al. 2012). This absent ADC increase is possibly related to diffusion restriction in the dense microstructure of persistent tumor. These promising results are currently still being validated, e.g., by the INSIGHT trial at the Royal Marsden (Wong et al. 2018). At the moment, no published data are available on the next logical step, i.e., actual treatment adaptation based on response on DWI.

6.3.2 Central Nervous System

In glioblastoma multiforme (GBM), posttreatment MRI is routinely used for decision on adjuvant treatment. GBM is the most common primary brain tumor in adults and has a dismal prognosis with an average survival of 14 months. The standard treatment for GBM is a maximal safe resection followed by fractionated radiotherapy and concurrent temozolomide, followed by six cycles of adjuvant temozolomide, the so-called Stupp regimen (Stupp et al. 2005, 2009). MRI plays a crucial role in response evaluation after CRT. Pre- and postoperative MRIs are routinely compared to an MRI obtained 1 month after the end of CRT which is then considered the new baseline. In the absence of disease progression, patients are referred for adjuvant temozolomide for 6 months. In case of clear progression, prognosis is poor and a palliative approach is indicated.

6.3.3 Gastrointestinal

6.3.3.1 Rectum

Locally advanced rectal cancer is typically treated by preoperative CRT followed by total mesorectal excision (Glynne-Jones et al. 2017). At the moment of surgery, it appears that the tumoral response to CRT is highly heterogeneous and up to 30% of patients achieve a pathological complete response (Maas et al. 2010; Vecchio et al. 2005).

In a study of 20 patients, it was demonstrated that the increase in ADC early during CRT for rectal cancer was significantly higher in patients achieving a complete response compared to those who did not, with an AUC of 100% at a cutoff point of 50% ADC increase (Lambrecht et al. 2012). Similarly, Cai et al. (2013) found that the mean ADC at the second week of neoadjuvant therapy was significantly increased in patients with T-downstaging and tumor regression according to Dworak.

The acknowledgment that response to CRT is heterogeneous and that well-responding rectal cancer patients have an excellent prognosis has led to the "watch-and-wait" policy, as introduced by the Brazilian surgeon Habr-Gama (Habr-Gama et al. 2004; Maas et al. 2011). *Using* a strict surveillance protocol, patients with a clinical complete remission based on digital rectal examination and endoscopic assessment and imaging are deferred from surgery. Adopting such a non-operative strategy in patients achieving a clinical complete response spares them the morbidity and mortality associated with invasive TME surgery. The concept of organ preservation for rectal cancer is currently further promoted via the International Watch and Wait database for rectal cancer (http://www.iwwd.org/).

It is clear that accurate imaging is crucial when a non-operative strategy is considered after end of CRT. Conventional imaging modalities such as computed tomography and endoscopic ultrasonography (EUS) cannot distinguish residual tumor from fibrosis, necrosis, or post-CRT edema and are therefore inaccurate in evaluating response to CRT. The superior soft-tissue contrast and the high image resolution make conventional MRI the cornerstone for response assessment after CRT. However, as discussed earlier, functional MRI provides insights into the tissue microstructure which can contribute to a more accurate evaluation of response to CRT. Recent studies focused on the role of DWI performed 4–6 weeks after the end of CRT. A higher increase in ADC reflects a higher diffusivity because of cellular breakdown and thus correlates with a better response to CRT. In a systematic review on rectal cancer, pooled analysis demonstrated a moderate performance of late ADC assessment in prediction of pathological complete response with overall accuracies of 74% and 78%. Volumetric DWI measurement after CRT however predicted a complete pathological response with overall accuracies of 83% and 85% (Joye et al. 2014).

Dynamic contrast-enhanced MRI is another functional MRI technique which potential in response assessment has been studied. DCE-MRI measures a volume transfer constant, which is dependent on the perfusion and the permeability of tumor vasculature. CRT causes a decreased blood flow and permeability of the tumor bed. Hence, lower values of blood flow and permeability are associated with a good tumor response after CRT (Gollub et al. 2017; Intven et al. 2015).

Currently, some groups focus on the predictive value of integrating the information from anatomical, perfusion, and diffusion MRI. In this "radiomics approach," models are built through systematic analysis of numerous multiparametric MRI features (Cusumano et al. 2018; Nie et al. 2016).

Although promising, it should be noted that studies reporting on the predictive role of functional imaging are mostly small single-center studies conducted in specialized centers. Before DWI or DCE could be clinically implemented for treatment individualization, validation in a multi-center setting and standardization of image acquisition and data analysis are necessary (Bulens et al. 2018; Wang et al. 2016a).

6.3.3.2 Esophagus

In esophageal cancer, the addition of CRT to surgery has shown to improve locoregional control and overall survival (Sjoquist et al. 2011; Van Hagen et al. 2012). Clearly, patients who respond well to the CRT could be offered less invasive surgery, while non-responders can be spared the toxicity of an ineffective treatment and can potentially benefit from early treatment intensification.

In a prospective study on 38 esophageal squamous cell carcinoma patients undergoing weekly DWI during CRT, only the ADC value after 15 fractions was shown to be an independent prognostic factor for RECIST tumor response (Wang et al. 2016a). Similarly, a Dutch group demonstrated that an increase in ADC during the first 2–3 weeks of CRT was highly predictive of histopathologic response (Van Rossum et al. 2015).

6.4 MRI for Objective Response After Radiation Treatment

Finally, MRI is used to objectively determine the successfulness of the radiation treatment as such. It is a frequently used tool in neuro-oncology.

6.4.1 Central Nervous System

6.4.1.1 Spine Stereotactic Body Radiotherapy (SBRT)

Spine stereotactic body radiotherapy (SBRT) is an emerging novel radiation technique to treat spinal bone metastases. Up to 40% of all cancer patients will ultimately develop spinal bone metastases (Thibault et al. 2015). The increased life expectancy of patients with metastatic disease and the focus on metastases-directed treatment since the recognition of the so-called oligometastatic state demand for strategies that allow local definitive treatment of metastatic sites (Spratt et al. 2017). In this way, spine SBRT has been developed to treat spinal metastases with ablative intent rather than palliative intent (see Fig. 6.1). Spine SBRT is a well-tolerated treatment technique with imaging-based 1-year local control rates of 80–90% (Katsoulakis et al. 2017). Conventional MRI is the most frequently used imaging modality for assessing tumor response after spine SBRT. Different patterns of signal changes on T1- and T2-weighted imaging have been reported with an increase in tumor volume and a homogeneous T2 hypointensity being suggestive for tumor progression (Thibault et al. 2015).

The international SPIne response assessment in Neuro-Oncology (SPINO) group advises the first spinal MRI after treatment should be done 2–3 months after SBRT, since iatrogenic fractures most frequently occur within this time period (Sahgal et al. 2013). Thereafter, an MRI every 8–12 weeks seems reasonable for response assessment. As is frequently the case after radiation treatment, pseudoprogression and necrosis should be considered, with sequential imaging and tissue diagnosis to confirm in case of doubt (Bahig et al. 2016). While conventional MRI only provides anatomical information, multiparametric functional MRI techniques may be helpful since they complement with insights in tumor pathophysiology and cell viability (Soliman et al. 2017). Although advanced MRI techniques such as DCE-MRI and DWI remain investigational in the response evaluation after spine SBRT, changes in perfusion on DCE-MRI have shown to be useful in assessing local control as early as

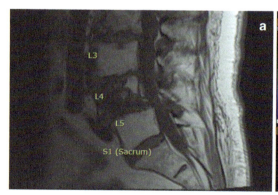
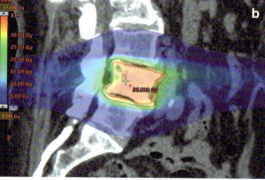

Fig. 6.1 SBRT spine treatment in patient with breast cancer. (**a**) T1-weighted MR image of the lumbar spine with metastatic involvement of lumbar 4. (**b**) Dose distribution of the stereotactic body radiotherapy with typical sharp dose gradients. (own data)

2 months post SBRT (Spratt et al. 2016). CT is not recommended for response assessment after spine SBRT, but it can be used in evaluating bone integrity and vertebral compression fractures.

6.4.1.2 Glioblastoma Multiforme (GBM)

After the end of CRT, patients with GBM are regularly followed with MRI. Within the first 3 months after the end of CRT, about 20% of the patients with GBM will develop increased contrast enhancement that ultimately will resolve on subsequent MRI scans (Brandsma et al. 2008). This phenomenon of pseudoprogression is believed to be caused by enhanced inflammation and disruption of the blood-brain barrier caused by the radiation itself (see Fig. 6.2). The recognition that contrast enhancement after CRT does not necessarily equal tumor progression, but that it can be due to the treatment itself, and the need to account for the non-enhancing component of the tumor are the basis of the Response Assessment in Neuro-Oncology (RANO) criteria (Wen et al. 2010). Findings on T1 and T2/FLAIR MRI sequences, the appearance of new lesions, the need for corticosteroids, and clinical assessment are defining the response to treatment according to RANO. However, as the RANO group excludes patients who progress within the first 12 weeks after CRT from clinical trials, further modification of the criteria is warranted to correctly identify early progressors and late pseudoprogressors. In this respect, advanced MR techniques have shown to be useful in distinguishing treatment necrosis from tumor progression (Maeda et al. 1993; Barajas Jr et al. 2009; Asao et al. 2005; Yoon et al. 2017; Zhang et al. 2014; Boonzaier et al. 2017; Fatterpekar et al. 2012).

Dynamic susceptibility contrast-enhanced (DSC) MRI can be used to make measurements of absolute cerebral blood flow (CBF) and volume (CBV) and relative CBV (rCBV). DCE-MRI yields estimates of additional parameters related to vascular permeability such as the vascular transfer constant (K^{trans}). As such, perfusion imaging reflects tissue vascularity and allows for a quantitative and qualitative response assessment (Fatterpekar et al. 2012). In a retrospective study on 57 patients, Barajas et al. found that the rCBV can be used to differentiate tumor recurrence from radionecrosis, with a higher rCBV in patients with recurrent GBM than in patients with radiation necrosis (Barajas Jr et al. 2009). In a prospective study using image-guided neuronavigation during surgical resection, specimen histopathology was directly correlated with localized DSC measurements (Hu et al. 2009). Forty tissue specimens from 13 subjects were investigated, and it

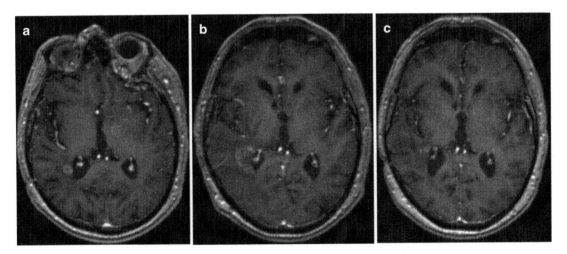

Fig. 6.2 Pseudoprogression after stereotactic radiosurgery (SRS) for glioblastoma on axial T1 contrast-enhanced MRI. (**a**) Prior to SRS; (**b**) 12 weeks after SRS showing increased enhancement, raising the possibility of progression; (**c**) 16 weeks after SRS showing significant reduction in contrast enhancement. (own data)

appeared that the treatment-related nontumoral specimens had a lower rCBV compared to those in which recurrent tumor was found.

DWI also yields insights in response to treatment as an increase in ADC after CRT suggests treatment response, pseudoprogression, or radionecrosis, while an ADC decrease indicates a higher cellularity which could indicate tumor progression (Hein et al. 2004; Mardor et al. 2003; Yoon et al. 2016). However, pitfalls exist as GBM are necrotic tumors, increasing the ADC, while treatment-induced changes such as necrosis and apoptosis induce initial cell swelling, leading to a potential decrease in ADC. Unfortunately, because of the relatively long diffusion times with moderate diffusion weightings, the sensitivity of conventional DWI methods is generally too low to clearly indicate radiation response in individual subjects in daily practice. Alternative DWI approaches are tested using oscillating gradients instead of the conventional pulsed gradient spin echo. A preclinical mice study demonstrated that the oscillating gradients better reflected histologically defined tumor areas and enabled earlier detection of microstructural radiation changes than conventional methods (Bongers et al. 2018). In a retrospective study on 30 glioblastoma patients treated with CRT, it was found that ADC histogram analysis performed at a high b-value of 3000 s/mm^2 was highly performant in differentiating true progression from pseudoprogression (Chu et al. 2013). DTI and diffusion kurtosis imaging are other advanced diffusion techniques which potential in response assessment is currently evaluated (Hyare et al. 2017).

MR spectroscopy (MRS) is another noninvasive functional imaging technique assessing cell and neuronal metabolites such as choline, n-acetylaspartate (NAA), lactate, lipid, and creatinine. MRS has its value in the distinction of glioma from nonneoplastic lesions as well as in glioma grading (Wang et al. 2016b). Different patterns are indicative for an increased cell turnover, and specifically the choline/NAA and choline/creatinine ratios are associated with malignancy. The usefulness of MRS in post-therapeutic glioma imaging is less well established. Although decreased choline/NAA and choline/creatinine ratios have been associated with worse treatment outcome, a meta-analysis concluded that MRS alone has moderate diagnostic performance in differentiating tumor recurrence from radionecrosis and suggests that MRS is best used in combination with other imaging modalities (Zhang et al. 2014).

It is clear that multiparametric imaging might improve the accuracy over single imaging modalities but is hampered by issues regarding validation and standardization. Incorporation of these newer functional imaging techniques into the response criteria, together with other end points such as neuropsychological testing and quality of life measures, will be considered by the RANO group during the upcoming years.

6.5 Normal Tissue Response

Imaging can provide quantitative assessment of radiation-induced normal tissue effects (Jeraj et al. 2010; Rafat et al. 2015). Identifying an early sign of normal tissue damage with imaging would have the potential to predict organ dysfunction, thereby allowing re-optimization of treatment strategies based upon individual patients' risks and benefits. Early detection with noninvasive imaging may enable interventions to mitigate therapy-associated injury prior to its clinical manifestation. Further, successive imaging may provide an objective assessment of the impact of such mitigation therapies.

6.5.1 Head and Neck Cancer

Xerostomia is thought to be the most prominent complication after radiotherapy for HNC. Radiation-induced damage to the salivary glands changes the volume, consistency, and pH of secreted saliva from thin secretions with a neutral pH to thick and tenacious secretions with increased acidity. Patients have oral discomfort or pain; find it difficult to speak, chew, or swallow; and run an increased risk of dental caries or oral infection. With conformal radiotherapy techniques, it is possible, in selected patients, to partly spare at least one parotid gland while still treating the target volumes in the bilateral neck with the prescribed doses. A high dose is administered to a small part of the parotid gland, positioned closest to the target volumes, while the rest of the gland receives a low dose or no dose at all (Dirix and Nuyts 2010).

Diffusion-weighted MRI has been investigated as a noninvasive tool to investigate major salivary gland function before and after radiotherapy for head and neck cancer. In normal salivary glands (i.e., before RT), the ADC value shows a decrease during the first 5 min of stimulation, followed by a steady increase until a peak ADC, significantly higher than the baseline value, is reached after a median of 17 min. After RT, the baseline ADC value at rest is significantly higher than before RT in the non-spared salivary glands but not in the spared parotid glands. In the spared parotid glands, the same biphasic response is seen as before RT. However, this pattern is completely lost in the non-spared glands (Dirix et al. 2008). These results were recently confirmed and elaborated on by a group from Helsinki, who also found that after gustatory stimulation with ascorbic acid, ADC showed a biphasic response with an initial increase and subsequent decrease. Again, post-RT ADC increased as a function of RT dose absorbed by the salivary glands (Loimu et al. 2017).

6.6 Conclusion

Imaging methods are decisive in the evaluation of tumor response. In this setting, MR imaging presents a great potential to be adopted as a technique of choice, although there are still important issues that need to be solved. Anatomic, molecular, and functional MR imaging data provide essential information regarding tumor biology and may offer biomarkers for an early evaluation of treatment effects.

There are still important issues that MR imaging needs to continue to address in tumor response evaluation, including (1) technical optimization, (2) evaluation of the reproducibility of the obtained parameters, (3) validation of these data as oncologic biomarkers, (4) biological correlation of these parameters with tumor biology and patients' outcomes, and (5) definition of adequate scenarios for their clinical use.

References

Ahmed HU, Bosaily AE, Brown LC, et al. Diagnostic accuracy of multi-parametric MRI and TRUS biopsy in prostate cancer (PROMIS): a paired validating confirmatory study. Lancet. 2017;389:815–22.

Aoyagi T, Shuto K, Okazumi S, Shimada H, Kazama T, Matsubara H. Apparent diffusion coefficient values measured by diffusion-weighted imaging predict chemoradiotherapeutic effect for advanced esophageal cancer. Dig Surg. 2011;28:252–7.

Arrayeh E, et al. Does local recurrence of prostate cancer after radiation therapy occur at the site of primary tumor? Results of a longitudinal MRI and MRSI study. Int J Radiat Oncol Biol Phys. 2012;82:e787–93.

Asao C, Korogi Y, Kitajima M, et al. Diffusion-weighted imaging of radiation-induced brain injury for differentiation from tumor recurrence. AJNR Am J Neuroradiol. 2005;26(6):1455–60.

Bahig H, Simard D, Létourneau L, Wong P, Roberge D, Filion E, et al. A study of pseudoprogression after spine stereotactic body radiation therapy. Int J Radiat Oncol Biol Phys. 2016;96(4):848–56.

Barajas RF Jr, Chang JS, Segal MR, et al. Differentiation of recurrent glioblastoma multiforme from radiation necrosis after external beam radiation therapy with dynamic susceptibility-weighted contrast-enhanced perfusion MR imaging. Radiology. 2009;253(2):486–96.

Barbaro B, Vitale R, Valentini V, et al. Diffusion-weighted magnetic resonance imaging in monitoring rectal cancer response to neoadjuvant chemoradiotherapy. Int J Radiat Oncol Biol Phys. 2012;83:594–9.

Bauman G, Haider M, Van der Heide U, Ménard C. Boosting imaging defined dominant prostatic tumors: a systematic review. Radiother Oncol. 2013;10:274–81.

Baumann M, Krause M, Overgaard J, et al. Radiation oncology in the era of precision medicine. Nat Rev Cancer. 2016;16:234–49.

Bongers A, Hau E, Shen H. Short diffusion time diffusion-weighted imaging with oscillating gradient preparation as an early magnetic resonance imaging biomarker for radiation therapy response monitoring in glioblastoma: a preclinical feasibility study. Int J Radiat Oncol Biol Phys. 2018;4:pii:S0360-3016(17)34506-6. https://doi.org/10.1016/j.ijrobp.2017.12.280.

Boonzaier NR, Larkin TJ, Matys T, van der Hoorn A, Yan J, Price SJ. Multiparametric MR imaging of diffusion and perfusion in contrast-enhancing and non-enhancing components in patients with glioblastoma. Radiology. 2017;284(1):180–90.

Brandsma D, Stalpers L, Taal W, Sminia P, van den Bent MJ. Clinical features, mechanisms, and management of pseudoprogression in malignant gliomas. Lancet Oncol. 2008;9(5):453–61.

Bulens P, Couwenberg A, Haustermans K, et al. Development and validation of an MRI-based model to predict response to chemoradiotherapy for rectal cancer. Radiother Oncol. 2018;126(3):437–42.

Cai G, Xu Y, Zhu J, et al. Diffusion-weighted magnetic resonance imaging for predicting the response of rectal cancer to neo-adjuvant concurrent chemoradiation. World J Gastroeneterol. 2013;19:5520–7.

Chopra S, et al. Pathological predictors for site of local recurrence after radiotherapy for prostate cancer. Int J Radiat Oncol Biol Phys. 2012;82:e441–8.

Chu HH, Choi SH, Ryoo I, et al. Differentiation of true progression from pseudoprogression in glioblastoma treated with radiation therapy and concomitant temozolomide: comparison study of standard and high-b-value diffusion-weighted imaging. Radiology. 2013;269(3):831–40.

Cusumano D, Dinapoli N, Boldrini L, et al. Fractal-based radiomic approach to predict complete pathological response after chemo-radiotherapy in rectal cancer. Radiol Med. 2018;123(4):286–95.

De Cobelli F, Giganti F, Orsenigo E, et al. Apparent diffusion coefficient modifications in assessing gastro-oesophageal cancer response to neoadjuvant treatment: comparison with tumour regression grade at histology. Eur Radiol. 2013;23:2165–74.

Dirix P, Nuyts S. Evidence-based organ-sparing radiotherapy in head and neck cancer. Lancet Oncol. 2010;11:85–91.

Dirix P, De Keyzer F, Vandecaveye V, et al. Diffusion-weighted magnetic resonance imaging to evaluate major salivary gland function before and after radiotherapy. Int J Radiat Oncol Biol Phys. 2008;71(5):1365–71.

Dirix P, Vandecaveye F, De Keyzer F, et al. Dose painting in radiotherapy for head and neck squamous cell carcinoma: value of repeated functional imaging with (18)F-FDG PET, (18)F-fluoromisonidazole PET, diffusion-weighted MRI, and dynamic contrast-enhanced MRI. J Nucl Med. 2009;50:1020–7.

Driessen JP, Caldas-Magalhaes J, Janssen LM, et al. Diffusion-weighted MRI imaging in laryngeal and hypopharyngeal carcinoma: association between apparent diffusion coefficient and histologic findings. Radiology. 2014;272:456–63.

Fatterpekar GM, Galheigo D, Narayana A, Johnson G, Knopp E. Treatment-related change versus tumor recurrence in high-grade gliomas: a diagnostic conundrum—use of dynamic susceptibility contrast-enhanced (DSC) perfusion MRI. AJR Am J Roentgenol. 2012;198(1):19–26.

Fuchsjager MH, et al. Predicting post-external beam radiation therapy PSA relapse of prostate cancer using pretreatment MRI. Int J Radiat Oncol Biol Phys. 2010;78:743–50.

Galvin J, De Neve W. Intensity modulating and other radiation therapy devices for dose painting. J Clin Oncol. 2007;25:924–30.

Glynne-Jones R, Wyrwicz L, Tiret E, et al. Rectal cancer: ESMO clinical practice guidelines for diagnosis, treatment and follow-up. Ann Oncol. 2017;28(suppl_4):iv22–40.

Gollub MJ, Tong T, Weiser M, Zheng J, Gonen M, Zakian KL. Limited accuracy of DCE-MRI in identification of pathological complete responders after chemoradiotherapy treatment for rectal cancer. Eur Radiol. 2017;27(4):1605–12.

Habr-Gama A, Perez RO, Nadalin W, et al. Operative versus nonoperative treatment for stage 0 distal rectal cancer following chemoradiation therapy: long-term results. Ann Surg. 2004;240(4):711–7; discussion 717–8.

Harrison L, Blackwell K. Hypoxia and anemia: factors in decreased sensitivity to radiation therapy and chemotherapy? Oncologist. 2004;5:31–40.

Hatakenaka M, et al. Pretreatment apparent diffusion coefficient of the primary lesion correlates with local failure in head-and-neck cancer treated with chemoradiotherapy or radiotherapy. Int J Radiat Oncol Biol Phys. 2011;81:339–45.

Hein PA, Eskey CJ, Dunn JF, Hug EB. Diffusion-weighted imaging in the follow-up of treated high-grade gliomas: tumor recurrence versus radiation injury. AJNR Am J Neuroradiol. 2004;25(2):201–9.

Hu LS, Baxter LC, Smith KA, et al. Relative cerebral blood volume values to differentiate high-grade glioma recurrence from posttreatment radiation effect: direct correlation between image-guided tissue histopathology and localized dynamic susceptibility-weighted contrast-enhanced perfusion MR imaging measurements. AJNR Am J Neuroradiol. 2009;30(3):552–8.

Hyare H, Thust S, Rees J. Advanced MRI techniques in the monitoring of treatment of gliomas. Curr Treat Options Neurol. 2017;19(3):11.

Intven M, Reerink O, Philippens ME. Diffusion-weighted MRI in locally advanced rectal cancer: pathological response prediction after neo-adjuvant radiochemotherapy. Strahlenther Onkol. 2013;189:117–22.

Intven M, Reerink O, Philippens ME. Dynamic contrast enhanced MR imaging for rectal cancer response assessment after neo-adjuvant chemoradiation. J Magn Reson Imaging. 2015;41(6):1646–53.

Jaffray D, Das S, Jacobs PM, Jeraj R, Lambin P. How advances in imaging will affect precision radiation oncology. Int J Radiat Oncol Biol Phys. 2018;101(2):292–8.

Jeraj R, Cao Y, Ten Haken R, Hahn C, Marks L. Imaging for assessment of radiation-induced normal tissue effects. Int J Radiat Oncol Biol Phys. 2010;76:S140–4.

Joseph T, et al. Pretreatment endorectal magnetic resonance imaging and magnetic resonance spectroscopic imaging features of prostate cancer as predictors of response to external beam radiotherapy. Int J Radiat Oncol Biol Phys. 2009;73:665–71.

Joye I, Deroose CM, Vandecaveye V, Haustermans K. The role of diffusion-weighted MRI and (18)F-FDG PET/CT in the prediction of pathologic complete response after radiochemotherapy for rectal cancer: a systematic review. Radiother Oncol. 2014;113(2):158–65.

Kasivisvanathan V, Rannikko AS, Borghi M, et al. MRI-targeted or standard biopsy for prostate-cancer diagnosis. N Engl J Med. 2018;378(19):1835–6.

Katsoulakis E, Kumae K, Laufer I, Yamada Y. Stereotactic body radiotherapy in the treatment of spinal metastases. Semin Radiat Oncol. 2017;27(3):209–17.

Kim S, Loevner L, Quon H, et al. Diffusion-weighted magnetic resonance imaging for predicting and detection of early response to chemoradiation therapy of squamous cell carcinomas of the head and neck. Clin Cancer Res. 2009;15:986–94.

Kim S, Loevner LA, Quon H, et al. Prediction of response to chemoradiation therapy in squamous cell carcinomas of the head and neck using dynamic contrast-enhanced MR imaging. AJNR Am J Neuroradiol. 2010;31:262–8.

Krishnan AP, Asher IM, Davis D, Okunieff P, O'Dell WG. Evidence that MR diffusion tensor imaging (tractography) predicts the natural history of regional progression in patients irradiated conformally for primary brain tumors. Int J Radiat Oncol Biol Phys. 2008;7:1553–62.

Lambin P, Rios-Velazquez E, Leijenaar R, et al. Radiomics: extracting more information from medical imaging using advanced feature analysis. Eur J Cancer. 2012;48:441–6.

Lambin P, Leijenaar R, Deist T, et al. Radiomics: the bridge between medical imaging and personalized medicine. Nat Rev Clin Oncol. 2017;14(12):749–62.

Lambrecht M, Vandecaveye V, De Keyzer F, et al. Value of diffusion-weighted magnetic resonance imaging for prediction and early assessment of response to neoadjuvant radiochemotherapy in rectal cancer: preliminary results. Int J Radiat Oncol Biol Phys. 2012;82:863–70.

Lambrecht M, Van Calster B, Vandecaveye V, et al. Integrating pretreatment diffusion weighted MRI into a multivariable prognostic model for head and neck squamous cell carcinoma. Radiother Oncol. 2014;110:429–34.

Ling C, Humm J, Larson S, et al. Towards multidimensional radiotherapy (MD-CRT): biological imaging and biological conformality. Int J Radiat Oncol Biol Phys. 2000;47:551–60.

Loimu V, Seppälä T, Kapanen M, et al. Diffusion-weighted magnetic resonance imaging for evaluation of salivary gland function in head and neck cancer patients treated with intensity-modulated radiotherapy. Radiother Oncol. 2017;122(2):178–84.

Maas M, Nelemans PJ, Valentini V, et al. Long-term outcome in patients with a pathological complete response after chemoradiation for rectal cancer: a pooled analysis of individual patient data. Lancet Oncol. 2010;11(9):835–44.

Maas M, Beets-Tan RG, Lambregts DM. Wait-and-see policy for clinical complete responders after chemoradiation for rectal cancer. J Clin Oncol. 2011;29(35):4633–40.

Maeda M, Itoh S, Kimura H, et al. Tumor vascularity in the brain: evaluation with dynamic susceptibility-contrast MR imaging. Radiology. 1993;189:233–8.

Mardor Y, Pfeffer R, Spiegelmann R, et al. Early detection of response to radiation therapy in patients with brain malignancies using conventional and high b-value diffusion-weighted magnetic resonance imaging. J Clin Oncol. 2003;21(6):1094–100.

Monninkhof EM, van Loon JWL, van Vulpen M, et al. Standard whole prostate gland radiotherapy with and without lesion boost in prostate cancer: toxicity in the FLAME randomized controlled trial. Radiother Oncol. 2018;127(1):74–80.

Nie K, Shi L, Chen O. Rectal cancer: assessment of neoadjuvant chemoradiation outcome based on radiomics of multiparametric MRI. Clin Cancer Res. 2016;22(21):5256–64.

Rafat M, Ali R, Graves E. Imaging radiation response in tumor and normal tissue. Am J Nucl Med Mol Imaging. 2015;5(4):317–32.

Sahgal A, Atenafu EG, Chao S, et al. Vertebral compression fracture after spine stereotactic body radiotherapy: a multi-institutional analysis with a focus on radiation dose and the spinal instability neoplastic score. J Clin Oncol. 2013;31(27):3426–31.

Shukla-Dave A, Lee NY, Jansen JF, et al. Dynamic contrast-enhanced magnetic resonance imaging as a predictor of outcome in head-and-neck squamous cell carcinoma patients with nodal metastases. Int J Radiat Oncol Biol Phys. 2012;82:1837–44.

Sjoquist K, Burmeister BH, Smithers BM, et al. Survival after neoadjuvant chemotherapy or chemoradiotherapy for resectable oesophageal carcinoma: an updated meta-analysis. Lancet Oncol. 2011;12(7):681–92.

Soliman M, Taunk N, Simons R, et al. Anatomic and functional imaging in the diagnosis of spine metastases and response assessment after spine radiosurgery. Neurosurg Focus. 2017;42(1):E5.

Spratt DE, Arevalo-Perez J, Leeman JE, et al. Early magnetic resonance imaging biomarkers to predict local control after high dose stereotactic body radiotherapy for patients with sarcoma spine metastases. Spine J. 2016;16(3):291–8.

Spratt DE, Beeler WH, de Moraes FY, et al. An integrated multidisciplinary algorithm for the management of spinal metastases: an International Spine Oncology Consortium report. Lancet Oncol. 2017;18(12):e720–30.

Stupp R, Mason WP, van den Bent MJ, et al. Radiotherapy plus concomitant and adjuvant temozolomide for glioblastoma. N Engl J Med. 2005;352(10):987–96.

Stupp R, Hegi ME, Mason WP, et al. Effects of radiotherapy with concomitant and adjuvant temozolomide versus radiotherapy alone on survival in glioblastoma in a randomised phase III study: 5-year analysis of the EORTC-NCIC trial. Lancet Oncol. 2009;10(5):459–66.

Sun YS, Zhang XP, Tang L, et al. Locally advanced rectal carcinoma treated with preoperative chemotherapy and radiation therapy: preliminary analysis of diffusion-weighted MR imaging of early detection of tumor histopathologic downstaging. Radiology. 2010;254:170–8.

Swartz JE, Driessen JP, van Kempen PMW, et al. Influence of tumor and microenvironment characteristics on diffusion-weighted imaging in oropharyngeal carcinoma: a pilot study. Oral Oncol. 2018;77:9–15.

Thibault I, Chang E, Sheehan J, et al. Response assessment after stereotactic body radiotherapy for spinal metastasis: a report from the SPIne response assessment in Neuro-Oncology (SPINO) group. Lancet Oncol. 2015;16:e595–603.

Van Hagen P, Hulshof MC, van Lanschot JJ, et al. Preoperative chemoradiotherapy for esophageal or junctional cancer. N Engl J Med. 2012;366(22):2074–84.

Van Rossum PS, van Lier AL, van Vulpen M, et al. Diffusion-weighted magnetic resonance imaging for the prediction of pathologic response to neoadjuvant chemoradiotherapy in esophageal cancer. Radiother Oncol. 2015;115:163–70.

Vandecaveye V, Dirix P, De Keyzer F, et al. Predictive value of diffusion-weighted magnetic resonance imaging during chemoradiotherapy for head and neck squamous cell carcinoma. Eur Radiol. 2010;20:1703–14.

Vandecaveye V, Dirix P, De Keyzer F, et al. Diffusion-weighted magnetic resonance imaging early after chemoradiotherapy to monitor treatment response in head-and-neck squamous cell carcinoma. Int J Radiat Oncol Biol Phys. 2012;82:1098–107.

Vecchio FM, Valentini V, Minsky BD. The relationship of pathologic tumor regression grade (TRG) and outcomes after preoperative therapy in rectal cancer. Int J Radiat Oncol Biol Phys. 2005;62(3):752–60.

Wang L, Liu L, Han C, et al. The diffusion-weighted magnetic resonance imaging (DWI) predicts the early response of esophageal squamous cell carcinoma to concurrent chemoradiotherapy. Radiother Oncol. 2016a;121(2):246–51.

Wang Q, Zhang H, Zhang J, et al. The diagnostic performance of magnetic resonance spectroscopy in differentiating high-from low-grade gliomas: a systematic review and meta-analysis. Eur Radiol. 2016b;26(8):2670–84.

Weinreb JC, et al. PI-RADS prostate imaging – reporting and data system: 2015, version 2. Eur Urol. 2016;69:16–40.

Wen PY, Macdonald DR, Reardon DA. Updated response assessment criteria for high-grade gliomas: response assessment in neuro-oncology working group. J Clin Oncol. 2010;28(11):1963–72.

Wong KH, Panek R, Dunlop A, et al. Changes in multimodality functional imaging parameters early during chemoradiation predict treatment response in patients with locally advanced head and neck cancer. Eur J Nucl Med Mol Imaging. 2018;45:759–67.

Wu J, Tha KK, Xing L, Li R. Radiomics and radiogenomics for precision radiotherapy. J Radiat Res. 2018;59:i25–31.

Yoon RG, Kim HS, Kim DY, Hong GS, Kim SJ. Apparent diffusion coefficient parametric response mapping MRI for follow-up of glioblastoma. Eur Radiol. 2016;26(4):1037–47.

Yoon RG, Kim HS, Paik W, Shim WH, Kim SJ, Kim JH. Different diagnostic values of imaging parameters to predict pseudoprogression in glioblastoma subgroups stratified by MGMT promotor methylation. Eur Radiol. 2017;27:255–66.

Zhang H, Ma L, Wang Q, Zheng X, Wu C, Xu BN. Role of magnetic resonance spectroscopy for the differentiation of recurrent glioma from radiation necrosis: a systematic review and meta-analysis. Eur J Radiol. 2014;83(12):2181–9.

Motion Management

Eric S. Paulson and Rob H. N. Tijssen

7.1 Introduction

Organ motion is an important source of uncertainty in radiotherapy. With the steep dose gradients typically employed to reduce doses to proximal organs at risk (OAR), organ motion can play a pivotal role in the efficacy of radiotherapy. Current CT-based techniques may result in suboptimal image guidance due to lack of soft-tissue contrast, motion degradation, and surrogate-based tracking assumptions and lack of real-time information about tumor location (Mittauer et al. 2018). MR-guided radiation therapy (MR-gRT) overcomes these challenges and is uniquely capable of managing motion during treatment. The goal of this chapter is to review the necessity of and strategies to perform motion management during MR-gRT.

For the purposes of discussion, it is instructive to define the phases of an MR-gRT treatment fraction. An MR-gRT fraction can be divided into three phases: (1) pre-beam, (2) beam-on, and (3) post-beam. In addition, MR-gRT involves the use of three subsystems: (1) imaging, (2) treatment planning, and (3) treatment delivery. Depending on the hardware implementation of the MR-gRT device (i.e., "nearby" or integrated) (Mutic and Dempsey 2014; Fallone 2014; Keall et al. 2014; Lagendijk et al. 2014; Jaffray et al. 2014), one or more subsystems may be executed individually or simultaneously. Figure 7.1 provides an example of a potential online MR-gRT treatment strategy for use on an integrated MR-gRT device.

7.2 Review of Motion Sources

7.2.1 Interfraction Motion

Interfraction motion describes the anatomical variations that occur between treatment fractions. This class of motion exhibits both systematic and random components (Van Herk 2004). Interfraction motion can result in severe translations, rotations, and deformations of targets and organs at risk (OAR). Classic examples of treatment sites susceptible to interfraction motions include the pelvis (e.g., bladder and rectum filling differences) and abdomen (e.g., stomach and small bowel filling differences). The combination of daily image guidance along with a safety margin is conventionally utilized to manage interfraction motion. All MR-gRT device implementations are capable of performing online adaptive replanning, based on

E. S. Paulson (✉)
Department of Radiation Oncology, Medical College of Wisconsin, Milwaukee, WI, USA

Department of Radiology, Medical College of Wisconsin, Milwaukee, WI, USA

Department of Biophysics, Medical College of Wisconsin, Milwaukee, WI, USA
e-mail: epaulson@mcw.edu

R. H. N. Tijssen
Department of Radiotherapy, University Medical Center Utrecht, Utrecht, The Netherlands
e-mail: R.Tijssen@umcutrecht.nl

© Springer Nature Switzerland AG 2019
G. Liney, U. van der Heide (eds.), *MRI for Radiotherapy*,
https://doi.org/10.1007/978-3-030-14442-5_7

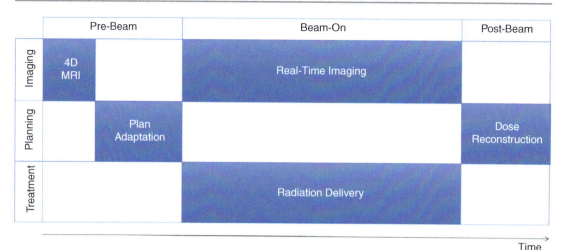

Fig. 7.1 Potential online MR-gRT treatment strategy for use on an integrated MR-gRT device. MR-gRT treatments are divided into pre-beam, beam-on, and post-beam phases. During each phase, imaging, planning, and treatment subsystems can be executed independently or in parallel. In this example, the treatment plan is updated with motion models obtain from a daily pre-beam 3D or 4D MRI, followed by real-time imaging during treatment delivery. After treatment, the dose is reconstructed and accumulated

the pre-beam image of the day, to manage interfraction motion.

7.2.2 Intrafraction Motion

Intrafraction motion describes the anatomical variations that occur within a treatment fraction. This class of motion largely exhibits random components. Intrafraction motion arises from a multitude of sources, including respiration, peristalsis, cardiac pulsations, organ filling, drifting (i.e., due to muscle relaxation), swallowing, and bulk motion. While these motions differ widely in terms of frequency and amplitude (see Table 7.1), respiratory motion typically dominates for targets in the upper abdomen and thorax. Respiration-induced displacements up to 4 cm have been reported for the pancreas (Feng et al. 2009). While all MR-gRT device implementations, including nearby implementations, are capable of managing interfraction motion, only integrated MR-gRT device implementations are additionally capable of managing intrafraction motion under MR guidance. Intrafraction motion can result in large deviations from planned dose distributions if not properly managed.

Table 7.1 Comparison of intrafraction motion frequencies and amplitudes (Feng et al. 2009; Guyton and Hall 2000; Trofimov et al. 2008; Paulson et al. 2011)

	Frequency (Hz)	Amplitude (cm)
Respiration	0.25	4 (pancreas)
Peristalsis:		
Stomach	0.05	
Duodenum	0.20	
Ileum	0.14	
Cardiac pulsations	1.2	
Organ filling	<0.01	
Drifts	<0.01	Arbitrary
Swallowing	0.02	2.8
Bulk motion	0.02	Arbitrary

7.3 Motion Management Strategies for Pre-beam Imaging

The goal of pre-beam motion management is to provide high-quality reference images for image guidance, online adaptive replanning, and dose accumulation and reporting. Control for effects of *interfraction* motion is the primary objective of pre-beam imaging. For treatment sites in the abdomen and thorax, motion management strategies must be employed during MR image acquisition to prevent contamination by motion artifacts due to respiration. Considerations of pre-beam motion management strategies are detailed in the following sections.

7.3.1 Requirements of Pre-beam Imaging

There are a number of requirements for pre-beam imaging. First, pre-beam imaging should be completed quickly but with sufficient time to prevent capture of anatomy at an arbitrary phase to avoid systematic errors (Van Herk 2004). Second, three-dimensional (3D) volumes must be acquired. The volumes can be obtained from true, 3D volumetric MR imaging or from multi-slice 2D imaging. Third, to reduce additional errors, the images must be free of motion artifacts and geometric distortions. Fourth, spatial resolution should be high enough to perform accurate image registration for image guidance. In addition, spatial resolution should be high enough to avoid errors during contour downsampling to the dose grid used for adaptive plan optimization and dose calculation. Finally, pre-beam image contrast resolution should provide sufficient landmarks to ensure accurate deformable image registration for contour transfers and dose accumulation.

7.3.2 Breath Holds

One straightforward approach for respiratory motion management during MR image acquisition is breath holds. Breath holds have the advantages of speed, ease of implementation, and provide flexibility in terms of which phase of the respiratory cycle is imaged. End-expiratory breath holds are often more consistent than inspiratory breath holds. However, deep inspiration breath holds offer the additional benefit of displacing the heart further from the chest wall, which may be particularly helpful in certain cancer sites (e.g., left-sided breast cancers) (Boda-Heggemann et al. 2016). The use of breath holds for pre-beam imaging implies that the treatment delivery be performed using breath holds performed at the same respiratory phase.

Despite these advantages, there are a number of challenges with breath hold acquisitions. First, pulse sequence parameters must be optimized to keep the acquisition duration around 15–20 s or less. This requirement often results in the need to compromise spatial resolution, coverage, and image contrast. High acceleration factors are also routinely utilized in breath hold acquisitions. For MR-gRT systems with limited radiofrequency receive coil array densities, higher acceleration factors can result in g-factor noise enhancement, reducing the overall SNR of the imaged volume. Second, even with short acquisition times, not all patients may be capable of performing breath holds. Residual motion artifacts may be introduced by patients that fail to maintain the breath hold over the full MRI acquisition. Finally, patients may get confused and perform breath holds at the wrong respiratory phase, resulting in severe anatomical displacement and/or deformation compared to the planned anatomy.

7.3.3 Respiratory Triggering or Gating

Respiratory motion can also be mitigated through the use of triggering or gating. In respiratory triggering, the image acquisition is initiated after an amplitude threshold on a respiratory waveform for the patient is exceeded. A trigger delay is often employed to adjust the phase of the image acquisition relative to the triggering point in the respiratory cycle. In respiratory gating, image acquisition is initiated only when the respiratory waveform falls within a predefined amplitude threshold. Figure 7.2 illustrates the differences between respiratory triggering and gating.

While respiratory gating involves optimization of the amplitude thresholds at a particular phase of the respiratory cycle, respiratory triggering is more complicated and involves additional sequence parameter optimization. First, if the trigger point is the end-inspiratory amplitude but desired acquisition phase is end-expiration, a trigger delay must be determined on a per-patient

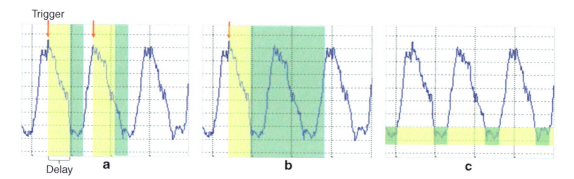

Fig. 7.2 Differences between respiratory triggering (optimized parameters (**a**); default parameters (**b**)) and respiratory gating (**c**). In all cases, the green-shaded regions indicate MR acquisition. In respiratory triggering, MR acquisition is initiated after an amplitude threshold on a respiratory surrogate is exceeded. A fixed trigger delay (yellow-shaded region in (**a**) and (**b**)) is introduced to adjust the phase of the MR acquisition relative to the trigger point. Variations in breathing can result in acquisition during inconsistent portions of the respiratory cycle (compare green-shaded regions in (**a**)). Optimization of concatenations/packages/acquisitions is required to ensure data is only acquired at specific respiratory phase, compared to the default parameters (compare green regions of (**a**) and (**b**)). In respiratory gating (**c**), MR acquisition is initiated only when the respiratory waveform falls within a predefined amplitude threshold

basis. Variations in respiratory rate may affect acquisition of images at a specific phase when a fixed trigger delay is employed (compare position of green-shaded regions in Fig. 7.2a). Second, the length of the acquisition window needs to be optimized to ensure that data is only acquired during the desired respiratory phase (compare green-shaded region of optimized parameters in Fig. 7.2a to default parameters in Fig. 7.2b). This optimization involves adjusting the number of concatenations, packages, or acquisitions based on the breathing pattern of each patient on Siemens, Philips, and GE scanners, respectively.

The respiratory waveform employed for triggering or gating can be obtained from a number of sources. Pneumatic respiratory bellows (Rohlfing et al. 2004), optical systems (Remmert et al. 2007), and tidal volume (Marx et al. 2014) measurements are examples of external respiratory surrogates. Alternatively, pencil beam navigators can be positioned to provide an internal surrogate. Pencil beam navigators utilize a 2D radiofrequency (RF) pulse to selectively excite a column of spins at a high-contrast interface (e.g., lung-liver interface or kidney/perirenal fat interface), as shown in Fig. 7.3 (Ehman and Felmlee 1989). A fast, parent pulse sequence samples the navigator and initiates acquisition of a child imaging sequence when trig-

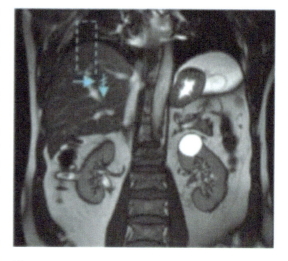

Fig. 7.3 Prescription of a 1D, pencil beam navigator (cyan box) at lung-liver interface for respiratory-triggered/respiratory-gated MR acquisition

gering or gating is performed. Finally, respiration-induced thermal noise variations in the RF receive coils during acquisition can be used as a respiratory surrogate (Andreychenko et al. 2017). Similar to breath holds, the use of respiratory-triggered or respiratory-gated sequences for pre-beam imaging requires that the treatment delivery also be performed using the same triggering or gating strategy.

7.3.4 Respiratory-Correlated 4D-MRI

While breath hold and respiratory-triggered/respiratory-gated acquisitions are effective at minimizing motion artifacts, information about the magnitude and direction of target and organ motion during respiration is lost with these approaches. This information can be obtained with respiratory-correlated four-dimensional MRI (RC-4D-MRI). In addition, RC-4D-MRI provides additional flexibility. Unlike breath holds or respiratory-triggered/respiratory-gated acquisitions, the output of pre-beam RC-4D-MRI can be used as reference images for non-gated or gated treatment deliveries. A multitude of RC-4D-MRI approaches have been introduced over the last decade, including prospective and retrospective multi-slice 2D (Celicanin et al. 2015; Tryggestad et al. 2013; Hu et al. 2013; Freedman et al. 2017; Breuer et al. 2018) and retrospective 3D approaches (Yang et al. 2015; Stemkens et al. 2015; Assländer et al. 2018; Han et al. 2017). The reader is referred to Stemkens et al. (2018) for a comprehensive review of RC-4D-MRI techniques.

RC-4D-MRI provides several pieces of information for respiratory motion management. First, individual image volumes at specific respiratory phases can be extracted from RC-4D-MRI (e.g., end-expiratory or mid-ventilation phases (van de Lindt et al. 2016)). Second, derived image volumes incorporating the geometric time-weighted mid-position of anatomy (Wolthaus et al. 2008) can be obtained from RC-4D-MRI. Finally, individualized internal target volumes (ITV) reflecting target motion of the day can be derived by dynamically propagating gross tumor volume contours across RC-4D-MRI phases.

7.3.5 Motion-Insensitive Pulse Sequences

An alternative motion management strategy is to employ MRI pulse sequences that are more robust against motion artifacts and acquire data over time scales longer than the motion sources. One family of pulse sequences that demonstrate good motion resilience is radial sequences, also known as projection imaging sequences. In radial sequences, the k-space sampling pattern is read out in spokes analogous to a bicycle wheel. Each spoke passes through the k-space center, which reduces the sensitivity of the sequence to motion. If a radial sequence is acquired over a time scale longer than the motion source, the motion will result in blurring. However, the overall position of anatomy is its time-averaged position.

7.3.6 Other Approaches

For some cancer sites such as head and neck, the majority of anatomy is static, and motion occurs by aperiodic, random events such as swallowing. In these cases, it may be useful to acquire 3D reference images for guidance along with a rapid cine MRI time series during deglutition to determine internal margins required to prevent a geographical miss (Paulson et al. 2011).

7.4 Motion Management Strategies for Beam-On Imaging

The goal of beam-on imaging is to provide support for online motion management strategies for MR-gRT delivery. Control for effects of *intrafraction* motion is the primary objective of beam-on imaging.

7.4.1 Review of Motion Management Strategies for Beam Delivery

It is instructive to review motion management strategies for beam delivery that may be employed in MR-gRT prior to discussing beam-on imaging.

7.4.1.1 Gating

Respiratory gating is an effective form of motion management for MR-gRT delivery

(Mittauer et al. 2018). Gating can be performed during free breathing or during manual breath holds at full inspiration or expiration. In free breathing, the treatment delivery is initiated only when the respiratory surrogate falls within a predetermined amplitude threshold. In breath hold deliveries, the treatment delivery is initiated only when the target falls within a predetermined tolerance. The patient is often coached while performing breath holds, which improves the consistency of anatomical position during multiple breath holds. The MRIdian system additionally offers video feedback, in which the cine MR images are presented to the patient during gated beam delivery, in order to increase the reproducibility of the breath holds (Tetar et al. 2018). Although gating can be effective at managing respiratory motion, gated treatment deliveries are less efficient because the treatment beam is paused a portion of the time that the patient is on the table.

7.4.1.2 Tracking

An alternative to gating is tracking, in which the multi-leaf collimator (MLC) apertures are dynamically conformed to the target as the target moves under free breathing (Keall et al. 2001). Tracking has the advantage of increased treatment efficiency, operating independent of patient compliance, and has the theoretical ability to handle abrupt irregular motions. However, the response rate of the MLC may reduce the ability to track abrupt, irregular motions. In addition, tracking in the presence of non-flat photon beams may also contribute to deviations between planned and delivered doses.

7.4.1.3 Trailing

Slower motions arising from drifts and organ filling can be handled with trailing. In the trailing strategy, intrafraction motion is considered to be a superposition of fast, periodic motions (e.g., respiration) and slow, ultracyclic motions (e.g., drifting and organ filling). Trailing aims to manage ultracyclic motion by performing setup adjustments whenever accumulated shifts exceed predefined tolerances (Trofimov et al. 2008). Because the time scale of drifting and organ filling is slow, rapid image acquisition is not required.

7.4.1.4 Dose Reconstruction

Estimation of the dose delivered during a treatment fraction is critical. Due to interplay (i.e., the start time of treatment and each segment with respect to the phase of motion and rate of dose delivery), the dosimetric outcome of each treatment fraction may be different from the plan or prior fractions (Trofimov et al. 2008). Dose reconstruction itself can serve as a motion management strategy. In this case, dose deposited to targets and OAR in the presence of motion is used as a bias dose to correct for errors during adaptive planning for the next treatment fraction.

7.4.1.5 Real-Time Plan Adaptation

Integrated MR-gRT devices are capable of supporting the ultimate motion management strategy, in which the treatment plan is continuously adapted based on each new anatomy update from the MRI (Kontaxis et al. 2017). One such approach utilizes an adaptive sequencer to perform segment-by-segment optimization based on an ideal dose fluence with direct update to the delivery hardware (Kontaxis et al. 2015a, b).

7.4.2 Requirements of Beam-On Imaging

The requirements of beam-on imaging will largely depend on the choice of motion management strategy employed for treatment delivery. Table 7.2 provides a comparison of basic imaging requirements for beam-on imaging. Gating and tracking require rapid, online imaging. Trailing requires online imaging, but a slower temporal resolution is permitted. Dose reconstruction requires volumetric images but can be performed offline. Real-time plan adaption requires online volumetric images acquired at a moderate temporal resolution.

Ideally, real-time volumetric MR imaging would be performed to fulfill the objectives of

7 Motion Management

Table 7.2 Comparison of imaging requirements for beam-on motion management strategies

	Temp res req'd	3D images req'd	Online acq req'd
Gating	Fast	No	Yes
Tracking	Fast	No	Yes
Trailing	Slow	No	Yes
Dose reconstruction	Slow	Yes	No
Real-time adaptive	Moderate	Yes	Yes

beam-on imaging. However, despite significant advancements in MR image acceleration over the past decade, it is still not possible to prospectively acquire and reconstruct volumetric MR images that meet the unique spatial, contrast, and temporal resolution requirements of radiotherapy. The following sections describe alternative approaches that have been proposed for beam-on imaging on integrated MR-gRT devices.

7.4.3 Cine MRI

MR fluoroscopy utilizing 2D cine MR imaging is a natural choice for real-time, prospective motion monitoring in gating and tracking beam-on motion management strategies. Cine MR images acquired in the sagittal plane at four frames per second have been successfully utilized for gated MR-gRT deliveries (Mittauer et al. 2018). The sequence of choice for 2D cine MR imaging is a balanced steady-state free precession sequence. 2D cine MR imaging is capable of resolving in-plane motion at high-temporal resolution. However, complex through-plane motion is not resolvable. This limitation can be overcome through acquisition of interleaved or simultaneous orthogonal plane cine imaging (Mickevicius and Paulson 2017).

7.4.4 Sequential 3D

Drifting and organ filling are slow motions that may be handled with trailing motion management strategies. Sequential 3D volumetric acquisition may be sufficient in these applications. Compared to pre-beam imaging, the beam-on 3D sequence prescription could utilize thinner, lower spatial resolution slabs positioned over the target and OAR.

7.4.5 Respiratory-Correlated 4D-MRI

Respiratory-correlated 4D-MRI can provide three-dimensional estimates of organ motion. However, several motion cycles are required to meet the data sufficiency conditions, which limit the utility of RC-4D-MRI for many motion management strategies requiring prospective, real-time imaging. One exception is the dose reconstruction strategy. In this approach, a 3D radial stack of stars sequence could be initiated prior to treatment and left acquiring data throughout the treatment course. The acquired data could then be retrospectively reconstructed into separate 4D phase bins for use in dose reconstruction. While this approach would handle effects of respiration, additional intrafraction motions (e.g., peristalsis) may result in blurring that could obscure reconstructed dose.

7.4.6 Hybrid Approaches

Although cine MR imaging can resolve in-plane motion with high-temporal resolution, 3D volumetric imaging is not available which limits its utility for dose calculation. Recently, several hybrid approaches have been introduced to fulfill the requirements of fast motion monitoring with simultaneous construction of volumetric images for dose reconstruction or real-time plan adaptation. In the method of Stemkens, statistical motion models, obtained from a pre-beam RC-4D-MRI, are driven with prospective, real-time 2D cine MR images obtained during beam-on to construct synthetic 3D volumes at the temporal resolution of the 2D cine images (Stemkens et al. 2016). The 2D cine MR images can be employed during motion management (e.g., gating or tracking), while the synthetic 3D volumes can be used for offline dose reconstruction or online plan adaptation. A similar approach was proposed by Harris et al. (2018). An alternative approach utilizes the simultaneous orthogonal plane imaging sequence. Navigator slices are kept fixed, while imaging slices are stepped through the patient volume. The navigator slices can be utilized for prospective, real-time motion monitoring and retrospective, self-navigated generation of serial RC-4D-MRI epochs for dose calculation (Mickevicius et al. 2018).

The advantage of the Stemkens and Harris methods is that the synthetic volumetric images are obtained prospectively, at the temporal resolution of the cine images. This permits the images to be used for both online real-time plan adaptation and offline dose reconstruction. However, both of these proposals rely on accurate deformable image registration (DIR) to synthesize the volumetric images. The advantage of the Mickevicius method is that DIR is not required to produce serial RC-4D-MRI epochs. However, the RC-4D-MRI epochs are obtained retrospectively and therefore can only be used for offline dose reconstruction.

7.4.7 Other Approaches

7.4.7.1 Pencil Beam Navigators

An alternative to using beam-on imaging for motion management may be to utilize 1D pencil beam navigators. The advantage of pencil beam navigators is their ability to resolve extremely fast and abrupt, irregular motions. Challenges of using pencil beam navigators include the need for a high-contrast interface and lack of spatial information for dose calculation.

7.4.7.2 Beam's Eye View Cine MR Imaging

An alternative to prescribing 2D cine images in static planes is to utilize beam's eye view (BEV) 2D cine imaging. In this approach, the cine imaging plane would rotate dynamically, remaining perpendicular to the treatment beam. BEV cine imaging permits direct visualization of targets and OAR within the prescribed slice. However, in comparison to x-ray fluoroscopy, the projection of anatomy is not obtained.

7.5 Emerging Acceleration Strategies

The ideal MR-gRT motion management strategy consists of continuous treatment plan adaptation with each new anatomy update from the MRI. Realization of this strategy will result in merging of the individual pre-beam, beam-on, and post-beam phases of MR-gRT. This section describes several emerging strategies to further accelerate MRI toward real-time volumetric imaging.

7.5.1 Simultaneous Multi-slice

One acceleration strategy is to excite more than one slice position within a repetition time. In simultaneous multi-slice (SMS) acquisitions, multiband radiofrequency pulses are employed to simultaneously sample two slice positions. Parallel imaging reconstruction algorithms are then used to separate the aliased slices. SMS approaches are a natural extension for 2D cine MR imaging and may be used to construct high-temporal resolution, prospective, and volumetric images using super-resolution reconstructions (Plenge et al. 2012; Van Reeth et al. 2015).

7.5.2 Compressed Sensing

Compressed sensing MRI is an approach to image acceleration based on the notion that medical images can be compressed by finding an appropriate transform domain, in which the image can be sparsely represented (e.g., spatial finite differences or wavelet domain) (Lustig et al. 2007). This, together with a random sampling pattern in k-space, allows images to be reconstructed from far fewer data than parallel imaging and partial Fourier acceleration techniques. Compressed sensing reconstruction is performed iteratively, minimizing the l_1 norm while maintaining data consistency. Although compressed sensing permits reconstruction of highly undersampled data, due to its iterative reconstruction, compressed sensing requires substantially longer reconstruction times than conventional MR reconstruction methods. The longer reconstruction times preclude the use of compressed sensing in prospective, real-time volumetric imaging.

7.5.3 Deep Learning

Recently deep learning approaches have begun being explored to reconstruct undersampled MR images (Hyun et al. 2017; Han et al. 2018; Qin et al. 2017; Hammernik et al. 2018). In this approach, models required to reconstruct MR images are trained in an offline environment. The advantage of this approach is that the time-consuming step of model training can be shifted to an offline setting, and then forward application of the trained models can be performed very quickly with each new frame of dynamic MRI data. Deep learning, combined with highly undersampled MR acquisition schemes, has the greatest potential of providing near real-time 3D volumetric images for MR-guided radiotherapy.

7.6 Summary

Effective management of organ motion is pivotal to the success of radiotherapy in many cancer sites. Control for interfraction motion is the primary objective of pre-beam imaging. Control for intrafraction motion is the primary objective of beam-on imaging. Deep learning-based image reconstruction, in combination with highly undersampled MR acquisition, offers the greatest potential to realize the ideal MR-gRT motion management strategy of continuous, real-time treatment plan adaptation with each new anatomy update from the MRI. Realization of this strategy will result in merging of the individual pre-beam, beam-on, and post-beam phases of MR-gRT.

References

Andreychenko A, et al. Thermal noise variance of a receive radiofrequency coil as a respiratory motion sensor. Magn Reson Med. 2017;77(1):221–8.

Assländer J, Cloos MA, Knoll F, Sodickson DK, Hennig J, Lattanzi R. Low rank alternating direction method of multipliers reconstruction for MR fingerprinting. Magn Reson Med. 2018;79(1):83–96.

Boda-Heggemann J, et al. Deep inspiration breath hold-based radiation therapy: a clinical review. Int J Radiat Oncol Biol Phys. 2016;94(3):478–92.

Breuer K, et al. Stable and efficient retrospective 4D-MRI using non-uniformly distributed quasi-random numbers. Phys Med Biol. 2018;63(7):075002.

Celicanin Z, Bieri O, Preiswerk F, Cattin P, Scheffler K, Santini F. Simultaneous acquisition of image and navigator slices using CAIPIRINHA for 4D MRI. Magn Reson Med. 2015;73(2):669–76.

van de Lindt TN, Schubert G, van der Heide UA, Sonke JJ. An MRI-based mid-ventilation approach for radiotherapy of the liver. Radiother Oncol. 2016;121(2):276–80.

Ehman RL, Felmlee JP. Adaptive technique for high-definition MR imaging of moving structures. Magn Reson Imaging. 1989;173:255–63.

Fallone BG. The rotating biplanar linac-magnetic resonance imaging system. Semin Radiat Oncol. 2014;24(3):200–2.

Feng M, et al. Characterization of pancreatic tumor motion using cine-mri: surrogates for tumor position should be used with caution. Int J Radiat Oncol Biol Phys. 2009;74(3):884–91.

Freedman JN, et al. T2-weighted 4D magnetic resonance imaging for application in magnetic resonance-guided radiotherapy treatment planning. Investig Radiol. 2017;52(10):563–73.

Guyton AC, Hall JE. Textbook of medical physiology. Philadelphia, PA: W. B. Saunders Company; 2000.

Hammernik K, et al. Learning a variational network for reconstruction of accelerated MRI data. Magn Reson Med. 2018;79(6):3055–71.

Han F, Zhou Z, Cao M, Yang Y, Sheng K, Hu P. Respiratory motion-resolved, self-gated 4D-MRI using rotating cartesian k-space (ROCK). Med Phys. 2017;44(4):1359–68.

Han Y, Yoo J, Kim HH, Shin HJ, Sung K, Ye JC. Deep learning with domain adaptation for accelerated projection-reconstruction MR. Magn Reson Med. 2018;80(3):1189–205.

Harris W, Yin FF, Wang C, Zhang Y, Cai J, Ren L. Accelerating volumetric cine MRI (VC-MRI) using undersampling for real-time 3D target localization/tracking in radiation therapy: a feasibility study. Phys Med Biol. 2018;63(1):01NT01.

Hu Y, Caruthers SD, Low DA, Parikh PJ, Mutic S. Respiratory amplitude guided 4D magnetic resonance imaging. Int J Radiat Oncol Biol Phys. 2013;86(1):198–204.

Hyun CM, et al. Deep learning for undersampled MRI reconstruction. arXiv. 2017;1:1–11.

Jaffray DA, et al. A facility for magnetic resonance-guided radiation therapy. Semin Radiat Oncol. 2014;24(3):193–5.

Keall PJ, Kini VR, Vedam SS, Mohan R. Motion adaptive x-ray therapy: a feasibility study. Phys Med Biol. 2001;46:1–10.

Keall PJ, Barton M, Crozier S. The Australian magnetic resonance imaging-linac program. Semin Radiat Oncol. 2014;24(3):203–6.

Kontaxis C, Bol GH, Lagendijk JJW, Raaymakers BW. A new methodology for inter- and intrafraction plan adaptation for the MR-linac. Phys Med Biol. 2015a;60(19):7485–97.

Kontaxis C, Bol GH, Lagendijk JJW, Raaymakers BW. Towards adaptive IMRT sequencing for the MR-linac. Phys Med Biol. 2015b;60(6):2493–509.

Kontaxis C, et al. Towards fast online intrafraction replanning for free-breathing stereotactic body radiation therapy with the MR-linac. Phys Med Biol. 2017;62(18):7233–48.

Lagendijk JJW, Raaymakers BW, van Vulpen M. The magnetic resonance imaging–linac system. Semin Radiat Oncol. 2014;24(3):207–9.

Lustig M, Donoho D, Pauly JM. Sparse MRI: the application of compressed sensing for rapid MR imaging. Magn Reson Med. 2007;58(6):1182–95.

Marx M, Ehrhardt J, Werner R, Schlemmer HP, Handels H. Simulation of spatiotemporal CT data sets using a 4D MRI-based lung motion model. Int J Comput Assist Radiol Surg. 2014;9(3):401–9.

Mickevicius NJ, Paulson ES. Simultaneous orthogonal plane imaging. Magn Reson Med. 2017;78(5):1700–10.

Mickevicius NJ, Chen X, Boyd Z, Lee HJ, Ibbott GS, Paulson ES. Simultaneous motion monitoring and truth-in-delivery analysis imaging framework for MR-guided radiotherapy. Phys Med Biol. 2018;63(23):235014.

Mittauer K, et al. A new era of image guidance with magnetic resonance-guided radiation therapy for abdominal and thoracic malignancies. Cureus. 2018;10(4):e2422.

Mutic S, Dempsey JF. The ViewRay System: magnetic resonance. Semin Radiat Oncol. 2014;24(3):196–9.

Paulson ES, Bradley JA, Wang D, Ahunbay EE, Schultz C, Li XA. Internal margin assessment using cine MRI analysis of deglutition in head and neck cancer radiotherapy. Med Phys. 2011;38(4):1740–7.

Plenge E, et al. Super-resolution methods in MRI: can they improve the trade-off between resolution, signal-to-noise ratio, and acquisition time? Magn Reson Med. 2012;68(6):1983–93.

Qin C, Schlemper J, Caballero J, Price A, Hajnal JV, Rueckert D. Convolutional recurrent neural networks for dynamic MR image reconstruction. IEEE Trans Med Imaging. 2017;38(1):280–90.

Remmert G, Biederer J, Lohberger F, Fabel M, Hartmann GH. Four-dimensional magnetic resonance imaging for the determination of tumour movement and its evaluation using a dynamic porcine lung phantom. Phys Med Biol. 2007;52(18):N401–15.

Rohlfing T, Maurer CR, O'Dell WG, Zhong J. Modeling liver motion and deformation during the respiratory cycle using intensity-based nonrigid registration of gated MR images. Med Phys. 2004;31(3):427–32.

Stemkens B, et al. Optimizing 4-dimensional magnetic resonance imaging data sampling for respiratory motion analysis of pancreatic tumors. Int J Radiat Oncol Biol Phys. 2015;91(3):571–8.

Stemkens B, Tijssen RHN, De Senneville BD, Lagendijk JJW, Van Den Berg CAT. Image-driven, model-based 3D abdominal motion estimation for MR-guided radiotherapy. Phys Med Biol. 2016;61(14):5335–55.

Stemkens B, Paulson ES, Tijssen RHN. Nuts and bolts of 4D-MRI for radiotherapy. Phys Med Biol. 2018;63(21):21TR01.

Tetar S, et al. Patient-reported outcome measurements on the tolerance of magnetic resonance imaging-guided radiation therapy. Cureus. 2018;10(2):e2236.

Trofimov A, Vrancic C, Chan TCY, Sharp GC, Bortfeld T. Tumor trailing strategy for intensity-modulated radiation therapy of moving targets. Med Phys. 2008;35(5):1718–33.

Tryggestad E, et al. Respiration-based sorting of dynamic MRI to derive representative 4D-MRI for radiotherapy planning. Med Phys. 2013;40(5):051909.

Van Herk M. Errors and margins in radiotherapy. Semin Radiat Oncol. 2004;14(1):52–64.

Van Reeth E, Tan CH, Tham IWK, Poh CL. Isotropic reconstruction of a 4-D MRI thoracic sequence using super-resolution. Magn Reson Med. 2015;73(2):784–93.

Wolthaus JWH, Sonke JJ, Van Herk M, Damen EMF. Reconstruction of a time-averaged midposition CT scan for radiotherapy planning of lung cancer patients using deformable registrationa. Med Phys. 2008;35(9):3998–4011.

Yang W, et al. Four dimensional magnetic resonance imaging with 3D radial sampling and self-gating based K-space sorting: early clinical experience on pancreatic cancer patients. Int J Radiat Oncol. 2015;93(3):S19.

Part III

MRI-Only Radiotherapy

Challenges and Requirements

Neelam Tyagi

8.1 Introduction

Radiation therapy requires images of high geometric fidelity with high spatial and contrast resolution to delineate disease extent and nearby organs at risk. Computed tomography (CT) is currently the gold standard with the most accurate geometrical information but poor soft tissue contrast. The results of multiple studies have shown the superiority of magnetic resonance imaging (MRI) soft tissue contrast for target and normal tissue segmentation in external beam radiotherapy. MRI has been an integral part of the radiotherapy process for more than a decade and has been shown to reduce interobserver variability in contouring on MR as compared with CT for multiple anatomical sites (Roach et al. 1996; Rasch et al. 1999; Weltens et al. 2001). The current radiotherapy simulation process relies on target and organ at risk segmentation on MRI followed by transfer of contours on CT via image registration. Although incorporating MRI decreases over-segmentation of structures as compared with CT-based segmentation, a wider transition to combined CT-MRI methods has been hampered by concerns about segmentation errors introduced by misregistration of the image sets and the changes to the shape and location of the soft tissues (e.g., the bladder, rectum, and seminal vesicles) that are inherent when acquiring multiple image sets. The uncertainties are further exacerbated when the anatomy has changed significantly due to surgery, or chemotherapy, or if the MRI is acquired in the diagnostic position (Hanvey et al. 2012). Geometric uncertainties between 2 and 5 mm have been reported for multiple disease sites (Ulin et al. 2010; Roberson et al. 2005; Dean et al. 2012; Brock and Deformable Registration Accuracy Consortium 2010). These registration errors are systematic and persist throughout the treatment course. In case of stereotactic body radiotherapy (SBRT) treatments where the steep dose gradients are advantageous for targeting tumor dose, these registration errors could lead to a geometric miss that may compromise tumor control.

To overcome these challenges, MR simulation platforms, including flat table tops, in-room lasers, and MR compatible immobilization, have been introduced that can reduce the image registration uncertainties between CT and MR. As discussed in previous chapters, these modern MR systems (or simulators) have been designed with tighter system-level distortions, primarily those relating to B0 inhomogeneity and gradient nonlinearity due to improved magnet design as well as higher-order corrections of gradient nonlinearity and high-order shimming. Although registration uncertainties are minimized, and higher geometric fidelity is achieved with MR simulation

N. Tyagi (✉)
Department of Medical Physics, Memorial Sloan-Kettering Cancer Center, New York, NY, USA
e-mail: tyagin@mskcc.org

platforms, changes in soft tissue anatomy between two imaging sessions, e.g., the bladder and rectum, are still a concern. By minimizing the time between CT and MR sessions, the consistency of normal soft tissue anatomy (bladder and rectal contents) can be maximized. Variation in organ positions can have an impact on radiotherapy planning for these sites because the position of nearby target structure (e.g., seminal vesicles) can differ on CT and MR, depending on rectum and bladder filling, as shown in Fig. 8.1 (Mak et al. 2012; Gill et al. 2014).

In addition to internal organ volume variation, there are also concerns about different tumor/target volumes on MR as compared with CT because of clear tumor boundaries (Prabhakar et al. 2007a; Fiorentino et al. 2013; Ahmed et al. 2010). For example, in the brain, tumor volumes are typically larger on MR potentially because of the surrounding edema. On the other hand, prostate volume is smaller on MR as compared with CT (Rasch et al. 1999). These volumes may also move freely compared to bones for some anatomical sites such as the prostate. Concerns then exist regarding how to register the two imaging modalities properly. The use of stable landmarks that can be observed on both image sets, such as the fiducials, is particularly helpful for this task and must be used.

Because of the challenges outlined above, in target delineation, registration uncertainties, and changes in anatomy due to temporal variations, surgery, or chemotherapy, a workflow in which MRI is the primary and sole imaging modality is preferred over a combined CT and MRI workflow. MR-only is defined as radiotherapy workflow where all components of treatment planning are based on MR. A complete MR-only workflow would also include MR-only delivery, but this chapter will only focus on the simulation and treatment planning aspect of MR-only. It is known that brachytherapy and brain stereotactic radiation therapy using a gamma knife have been using an MR-only workflow for quite some time by assuming a water-equivalent patient model. This section will focus on a MR-only solution for external beam radiotherapy that can also have applicability for brachytherapy and MR-guided radiation therapy. Figure 8.2 shows a typical MR-only workflow where simulation, contouring, planning, and treatment localization are performed based on MR images only.

In addition to minimizing segmentation and dosimetric errors introduced by misregistration between the CT and MR, a MR-only workflow improves efficiency by reducing the number of imaging sessions and CT exposures and may potentially reduce patient costs and resources

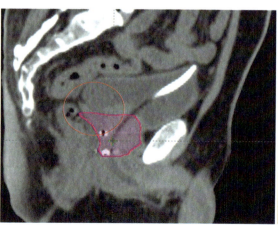
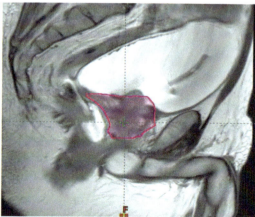

Fig. 8.1 An example case when magnetic resonance (MR) is used as a secondary imaging modality. Variations in the bladder and rectum between computed tomography (CT) and MR resulted in different seminal vesicle positions. A target drawn based on MR shows the seminal vesicle position outside the clinical target volume on the CT scan

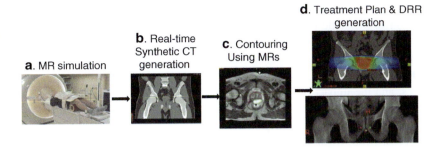

Fig. 8.2 A typical magnetic resonance (MR)-only workflow. (**a**) MR simulation. (**b**) Real-time synthetic CT generation. (**c**) Contouring using MRs. (**d**) Treatment plan and DRR generation

such as employee workload. For clinics where CT and MR resources are shared with radiology, MR-only can further improve patient throughput. MR-only also reduces inconveniences to the patient and is particularly helpful for pediatric patients or patients that are undergoing palliative treatment. Finally, in addition to accurate target and normal tissue volume, MR-only allows easy translation to a MR-linac platform and enables online MR-guided adaptive planning that may potentially reduce planning margin and treatment-related toxicity. Technically most sites that routinely use MRI as a secondary imaging modality can benefit from MR-only planning. Some of these sites include the brain, head and neck, prostate, and gynecology. Brachytherapy also benefits from MR-only planning but is not a focus of this chapter. In the future, MR-only planning would also be beneficial for patients with metal implants due to the advantage of soft tissue visualization and contouring based on MRI in the presence of dental and hip implants.

Although MR-only workflow has several advantages, there are also some challenges in implementing such workflows in the clinic. MR data sets do not contain the electron density and electron stopping power information that is required for dose calculation. MR intensities on a MR image are related to proton density, and magnetic relaxation properties of the imaged tissue are relative and show no correspondence to tissue electron density as CT. Hence, synthetic CTs, or pseudo-CTs, with electron density information will need to be generated directly from MR images for accurate dose calculation. At the same time, 2D digitally reconstructed radiographs (DRRs) or 3D reference images with sufficient bone, soft tissue, and/or implanted fiducial visualization are needed to guide image-based patient setup and treatment verification. Position verification using synthetic CTs can be achieved by generating DRRs from synthetic CTs and registering them to the orthogonal projection images prior to treatment or by matching the synthetic CTs with the onboard cone beam CT images.

In addition to synthetic CT generation, some thought should be given to MR images with sufficient soft tissue contrast and field of view for contouring both target and normal tissues for MR-only planning. For an efficient MR-only workflow, a single MR to generate both synthetic CTs and target and soft tissue delineation is ideal. The use of multiple MRs may introduce registration uncertainties due to intrafraction motion. It can be argued that although MR-only has the potential to reduce systematic misregistration error between CT and MR, it can also introduce systematic errors if care is not taken to remove intrafraction uncertainties when multiple MRs are acquired or, e.g., if the implanted fiducial location is misidentified on the MR. Performing an end-to-end test using dedicated MR simulation phantoms is helpful to verify and integrate MR-only workflows in the clinic (Sun et al. 2015).

Clinical implementation and robust, streamlined workflows for MR-only will depend on various factors, including a dedicated MR simulator in the radiation oncology and may need to be adapted accordingly for a busy clinic. Other factors that can help with a streamlined clinical workflow implementation include (a) clear indication of patient-specific contraindications such as size, implants, etc.; (b) dedicated water bath for making immobilizations in MR, (c) MR compatible immobilization and tattoo marking; (d) isocenter marking (relative or absolute); (e) real-time generation of synthetic CTs and assessment of MR image quality used for target and normal tissue delineation; (f) site-specific considerations such as fiducial identification, bowel preparation guidelines, and the impact of MR acquisition time on the contents of bladder and rectum filling; (g) automated scripts to verify registrations between different MRs, break dicom frame of reference, and allow independent adjustment if needed; and (h) physician-friendly layouts if multiple MRs are used . It is also important that multiple QA checks are implemented at various stages of simulation, contouring, planning, and delivery to ensure accuracy of MR-only workflow (Tyagi et al. 2017a). Further updates on clinical implementation of MR-only planning are discussed in the next chapter. This chapter will review the background and history of synthetic CT methods and provide a brief overview of bulk density methods of generating synthetic CTs. Other methodologies, clinical integration, implementation, and workflows for MR-only are discussed in the next chapter.

8.2 Background/History of Synthetic CT

A crucial requirement for MR-only simulation and planning is the ability to perform dose calculation and patient positioning using MR images. A synthetic CT image is one created directly from an underlying base MR image through a method of tissue classification and subsequent assignment of CT or Hounsfield number, which can then be used to describe the X-ray attenuation properties of the tissue. The development of synthetic CT was spurred by the growth of PET-MR and, recently, MR simulators and MR-linacs. A systematic review of synthetic CT generation methods for a MR-only workflow has been recently reported (Edmund and Nyholm 2017; Johnstone et al. 2018). Regardless of the synthetic CT method used, the synthetic CT images should be thoroughly commissioned for their geometric and dosimetric accuracy before using them clinically for an MR-only workflow (Korhonen et al. 2014, 2015; Persson et al. 2017;

Tyagi et al. 2017b). Ideally, the synthetic CT generation method should be real-time, and, if possible, scanner and sequence-independent for wide adoption in the clinic. The methods for generating synthetic CTs for MR-guided radiotherapy can be broadly classified into bulk density assignment, atlas-based, voxel-based, and hybrid methods.

To date, there are only two commercial synthetic CT software solutions that are available for MR-only planning for the prostate for clinical use. One of them is a classification-based method called MRCAT,[1] or *MR for Calculating Attenuation*, which is currently limited to a Philips MR scanner (Köhler et al. 2015). The method uses a Dixon-based MR sequence along with a constrained shape model for bones to generate synthetic CT by assigning bulk HU for water, fat, and spongy and cortical bones. The method has been clinically implemented (Tyagi et al. 2017a, b). The other method (MRI planner[2]) is scanner-independent and currently CE marked for clinical use in Europe (Persson et al. 2017). MRI planner uses a statistical decomposition algorithm for generating synthetic CT and has been evaluated for dosimetric accuracy within a multicenter/multivendor validation where accuracy was within 1% of CT-based plans (Persson et al. 2017). Both methods will be described in further detail in the next chapter.

8.3 Review of Bulk Density Assignment Methods

Bulk density assignment methods are the simplest synthetic CT generation methods. They rely on contouring of relevant tissues and assigning a bulk electron density to the segmented tissues. The accuracy of these methods depends on how many different tissue types (such as bone, soft tissues, lung, air, etc.) are segmented, and, subsequently, which tissue densities are applied to these segmented structures to attain clinically acceptable dose distributions. The simplest

---

[1]Philips Healthcare NA, Cleveland, OH.

[2]Spectronic Medical AB.

approach is assuming a homogeneous water-equivalent geometry and assigning a uniform bulk electron density of water that has traditionally been done for brachytherapy and stereotactic radiosurgery applications.

8.3.1 Assuming Homogeneous Water-Equivalent Geometry

Several groups have evaluated MR-only planning for various anatomical sites by assuming a homogeneous water-equivalent geometry. The studies vary in the method of planning and dose calculation algorithm used. In radiotherapy of brain tumors, MRI has been deemed the imaging modality of choice due to its superior soft tissue contrast. Several authors have reported that the lack of electron density information from MRI has been shown not to cause discrepancies, including radiosurgeries of the brain, because the dose distribution was not significantly altered (within 2% of CT-based dose calculation) by tissue inhomogeneities in the brain and is hence clinically acceptable (Gademann et al. 1993; Schad et al. 1994; Weber et al. 2008; Beavis et al. 1998). Prabhakar et al. found that the difference in dose volume parameters between CT- and MRI-based planning using three-field pencil beam plans was not statistically significant, and the dosimetric variations were within ±2% (Prabhakar et al. 2007b). Most of the tumors in their study were treated with two lateral fields and one vertex field, and none of the fields passed through large air cavities such as maxillary sinus. In the case of pituitary tumors, a portion of the two lateral fields passed through the posterior ethmoid sinus, and even in those cases, the dosimetric parameters were within 2% for all three plans. Ramsey et al. used the RANDO head phantom to compare CT- and MRI-based treatment planning (Ramsey et al. 1999). MR-based treatment planning of the head phantom produced a 0–2% decrease in absorbed dose for treatment fields passing through the cranium due to the increased attenuation of the skull. For situations where the treatment field passed through a large air cavity, such as the maxillary sinus, differences up to 4% were observed, and heterogeneity corrections were necessary to account for decreased attenuation of the air cavity to accurately determine the spatial distribution of absorbed dose. Dosimetric error of this magnitude is obviously clinically unacceptable, but contouring air cavities and manually assigning them, densities can easily circumvent the problem. This procedure, which takes less than 5 min, reduces the dosimetric error of MR-based treatment planning to less than 2%. In another study, dose errors above 2% were observed in low-dose areas on unit density mediums. Monte Carlo simulations with 4 MV photons showed large deviations in dose (>2%) just behind the skull if the bone was not segmented (Kristensen et al. 2008). Similar large dosimetric errors of 3–5% were also seen by others when MRI-based calculations were performed using intensity-modulated radiotherapy (IMRT) with voxel values assigned with water density (Wang et al. 2008).

Dose calculation is more challenging in the head and neck region and contains heterogeneities ranging from airways to cortical bone. The accuracy of dose calculation in this region will depend on the tumor and organs at risk (OAR) location. Differences between 15% and 30% have been reported for nasopharyngeal tumors when the dose calculation is performed assuming water-equivalent medium (Chin et al. 2014). In the same study, differences as large as 65% were reported due to dental implants. In another study, homogeneous anatomy resulted in 4–5% deviations in dose distribution as compared with CT-derived electron density calculations due to underestimation of attenuation in the bones (Karotki et al. 2011). Trends for OAR were similar to those observed in target volume with the largest deviations exceeding 5% (the spinal cord, eye, and optic nerve). Another study by Korsholm et al. showed the mean difference between homogeneous and CT-based dose calculation is less than 2% for both planning tumor volume (PTV) and OAR but also a large standard deviation of 7.4% for the parotids (Korsholm et al. 2014). This was due to the difference in body outline in the area around the ears, which affected the calculated dose to the parotids. Small variations in setup between CT and MRI scans can result in differences in external contours between CT and MRI. Also, some of the internal contours could occasionally extend beyond the MRI body because of these setup differences. Therefore, to exclude the effects of body contour differences on the dosimetric comparison, MRI and CT external contours were typically matched, and all internal contours were cropped 5 mm within the MRI external contour and used in both CT and MRI (Chin et al. 2014).

Only one study has shown the effect of applying homogeneous electron density to the thorax in the context of synthetic CT dose calculation accuracy (Jonsson et al. 2010). The mean dosimetric deviation was 1.4% with a standard deviation of 2.1%. Similar to the head and neck and lung, the pelvis area contains pelvic bones, which constitute a large part of the irradiated volume. It is implied that the dose distribution will be altered by the inhomogeneity of tissues in the pelvic region. For prostate cases, the target volumes drawn on CT and MRI differed by more than 30% in some cases (Lee et al. 2003). Most studies have indicated that accurate target delineation based on MRI has a significant clinical impact for prostate treatment, whereas dose calculation using homogeneous geometry based on MRI data is reasonable (Lee et al. 2003). Lee et al. showed that by assigning a homogeneous density of water, greater than 2% difference in dose was noted in the high-dose regions when compared to the CT dose distribution (Lee et al. 2003). Overall, the difference was small in target and critical structure doses for five prostate cases planned separately using CT and MRI. The maximum difference was less than 3.2% in the maximum, minimum, and mean target doses. Another study showed that dose distributions between CT- and MRI-based plans were equally acceptable based on their institution's clinical criteria (Chen et al. 2004a, b). The difference in the target dose between CT- and MRI-based plans using homogeneous geometry was within 2.5%. No clinically significant differences were found between MRI- and CT-based treatment plans using the same beam arrangements, dose constraints, and optimization parameters. Similar dose discrepancies with 2% were observed for other studies (Eilertsen et al. 2008; Pasquier et al. 2006).

8.3.1.1 Limitations of Homogeneous Bulk Density Methods

Although homogenous, the bulk density method gives acceptable dosimetric results for prostate and intracranial anatomies. The head and neck and thorax, due to increased heterogeneities, show much larger differences that could be clinically significant. In addition to dose calculation accuracy, positional verification based on DRRs is limited, or not possible, with this method because the bones cannot be generated or classified when assigning a uniform water-equivalent electron density. This may not be an issue for anatomical sites that require soft tissue matching, such as the prostate, where MR images can be used for daily positioning if appropriate landmarks, e.g., implanted fiducials, are identified.

8.3.2 Bulk Density Assignment Manual Contouring of Relevant Tissues Like Bones, Air, and Soft Tissues

Synthetic CT accuracy can be improved from a homogeneous geometry by contouring structures on CT, or on MR, and assigning a bulk electron density. The structures are either manually delineated or some form of auto- or semiautosegmentation method is used on CT and MR to automatically delineate various relevant tissue types. The accuracy of bulk density assignment-based synthetic CT studies reported in the literature varies based on the treatment planning technique (3D conformal radiation therapy, IMRT, or arc), dose calculation algorithm, and bulk density (or mass density) assignments used to generate the synthetic CTs.

(a) *Brain and head and neck*

Several authors have reported dose differences <2% between CT-based dose calculation and MR-based dose calculation when bones are added with a bulk density assignment in the brain (Kristensen et al. 2008; Jonsson et al. 2010; Stanescu et al. 2008). For head and neck anatomy, authors have reported synthetic CT dose calculation accuracy by segmenting either the bone alone or bone and air tissue. Bulk value bone density assignment sufficiently accounted for most heterogeneity effects. Further, segmentation of air in addition to bone did not produce substantial improvement of target coverage over bone alone. But isodose distributions near air pockets, such as sinonasal air, resembled the CT-based plan closely when air was also segmented (Chin et al. 2014). Most studies have reported dosimetric accuracy of <2% between CT- and bulk density assignment-based plans in the head and neck using different thresholding methods on CT or MR. Karotki et al. have shown that by contouring bone and air cavities and assigning bulk electron density of 1.5 and 0 g/cm^3, respectively, all the dosimetric parameters were within 2% of the heterogeneous dose calculations, with most of the parameters being within 1%. The authors used an autothreshold tool in pinnacle to set the threshold to 200 HU for bone and [−1000 to 900] HU for air. In another study, Chang et al. (2010) used an automated segmentation-based algorithm with thresholding to derive a heterogeneous pseudo-CT image from a T1-weighted MRI volume with four distinct types: air, lung, tissue, and bone. Each class was assigned a CT number corresponding to fixed relative electron densities of 0, 0.25, 1.0, and 2.0, respectively. For T1-weighted MRI, they also found a good one-to-one correspondence for air, lung, and tissue between CT and MRI numbers. This correspondence is 0–15 for air, 15–60 for the lung, and 60–500 for tissue. There was an overlap between the lung and bone, 40–60 for the bone and 15–60 for the lung, probably due to the similarly decreased hydrogen contents in these materials compared with tissue. The mean and maximum dose values of the structures were typically less than 2% between the two methods. Korsholm et al. showed an uncertainty of 2% or less on the PTV coverage for the bulk density-corrected plans. Similar to homogeneous distribution, the standard deviation in the OAR distribution was large (up to 7%) due to the proximity of parotids near the outer body. In addition to bones, when air was also segmented and assigned a bulk density, the percentage deviation in the tumor bed area close to the trachea decreased from 2.3% to 0.6%, indicating the importance of including air segmentation for head and neck synthetic CT dose calculation.

In some studies where MR images were not acquired in the treatment position, CT images were used to identify and assign bulk density structures such as patient outline, skull bone, and air cavities (Jonsson et al. 2010). The treatment plans that were investigated yielded good results and suggested that the use of MR-based synthetic CT may be used to decrease the impact of dental filling artifacts in head and neck cases.

(b) *Thorax and abdomen*

In addition to the brain and head and neck, Jonsson et al. also performed a study of assigning bulk electron density to thorax patients and showed very good agreement between CT and the bulk density approach (Jonsson et al. 2010). The ribcage was not segmented in their study because of the very troublesome and time-consuming task of manual segmentation. It was implied that the effect on the radiation beam caused by the bone should be minor compared to the impact of lung tissue. The distortions in the dose distributions were relatively small even in this inhomogeneous PTV that included pulmonary tissue and air gaps. Only one study has been carried out in the abdomen/pancreas in the context of MR-guided RT. Prior et al. investigated the effects of bulk ED assignment on plan quality for representative pancreas and prostate cancers treated with step-and-shoot IMRT and examined the dosimetric variation with and without a magnetic field. This is a first study that performed a dosimetric analysis on pancreas patients. The effects of using different electron density assignments and the presence of 1.5 T transverse magnetic field for pancreas and prostate IMRT plans were generally within 3% and 5% of PTV and OAR CT-based values. There were noticeable dosimetric differences between the CT- and MRI-based IMRT plans caused by a combination of anatomical changes between the two image acquisition times, uniform electron density assignment, and the effect of a magnetic field.

(c) *Prostate*

Synthetic CTs for the prostate have been extensively studied by assigning bulk electron densities to the pelvic bones; the results have shown a good dosimetric accuracy of <2% with CT-based plans. Different authors have used different electron density assignment values to the pelvic bones. In a study by Lee et al., a bone and water bulk-assigned image was created on the CT image. The average bone-electron-density-equivalent value of 320 HU was used instead of the electron-density-equivalent values given in the international standard ICRU 46 that would require outlining different components of the bone (cortical bone and bone marrow) (Lee et al. 2003). This was not possible because bone cannot be segmented reliably based on contrast of the images. The differences between dose-plans on bulk density-assigned images when compared to CT were less than 2%. Another study assigned a HU of 480 HU to the bones by contouring bony tissues on CT and measuring the average CT number (Doemer et al. 2015). No air pockets were present in the treated area; otherwise a value of −1000 HU would have been used. The global maximum dose differed by 1.01% between MRI and CT plans for the patient cohort, and both the D99 and D95 were within 0.2% of the CT-based dose calculation. In another study, electron density values ranging from 1.02, 1.3, and 2.1 g/cm^3 were assigned to the pelvic bones on the MR to generate three different synthetic CT images. A dose discrepancy of <1% was noted when bones were assigned an electron density of 1.3 g/cm^3. Setting the bone density to 2.1 g/cm^3 significantly increased the dose inhomogeneity in the CTV as well as leading to deviations from the clinically approved plans in all aspects. Even though a density of 2.1 g/cm^3 is representative for some bony details, applying this density led to an overestimation of the attenuation that takes place in the bone tissue in the pelvic region. Bulk density of 1.3 g/cm^3 was also used by other authors who reported mean differences in monitor units (MUs) of 0.2% with a standard deviation of 0.5% for the prescription point for different MRI bulk density-corrected geometries of prostate patients (Jonsson et al. 2010).

Lambert et al. calculated the effective density assignment to the bone using effective depth calculation (Lambert et al. 2011). The effective density for the bone was calculated by dividing the water-equivalent width of the bone by the physical width of the bone. A dose discrepancy of 1.3 ± 0.8% with the CT-based plans was observed when effective bone density was assigned on the MR images and the dose was recalculated.

8.3.2.1 Positional Verification: DRR Generation

In addition to the dosimetric accuracy, geometric accuracy of synthetic CTs for patient positioning is also very crucial for MR-only planning. Planar and volumetric IGRT for prostate patients is performed using 2D DRRs and 3D CBCTs. There are two studies that attempted to generate MR-based DRRs by thresholding MR intensities that corresponded to different anatomical structures such as bones, or relevant target, and critical structures (Ramsey and Oliver 1998; Yin et al. 1998). Misalignment errors of 3–10 mm were visually detected during verification simulation using this technique, which was noted to be comparable to CT-based DRRs with the same imaging parameters. In another study by Weber et al. (2008), MRI-derived DRRs were generated using the AcQPlan treatment planning system. The mean setup differences observed with the CT and MRI DRRs ranged from 1.0 to 4.0 mm (mean 1.5 mm; standard deviation ±1.4 mm). The precision of setup verification using MRI-derived DRRs was within 1–2 mm and thus seemed similar to that achieved by using conventional CT-based DRRs. The above studies generated MR-based DRRs without explicitly assigning electron density to bones. In a study by Chen et al., MRI-based DRRs were generated for pelvis anatomy that included structure outlines for relevant bony landmarks, such as pubic symphysis, acetabulum, femoral heads, and sacrum, assigned a bulk density of 2.0 g/cm^3. The accuracy of MR-based DRRs was verified by comparing to CT-derived DRRs, and the agreement between the two methods was estimated to be 2–3 mm based on 18 patients (Chen et al. 2004b).

In addition to DRR, 3D CBCT-MRI matching studies have been performed. Buhl et al. have reported on CBCT shifts compared to reference MRI images of the brain and have shown mean and standard deviation values of 0.8 ± 0.6, 1.5 ± 1.2, and 1.2 ± 1.2 mm differences in the anterior-posterior, superior-inferior, and left-right directions, respectively (Buhl et al. 2010). MRI-CBCT registration was reported for the prostate by manually prioritizing alignment of the prostate-rectum interface correctly. The differences in shift positions for the entire cohort between CBCT-to-CT registration and CBCT-to-MRI registration were −0.15 ± 0.25 cm in the anterior-posterior direction, 0.07 ± 0.19 cm in the superior-inferior direction, and −0.01 ± 0.14 cm in the left-right direction. CBCT-MRI registration is within 2 mm of those between CBCT-CT (Doemer et al. 2015).

8.4 Drawbacks/Challenges of Bulk Density Assignment Methods

Studies have shown that dose calculation accuracy is not a limiting factor for radiotherapy treatment planning solely using MR images when using a bulk density approach, even in the case of tissues that differ largely from water such as bones and the lung. Although bulk density assignment methods have been extensively studied, the method is not clinically acceptable because of the time-consuming task of defining specific structures, especially bones and air. Manual contouring is laborious and subjective in nature. For MR-only radiotherapy to be feasible, automated methods of MR conversion to synthetic CT data are necessary. In the future, the development of auto-segmentation of bones and air on MR images may overcome the challenge of manual contouring of these relevant structures. Once validated for different anatomical sites, auto-segmentation-based bulk density assignment methods may be suitable for MR-only planning. Automatic contouring of tissues on MR images has been an active area of research, but few studies have focused on contouring the bone (Boettger et al. 2008). Automatic segmentation of the bone, e.g., by using deformable atlas-to-patient image registration, (Ellingsen et al. 2010) eliminates the need for manual segmentation and may improve the efficiency of the workflow.

It is also argued that to improve the accuracy of bulk density-based synthetic CT methods, it is preferable to segment as many tissue types as possible and assign the appropriate density. Unfortunately, such an approach is not practical. With multiple beams used in IMRT, the impact of various heterogeneities encountered, for example, in the head and neck region, on the overall dose is reduced. Hence, high dosimetric accuracy may be achieved by using a limited number of bulk densities. The other challenge is to figure out the appropriate electron density to assign to various structures. Jonsson et al. reported that for the prostate, changing the relative mass density of pelvic and femur bone density from 1.2 to 1.4 g/cm^3, an increase of 15%, changes the dose by only 1–2% (Jonsson et al. 2010).

Bulk density-based methods are the simplest approach used to generate synthetic CT. But some caution should be used in applying uniform electron assignment to all cases, especially affected tumor volumes, where realistic values are important for accurate dosimetry. Recently, Hoogcarspel et al. demonstrated this in the inability of uniform electron density assignment to generate a clinically acceptable plan for spinal bone metastases (Hoogcarspel et al. 2014). The results presented in this study show that a simple "bulk density" pseudo-CT strategy may not be feasible for online MRI-based treatment plan adaptation for spinal bone metastases. However, a clinically acceptable result is generated if the information on the heterogeneous electron density distribution within the affected vertebral bone is available. Therefore, any synthetic CT strategy for this tumor site should include a method that can estimate the heterogeneous electron density of the affected vertebral bone. The next chapter will focus on more advanced methods for synthetic CT generation that can overcome some of the challenges posed by bulk density-based methods.

References

Ahmed M, et al. The value of magnetic resonance imaging in target volume delineation of base of tongue tumours—a study using flexible surface coils. Radiother Oncol. 2010;94(2):161–7.

Beavis AW, et al. Radiotherapy treatment planning of brain tumours using MRI alone. Br J Radiol. 1998;71(845):544–8.

Boettger T, et al. Radiation therapy planning and simulation with magnetic resonance images. In Medical imaging. SPIE. 2008.

Brock KK, Deformable Registration Accuracy Consortium. Results of a multi-institution deformable registration accuracy study (MIDRAS). Int J Radiat Oncol Biol Phys. 2010;76(2):583–96.

Buhl SK, et al. Clinical evaluation of 3D/3D MRI-CBCT automatching on brain tumors for online patient setup verification – a step towards MRI-based treatment planning. Acta Oncol. 2010;49(7):1085–91.

Chang C, et al. Dosimetric evaluation of a volume segmentation algorithm for MRI-based treatment planning for head and neck cancer. Int J Radiat Oncol Biol Phys. 2010;78(3):S70.

Chen L, et al. Dosimetric evaluation of MRI-based treatment planning for prostate cancer. Phys Med Biol. 2004a;49(22):5157–70.

Chen L, et al. MRI-based treatment planning for radiotherapy: dosimetric verification for prostate IMRT. Int J Radiat Oncol Biol Phys. 2004b;60(2):636–47.

Chin AL, et al. Feasibility and limitations of bulk density assignment in MRI for head and neck IMRT treatment planning. J Appl Clin Med Phys. 2014;15(5):4851.

Dean CJ, et al. An evaluation of four CT-MRI co-registration techniques for radiotherapy treatment planning of prone rectal cancer patients. Br J Radiol. 2012;85(1009):61–8.

Doemer A, et al. Evaluating organ delineation, dose calculation and daily localization in an open-MRI simulation workflow for prostate cancer patients. Radiat Oncol. 2015;10:37.

Edmund JM, Nyholm T. A review of substitute CT generation for MRI-only radiation therapy. Radiat Oncol. 2017;12(1):28.

Eilertsen K, et al. A simulation of MRI based dose calculations on the basis of radiotherapy planning CT images. Acta Oncol. 2008;47(7):1294–302.

Ellingsen LM, et al. Robust deformable image registration using prior shape information for atlas to patient registration. Comput Med Imaging Graph. 2010;34(1):79–90.

Fiorentino A, et al. Clinical target volume definition for glioblastoma radiotherapy planning: magnetic resonance imaging and computed tomography. Clin Transl Oncol. 2013;15(9):754–8.

Gademann G, et al. Fractionated stereotactically guided radiotherapy of head and neck tumors: a report on clinical use of a new system in 195 cases. Radiother Oncol. 1993;29(2):205–13.

Gill S, et al. Seminal vesicle intrafraction motion analysed with cinematic magnetic resonance imaging. Radiat Oncol. 2014;9:174.

Hanvey S, et al. The influence of MRI scan position on image registration accuracy, target delineation and calculated dose in prostatic radiotherapy. Br J Radiol. 2012;85(1020):e1256–62.

Hoogcarspel SJ, et al. The feasibility of utilizing pseudo CT-data for online MRI based treatment plan adaptation for a stereotactic radiotherapy treatment of spinal bone metastases. Phys Med Biol. 2014;59(23):7383–91.

Johnstone E, et al. Systematic review of synthetic computed tomography generation methodologies for use in magnetic resonance imaging-only radiation therapy. Int J Radiat Oncol Biol Phys. 2018;100(1):199–217.

Jonsson JH, et al. Treatment planning using MRI data: an analysis of the dose calculation accuracy for different treatment regions. Radiat Oncol. 2010;5:62.

Karotki A, et al. Comparison of bulk electron density and voxel-based electron density treatment planning. J Appl Clin Med Phys. 2011;12(4):3522.

Köhler M, et al. MR-only simulation for radiotherapy planning. Philips White Paper. 2015.

Korhonen J, et al. A dual model HU conversion from MRI intensity values within and outside of bone segment for MRI-based radiotherapy treatment planning of prostate cancer. Med Phys. 2014;41(1):011704.

Korhonen J, et al. Feasibility of MRI-based reference images for image-guided radiotherapy of the pelvis with either cone-beam computed tomography or planar localization images. Acta Oncol. 2015;54(6):889–95.

Korsholm ME, Waring LW, Edmund JM. A criterion for the reliable use of MRI-only radiotherapy. Radiat Oncol. 2014;9:16.

Kristensen BH, et al. Dosimetric and geometric evaluation of an open low-field magnetic resonance simulator for radiotherapy treatment planning of brain tumours. Radiother Oncol. 2008;87(1):100–9.

Lambert J, et al. MRI-guided prostate radiation therapy planning: investigation of dosimetric accuracy of MRI-based dose planning. Radiother Oncol. 2011;98(3):330–4.

Lee YK, et al. Radiotherapy treatment planning of prostate cancer using magnetic resonance imaging alone. Radiother Oncol. 2003;66(2):203–16.

Mak D, et al. Seminal vesicle interfraction displacement and margins in image guided radiotherapy for prostate cancer. Radiat Oncol. 2012;7:139.

Pasquier D, et al. MRI alone simulation for conformal radiation therapy of prostate cancer: technical aspects. Conf Proc IEEE Eng Med Biol Soc. 2006;1:160–3.

Persson E, et al. MR-OPERA: a multicenter/multivendor validation of magnetic resonance imaging-only prostate treatment planning using synthetic computed tomography images. Int J Radiat Oncol Biol Phys. 2017;99(3):692–700.

Prabhakar R, et al. Comparison of computed tomography and magnetic resonance based target volume in brain tumors. J Cancer Res Ther. 2007a;3(2):121–3.

Prabhakar R, et al. Feasibility of using MRI alone for 3D radiation treatment planning in brain tumors. Jpn J Clin Oncol. 2007b;37(6):405–11.

Ramsey CR, Oliver AL. Magnetic resonance imaging based digitally reconstructed radiographs, virtual simulation, and three-dimensional treatment planning for brain neoplasms. Med Phys. 1998;25(10):1928–34.

Ramsey CR, et al. Clinical application of digitally-reconstructed radiographs generated from magnetic resonance imaging for intracranial lesions. Int J Radiat Oncol Biol Phys. 1999;45(3):797–802.

Rasch C, et al. Definition of the prostate in CT and MRI: a multi-observer study. Int J Radiat Oncol Biol Phys. 1999;43(1):57–66.

Roach M III, et al. Prostate volumes defined by magnetic resonance imaging and computerized tomographic scans for three-dimensional conformal radiotherapy. Int J Radiat Oncol Biol Phys. 1996;35(5):1011–8.

Roberson PL, et al. Use and uncertainties of mutual information for computed tomography/ magnetic resonance (CT/MR) registration post permanent implant of the prostate. Med Phys. 2005;32(2):473–82.

Schad LR, et al. Radiosurgical treatment planning of brain metastases based on a fast, three-dimensional MR imaging technique. Magn Reson Imaging. 1994;12(5):811–9.

Stanescu T, et al. A study on the magnetic resonance imaging (MRI)-based radiation treatment planning of intracranial lesions. Phys Med Biol. 2008;53(13):3579–93.

Sun J, et al. Investigation on the performance of dedicated radiotherapy positioning devices for MR scanning for prostate planning. J Appl Clin Med Phys. 2015;16(2):4848.

Tyagi N, et al. Clinical workflow for MR-only simulation and planning in prostate. Radiat Oncol. 2017a;12(1):119.

Tyagi N, et al. Dosimetric and workflow evaluation of first commercial synthetic CT software for clinical use in pelvis. Phys Med Biol. 2017b;62(8):2961–75.

Ulin K, Urie MM, Cherlow JM. Results of a multi-institutional benchmark test for cranial CT/MR image registration. Int J Radiat Oncol Biol Phys. 2010;77(5):1584–9.

Wang C, et al. MRI-based treatment planning with electron density information mapped from CT images: a preliminary study. Technol Cancer Res Treat. 2008;7(5):341–8.

Weber DC, et al. Open low-field magnetic resonance imaging for target definition, dose calculations and set-up verification during three-dimensional CRT for glioblastoma multiforme. Clin Oncol (R Coll Radiol). 2008;20(2):157–67.

Weltens C, et al. Interobserver variations in gross tumor volume delineation of brain tumors on computed tomography and impact of magnetic resonance imaging. Radiother Oncol. 2001;60(1):49–59.

Yin FF, et al. MR image-guided portal verification for brain treatment field. Int J Radiat Oncol Biol Phys. 1998;40(3):703–11.

MR-Only Methodology

Jason A. Dowling and Juha Korhonen

9.1 Introduction

Computed tomography (CT) is currently an essential component of modern radiation therapy planning, providing a geometrically accurate three-dimensional representation of a patient's body. The information for each voxel (acquired in the transverse plan) represents the relative linear attenuation coefficient at that location. These values, quantified as Hounsfield units, can then be extrapolated to electron density values which can then be used for dose calculation (Khan 2007). CT-based workflows are well established and ubiquitous in radiation oncology departments (Brock and Dawson 2014). CT scans also enable the generation of digitally reconstructed radiographs enabling treatment verification (with electronic portal imaging devices) of the patient setup and target location at each treatment fraction (Herman et al. 2001).

Magnetic resonance imaging (MRI) has a number of advantages (and disadvantages) over CT. Of particularly importance is that the superior soft tissue contrast from MRI improves the delineation of both target volumes and organs at risk. For this reason, it is currently common for MR images to be used in treatment planning for structure delineation. These images are then registered to the corresponding patient's CT scan (sometimes with the assistance of fiducial markers) allowing any manual contouring from the MRI to be mapped across to the planning CT. This step has been shown to introduce systematic registration error which can be as large as 5 mm (Herman et al. 2001).

The aim of MRI-only radiotherapy is to remove the planning CT from the workflow to eliminate this registration uncertainty. Additional support for the use of MRI-alone workflow is the lack of patient exposure to ionising radiation, the ability to also acquire a range of functional imaging sequences, and potential cost savings from the use of a single imaging modality. Hybrid MRI-linear accelerator devices and MRI-positron emission tomography attenuation correction provide additional motivation (Lagendijk et al. 2014; Karlsson et al. 2009; Lee et al. 2003; Glide-Hurst et al. 2015; Greer et al. 2011).

The main technical challenge when moving to an MRI-alone workflow is that MR intensities cannot be easily calibrated to electron density, and therefore dose calculations cannot be performed. To address this, there is a need for methods to generate substitute CT (sCT) from MRI (these are also frequently referred to as pseudo-CT or synthetic-CT). This chapter aims to provide

J. A. Dowling (✉)
CSIRO Australian e-Health Research Centre,
Royal Brisbane and Women's Hospital, Herston,
QLD, Australia
e-mail: Jason.Dowling@csiro.au

J. Korhonen
Kymenlaakso Central Hospital and Aalto University,
Kotka, Finland
e-mail: juha.korhonen@kymsote.fi

© Springer Nature Switzerland AG 2019
G. Liney, U. van der Heide (eds.), *MRI for Radiotherapy*,
https://doi.org/10.1007/978-3-030-14442-5_9

an overview of the main current methods for sCT generation (based on the main categories suggested by Han (2017): tissue class segmentation, learning-based methods and atlases). For exhaustive lists of sCT methods and performance comparisons, the reader is referred to recent reviews by Kerkmeijer et al. (2018), Johnstone et al. (2018), Edmund and Nyholm (2017) and Owrangi et al. (2018). Note that the sCT methods described can also be applied to attenuation correction in PET-MRI (recent reviews are provided in Ladefoged et al. (2017) and Mehranian et al. (2016)).

9.2 Image Acquisition and Processing for sCT

The quality of generated sCT is reliant on the quality of the input MR information. Some of the issues that may be encountered when acquiring MR volumes with the aim of generating matching MR and CT volumes (for training an sCT algorithm) or for converting a new MRI into an sCT include:

- *Anisotropic voxels* (ideally voxels should be near-isotropic to enable 3D image processing).
- *Insufficient coverage* from the MRI (if the superior-inferior extent is inadequate or the skin boundary is truncated, meaning the sCT cannot be used for treatment planning. In addition the sCT field of view might need to be padded for some treatment planning systems to enable the couch structure to be inserted).
- *Too much coverage* from the MRI (a superior-inferior extent greater than the training set may cause problems with some methods. An example is shown in Fig. 9.1).
- *Geometric distortion* (vendor-supplied correction is usually required).
- *Patient positioning* and setup (the patient needs to be on a treatment position).
- *Interleaving artefacts* from multi-shot acquisitions (see Fig. 9.2).

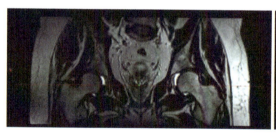
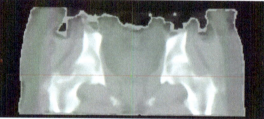

Fig. 9.1 sCT generation where the superior extent on a target patient's scan (left) is larger than the MRIs in a training set (this can be a problem with atlas-based methods

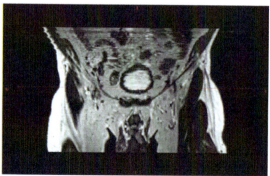
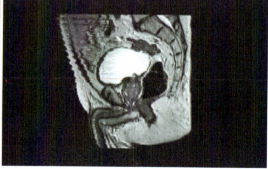

Fig. 9.2 Example of transverse multi-shot acquisition leading to artefacts (breathing motion). The figure shows coronal (left) and sagittal (right) MRI of the male pelvis

- *Motion* (this includes the risk of patient motion through lack of cooperation or discomfort, in addition to intra-treatment internal motion such as peristalsis which may increase with scanner session duration).
- *Intensity inhomogeneity* (post-processing may be required. See Fig. 9.3).
- *Metallic implants* (blooming artefacts may be produced).
- *Anatomical deformation* caused by MRI surface coil position (coil mounts may be required).
- *MRI orientation* should ideally be identified to prevent errors when importing sCT DICOMs into treatment planning systems (particularly for DICOM-RT structures). Similarly MRs acquired in a non-axial plane, such as sagittal lung MRI, may require re-slicing to an axial orientation.
- *DICOM tags* will need updating (to reflect the change in modality).

As discussed in Chap. 1, an MRI-simulator setup is preferred for MRI acquisition, particularly the use of a flat couch top and coil mounts to replicate the external body contour used for treatment. Geometric distortion (discussed in Chap. 3) may be required to correct MR scans used for sCT generation.

The most frequently used MRI sequences in the field to date for sCT generation appear to be T1w sequences for the brain region and T2w for the pelvis. The Dixon method has been widely used with these weightings, as it's fast and provides separate fat and water volumes. Ultrashort echo time and zero echo time sequences have been investigated as they enable imaging of tissue with short $T2^*$ relaxation time (such as cortical bone); however, they may not be currently available on all scanners, but can be prohibitively time-consuming and sensitive to magnetic field inhomogeneities.

A frequent artefact which can affect registration, classification and clustering of MRI information is intensity inhomogeneity. The artefact results in a smooth low-frequency field that is notifiable in homogenous regions of an MR image. This artefact can result in poor classification or registration of images. An example of an MR image before and after bias field correction is shown in Fig. 9.3. Two popular open-source algorithms are commonly used to correct this artefact. The first is the Non-parametric Non-uniformity Normalisation (N3) package available from https://github.com/BIC-MNI/N3 . The second, and more recent, is the N4 extension to N3 written by Tustison et al. (2010) available as part of the Insight Toolkit (Ibanez and Schroeder 2005).

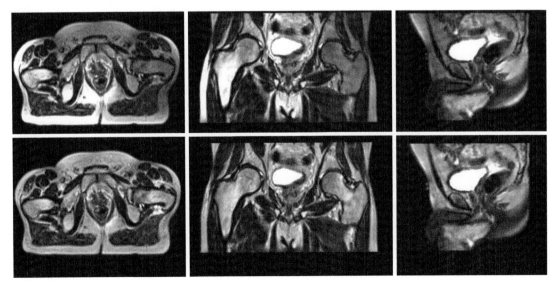

Fig. 9.3 Axial, coronal and sagittal views of an original T2w MRI of the male pelvis (top row). Bias-field-corrected version (lower row). No improvement on left and right side of axial image and greater consistency in femoral heads

Image processing steps may also include masking background voxel intensities outside the patient's body. Image smoothing may also be applied to reduce image noise. Histogram matching (Nyul et al. 2000) is also frequently used to standardise MR image intensities to a base image.

The steps involved in obtaining a co-registered CT-MR dataset suitable for training an sCT method are summarised in Fig. 9.4. The original MR image in row (A) has been bias-field-corrected with N4, histogram matched to a standard MR image and smoothed with anisotropic diffusion (which attempts to reduce noise while maintaining edges). The same patient's CT scan is shown in (C) and with the couch automatically removed in (D).

Virtually all methods for sCT generation require a co-registered set of MR and CT volumes, both for training and validation. An overview of MRI to CT registration is provided in Chap. 2. sCT generation methods require highly accurate CT to MR registration for training set generation (particularly for atlas-based methods). Figure 9.4e shows the result of rigid followed by structure-guided registration to match the planning CT to MRI. The method from (Rivest-Hénault et al. 2014) was used to achieve this result; other algorithms include (Weistrand and Svensson 2014; Lu et al. 2012; Burgos et al. 2017).

9.3 Validation

There is currently no comprehensive consensus on how to evaluate sCT compared with CT. The most common reported evaluation metrics are differences in HU values between (either rigid or nonrigidly depending on anatomy) co-registered sCT and CT (mean, mean absolute errors and voxel-to-voxel comparisons), dose-volume histogram comparison, percent difference in point dose and gamma pass rate (usually 2 mm/2%). Conversion methods which generate automatic contours (such as advanced atlas methods) can also use these contours for validation (e.g. external body or bone contours). Contour validation is generally performed with a voxel-wise overlap metric (usually the Dice similarity coefficient (Dice 1945)) and a surface distance metric (such as mean absolute surface distance).

A leave-one-out approach is frequently used in the literature to assess sCT generation results, particularly with smaller sets of matching CT and MRI data. In this testing methodology, to avoid biasing results, each sCT is generated without data from the patient being tested. In this case n-1 patient scans are used to generate each sCT. A related approach is to use k-fold cross-validation, where the dataset is divided into k different groups which one of these groups is used for testing and the remainder used for training.

A thorough review of validation metrics is provided by Edmund and Nyholm (2017).

9.4 Image Segmentation

Image segmentation (or automatic contouring) involves the identification and labelling of regions of interest from images. A very brief overview is given here as a number of sCT generation methods rely on segmentation, particularly for bone localisation in atlas-based methods. In addition for most non-atlas methods, the accurate segmentation of different tissue classes is very important, especially in the presence of noise and partial volume effects in MRI (Mehranian et al. 2016).

Medical image segmentation is generally performed in 3D (providing further motivation for isotropic voxels). Most of the methods used for sCT generation are fully automatic, although some semiautomatic algorithms are used (e.g. manually selected points being used to seed region growing algorithms). Medical image segmentation is difficult due to patient anatomical variability, pathology, complexity of medical image data and the need for accurate, reproducible and robust methods. This is a very active research field, and only a general introduction will be provided here (good overviews can be found in Toennies (2012), Bankman (2009) and Brock (2014)).

The simplest segmentation methods use low-level image processing techniques such as grey-level thresholding to separate voxel intensities within a defined intensity range into different regions of interest. This can work well on CT;

9 MR-Only Methodology

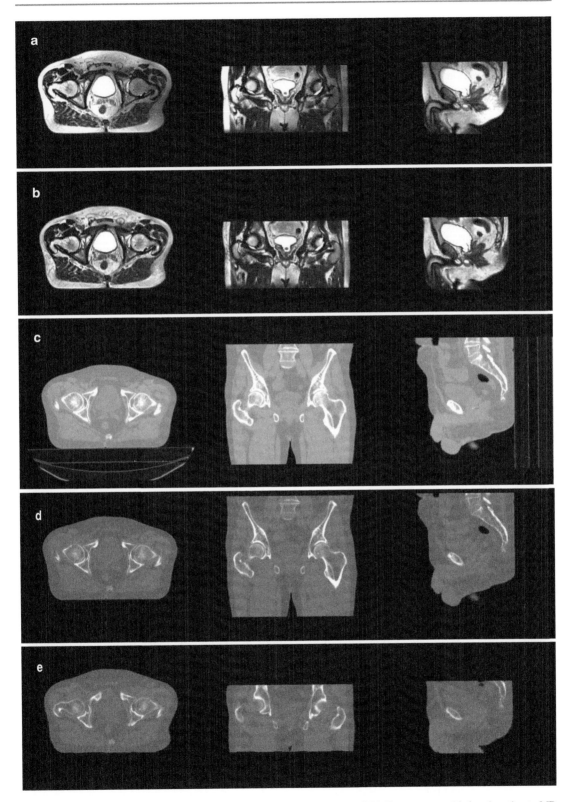

Fig. 9.4 Example preprocessing for CT and MR training set. (**a**) Original MRI. (**b**) Preprocessed MRI (histogram and bias field correction). (**c**) Original CT with couch removed (**d**). CT-MR structure-guided registration to MR in (**a**) is shown in (**e**)

however noise, intensity inhomogeneity and overlapping tissue classes limit its usefulness on MRI. Other simple methods can include edge detection and region growing from seed points. These methods are generally efficient and easy to implement.

The second group of methods apply machine learning techniques which remove the reliance of heuristics and apply more advanced optimisation and uncertainty models. One disadvantage of these methods can be the lack of spatial information in voxel locations. Unsupervised methods (which don't require labelled training data for segmentation) include fuzzy c-means, k-means or the mean-shift algorithm. These methods also include mixture models which can either be trained or estimated from a new image to provide a probabilistic estimate of which class image voxels belong to. Gaussian mixture models are often used for unsupervised segmentation, with the assumption that intensities in each class are normally distributed. The output from k-means can be used to initialise Expectation-Maximisation models to provide a voxel-wise probability of belonging to each class (this can be then used to train tissue-specific regression models, for example, in Ghose et al. (2017a)). Supervised methods also include k-nearest neighbour classification and Bayesian classifiers. These methods may be applied to different image features (such as patches of texture rather than individual voxels). Recently deep learning methods have become increasingly important for segmentation due to both accuracy and segmentation speed. These methods (which may require large amounts of training data) use multiple layers of data processing which make it possible to learn through many layers of abstraction. One disadvantage is that the underlying model is usually composed of millions of parameters and the mechanism of how a model works can be a mystery (Meyer et al. 2018).

A third group of methods use higher-level knowledge in the form of a priori information such as organ shape (based on expert observer contours) into the segmentation approach to improve accuracy and robustness. Earlier classical deformable models (e.g. snakes or level sets)

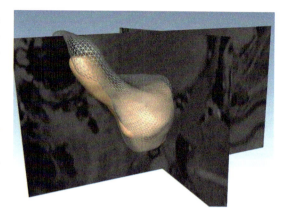

Fig. 9.5 Sagittal and coronal views showing a prostate deformable model in action after initialisation. The wireframe represents the deformable model, and the coloured surface represents the manual surface. Further details can be found in Chandra et al. (2012)

typically used limited prior knowledge (they might have included smoothness constraints) and do not appear to have been used in sCT generation pipelines; however, they evolved into shape models which can learn shape, appearance, motion or deformation information from a set of training examples and express this a mean shape and a set of characteristic variations (Cootes et al. 1995) which can be utilised for advanced segmentation (e.g. pelvic bone segmentation (Tyagi et al. 2017a) or the prostate shown in Fig. 9.5). Atlas-based segmentation involves registering one or more labelled images onto a new image (Rohlfing et al. 2004). If multiple images and labels are propagated to the new image, they can be fused together with a variety of methods (e.g. using voting or STAPLE). Usually rigid followed by nonrigid registration is used to account for anatomical deformation. Atlas-based segmentation can be slow (as many registrations may be required), but the results can be very good (e.g. automatically segmented bones in Fig. 9.6).

9.5 Bulk Density Methods

The simplest approach to sCT generation is to assume the patient is water-equivalent and assign the same electron density value to all voxels within the patient's body contour. The advantage

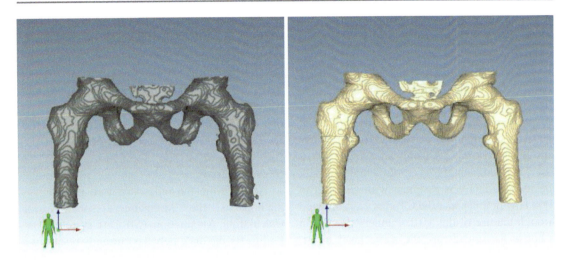

Fig. 9.6 Automatic (left) and manual (right) bones from MRI (T2w SPACE) generated through multi-atlas segmentation using local-weighted vote

of this approach, which is frequently used in MRI planning for brachytherapy, is that of its simplicity and speed (assuming the body contour is available). There is no image registration required. However, the approach is not very accurate as tissue heterogeneity is ignored, and it is impossible to generate realistic digitally reconstructed radiographs (DRRs). Bone contouring would be required for DRR generation, and the use of an MRI simulation image would be needed as a reference for cone beam CT guidance. A thorough review of bulk density methods is provided in the previous chapter.

9.6 Tissue Class Segmentation Methods

The first of the three main approaches to generating accurate sCT is to extend the bulk density approach to identify classes of segmented tissues which can then be assigned the same HU. Unlike atlas methods, this approach is robust to abnormal anatomy and does not rely on the training set having the same field of view as the target MR image, and the conversion to sCT is time efficient (there is no registration required). In practice tissue classification errors can occur, increasing the need for multiple sequences to be acquired (adding to acquisition time and increasing patient discomfort and motion). There may also be a need for nonstandard sequences (e.g. ultrashort echo (UTE) time sequence for the separation of cortical bone and air cavities may be required). In addition the methods may need calibration before generalising to different MR scanners. Generally a minimum of three tissue classes (soft tissue, air and bone) are required; however, water and fat may also be added for increased accuracy. Most commercial PET/MR systems compute the attenuation map from MRI using a four-tissue segmentation approach (Marshall et al. 2013).

To illustrate the tissue segmentation approach, five different methods, with increasing complexity, will be described. An early paper by Chen et al. (2007)) is a simple example of this method for creating an sCT-based digitally reconstructed radiograph (DRR) for prostate external beam radiation therapy. The pelvic bony structures, including femoral heads, pubic rami, ischium and ischial tuberosity, all relevant for routine clinical patient setup were manually contoured on axial MR images from 20 patients. The contoured bony structures were then assigned a bulk density of 2.0 g/cm³. The accuracy of the MR-based DDRs was quantitatively evaluated by comparing MR-based DRRs with CT-based DRRs for these patients. For each patient, eight measuring points on both coronal and sagittal DRRs were used for quantitative evaluation (the maximum difference in absolute positions being 3 mm).

Stanescu et al. (2008) published an early method for brain sCT generation from T1-weighted MRIs from a 3 T scanner in 2008, which used four classes (bone, scalp, brain and air). Segmentation was performed on 3D distortion correction images using an average atlas-based method. For the scalp and brain, a bulk density of 0 HU was assigned with bone set to 1000 HU. In this paper the CT-sim was emulated through the use of the MRI scanners' lasers, an in-house flat couch top, the same head insert, plastic shells and fiducial markers. The results from four glioma patients suggested that sCT-based plans generated from corrected MRI were more accurate than CTs with registered uncorrected MRI.

A three-class (air, bone and soft tissue) approach for the male pelvis was assessed on 39 localised prostate cancer patients by Lambert et al. (2011) who found that (T2-weighted) MRI bulk bone and tissue density plans were 1.3 ± 0.8% lower than the full density CT plan. Bone was manually contoured and assigned an average bulk density of 1.19 g/cm^3, equating to 288 HU. The major dose differences for the MR bulk density plans were hypothesised to be from patient external contour differences (from the MR couch top and deformation caused from the surface coil).

The main extension to these early tissue class approaches has been the incorporation of information from multiple MRI sequences. This approach was illustrated in 2013, in a paper from the University of Michigan (Hsu et al. 2013), where T1-weighted, T2-weighted and an ultra-short echo time (UTE, TE = 0.06) in addition to the water and fat volumes from a two-point Dixon sequence) were acquired from ten patients on a 3 T Siemens Skyra. Probabilistic classification was then performed using a fuzzy c-means clustering with a spatial constraint to identify the major tissue types and assign bulk density HU values: fluid (−98 HU), fat (−12 HU), white matter (14 HU), grey matter (14 HU) and bone (1139 HU). The same group later adapted this method to the generation of sCT for the female pelvis by removing the UTE sequence and fitting a pelvic bone shape model then assigning densities to fat (−100 HU), muscle (30 HU), bone marrow (50 HU) and bone (800). The method was validated on nine patients resulting in MAE of 13.7 (SD 1.8 HU) for muscle, 15.9 (2.8 HU) for fat, 49.1(17.8 HU) for intra-pelvic soft tissues, 129.1 (29.2 HU) for marrow and 274.4 (26.9 HU) for bones.

At this time the most advanced tissue class method is the Magnetic Resonance for Calculating Attenuation (MRCat) system from Philips for the male pelvis is currently one of two FDA cleared commercial systems. This method is based on a dual-echo 3D mDIXON fast field echo (FFE) sequence resulting in in-phase, fat and water images. Tissues are classified as air, adipose, water, trabecular/spongy bone and compact/cortical bone and assigned bulk HU values. As with most methods, the body is automatically contoured based on the mDIXON water and in-phase images, and everything outside the body mask is classified as air. A pelvic bone shape model is then fitted to the in-phase image, and voxels within this segmentation result are classified as compact or spongy bone depending on intensity (Tyagi et al. 2017a) (Fig. 9.7). Clinical workflow implementation and experience are described in Tyagi et al. (2017b) and in the clinical translation section below.

9.7 Learning-Based Methods

9.7.1 Regression

Learning-based approaches involve the assignment of CT numbers for each MRI voxel based on regression or more advanced machine learning methods. The advantages of this approach include speed (as there is a need for image registration), a reduction in registration error and robustness to abnormal anatomy. Potential disadvantages of the method include a possible need for multiple sequences, a lack of spatial information to help guide the regression and contouring of the bone. The methods can also be vulnerable

9 MR-Only Methodology

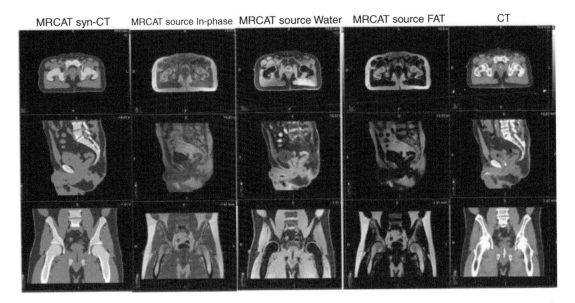

Fig. 9.7 MRCAT input MR images (middle three columns), with the sCT output shown in the left-hand column and patient planning CT in the final column). Image source: Neelam Tyagi

to the effects on MR signal from different MRI platforms and may require calibration before they can generalise across different MRI scanners. This section will provide a brief overview of single-sequence, multiple-sequence and deep learning approaches.

There is no direct relationship between MR intensity across a volume and HU. An approach to overcome this is to apply a segmentation method and generate separate regression models for different regions within MRI. One approach, used to treat prostate patients in Helsinki, Finland (see the clinical translation section below), is to have different regression models within and outside of contoured pelvic bones (Korhonen et al. 2014). Within the bone segment, local MRI intensity values from a Dixon in-phase T1-weighted image are converted to HUs by applying a second-order polynomial model. The soft tissue HU conversion model is generated by a piecewise MR image intensity scale into threshold-based sections representing signals from urine, muscle and fat. Example outputs of the model for the pelvis and lungs are shown in Fig. 9.8. To overcome the dual model's reliance on absolute MR image intensity values, a generalised method was developed (Koivula et al. 2017) and validated on data from four different centres. This generalised method incorporates a scaling of the original MR intensities to a base level, prior to the MR intensity value to HU value conversion with the dual model method. Additionally, the method has been applied for several body sites (Korhonen et al. 2016a). Figure 9.9 shows an example of a torso sCT. To generate this sCT at the sites including air cavities, the method applies additional automatic segmentation, followed by a separate conversion model also for this segment (e.g. for lung tissues).

An effective hybrid regression model approach was proposed by Ghose et al. (2017b) based on a single 3 T T2-weighted isotropic patient image. This method incorporated automatic bone and bladder statistical and appearance-shape models, while other soft tissues were separated using an Expectation-Maximisation-based clustering model. The closest matching CT bone to the MRI bone segmentation was selected from a training database and was transformed with deformable registration to the sCT. Predictions for the bone, air and soft tissue from the separate regression models were successively combined to generate the whole pelvis sCT.

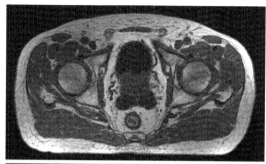
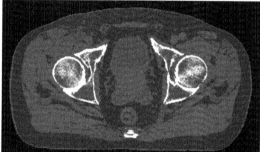
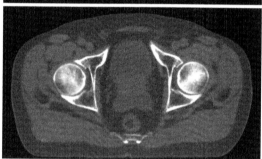

Fig. 9.8 Dual model conversion method of Korhonen et al. applied to Dixon in-phase prostate MRI (top). sCT (middle) and actual CT (bottom). Source: Lauri Koivula (Helsinki University Hospital)

9.7.2 Learning with Multiple Sequences

Standard MR imaging sequences do not enable the separation of cortical bone and air. There is lack of signal in cortical bone due to the low proton density and short T2 relaxation time. Ultrashort echo (UTE) and zero echo time (ZTE) sequences may allow voxels from these two classes to be separated.

Johansson et al. (2011) developed a brain sCT method based on Gaussian mixture regression model which linked HU values with intensities from three different MRI sequences: a T2-weighted 3D spin-echo sequence and two dual-echo UTE MRI sequences (with different echo times and flip angles). An additional method was later developed for uncertainty estimation which was shown to accurately predict voxel-wise in generated sCT volumes (Johansson et al. 2012). Spatial information (3D voxel coordinate distance from the mean coordinate value inside the head, in addition to the shortest Euclidean distance from each voxel to the patient external contour) was included in later work which improved the accuracy of the estimated sCT, particularly in smaller, complicated anatomical regions (Johansson et al. 2013). Edmund et al. (2014) also used a statistical regression method for generating brain sCT from a 1 T scanner. Their method was similar to the previous method (Johansson et al. 2011) and utilised two different UTE sequences in addition to a T1-weighted isotropic volume.

An alternate approach was proposed by Kim et al. (2015) for prostate planning which generated sCT voxels as a weighted summation of normalised MR voxel intensities. The method combined intensities from a 3D T1-weighted, T2-weighted and a 3D balanced turbo field echo sequence acquired on a 1 T scanner. The total acquisition time was 18 min. Bones were manually contoured on the T2-weighted image. Image voxels were then sorted into five material classifications: air, bone, fat, soft tissue and fluid. A truth table was used (based on voxel intensity in the acquired MR images) to determine class assignment for each voxel. Low-intensity voxels not within the bone contour were classified as air and assigned a bulk density; all other voxels were calculated using a weighted sum of the acquired and derived MR images. The weights used for these classes were optimised by minimising the Euclidean distance of voxel value differences between sCT and the actual CT.

9.7.3 Deep Learning-Based Approaches

Typical approaches to machine learning require careful selection of features to include in feature

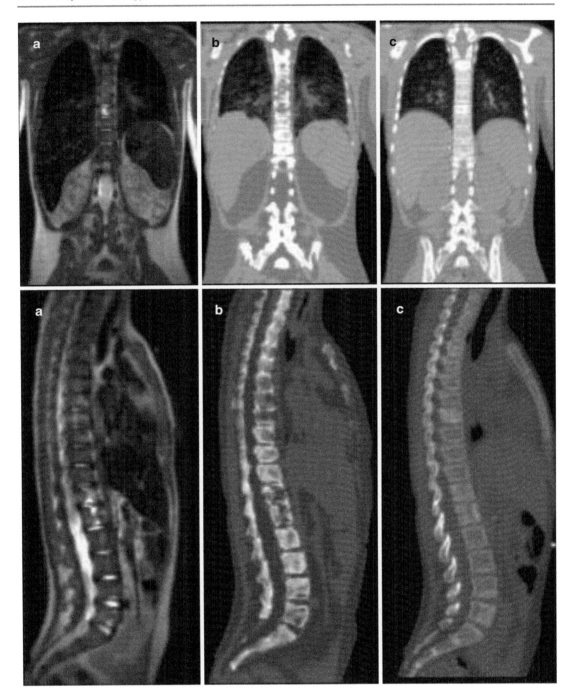

Fig. 9.9 Coronal (top) and sagittal (bottom) view of a lung sCT produced from the generalised dual method. A is the original MRI, B is the sCT, C is the actual CT. Source: Lauri Koivula (Helsinki University Hospital)

vectors. Selecting these features can often be the most time-consuming part of developing machine learning systems. One advantage of deep learning approaches is that these systems can learn their own features. Currently the most common type of deep learning models for image analysis is convolutional neural networks which contain many layers, at least one of which uses convolution instead of general matrix multiplication (Litjens et al. 2017). A significant advantage of these approaches over other methods for sCT generation is that although training can take a long time (up to days (Xiang et al. 2018)), once this is done, they are capable of rapid sCT conversion (less than a minute compared to approximately an hour for multi-atlas approaches) which can open new opportunities (such as daily online replanning). This is a rapidly developing field, and this section will only present an overview. A good summary of deep learning in radiation therapy is provided in Meyer et al. (2018).

Han (2017) has proposed a deep convolutional neural network (DCNN) using a novel U-net-based architecture to generate brain sCT in around 9 s with higher accuracy than a multi-atlas approach (Fig. 9.10). The model was trained on real image data from 18 patients, using each patient's CT rigidly registered to a single 1 mm isotropic T1-weighted 3D-spoiled gradient-recalled echo sequence. One potential limitation of the approach is that the sCT is generated using a 2D approach, which may result in discontinuities in the sCT. This limitation was addressed through a novel deep embedding convolutional neural network proposed by Xiang et al. (2018) which achieved similar results to multi-atlas methods for the brain and prostate in rapid time (46 s for the brain and 28 s for the prostate). Generative adversarial networks (GANs) have also been recently investigated and dosimetrically validated for prostate sCT (Maspero et al. 2018).

9.8 Atlas and Patch-Based Methods

Another approach to sCT generation is to utilise image registration (covered in Chap. 2). Rigid and affine registration methods typically generate two output files: a resampled moving image aligned to the target image, along with a transformation matrix (representing global translation, rotation, shearing and scaling). Nonrigid (or deformable) image registration typically takes the result of rigid or affine registration and maps each voxel from this moving image to a target, resulting in a deformation field, along with a resampled moving image. Atlas-based methods reuse the transformation matrix (and usually the deformation field). An atlas (or training) set consists of co-registered CT-MR from one or more patients. For segmentation these are used to propagate labels across to the target image (Rohlfing et al. 2001). For sCT generation, there is the requirement for an atlas set of at least one co-registered patient CT-MR pair. After the atlas MR image is registered to a target MR image, this CT-MR image can then be propagated to the MR image target.

9.8.1 Single-Atlas Registration

A simple atlas approach is to use a single registration from a CT-MR pair to a new target MRI. This has been explored using images acquired from the same patient (Wang et al. 2008) and also where the target MRI is from a different patient. A disadvantage of a single-atlas approach is that the MRI and CT scans may be acquired in significantly different patient positions, a calibration to electron density may not be available and registration is unlikely to account for differences in patient anatomy (even for the same patient).

An extension of the approach is to select the most similar atlas from a set of atlas images (e.g. by running an initial rigid registration between a number of atlas volumes and then selecting the closest matching image based on a global metric such as voxel-wise mean squared error). A similar method is to incorporate metadata to select the best matching volume: Marshall et al. (2013) used heuristic measures (such as the BMI of atlas patients) to try and find the most similar CT in terms of body geometry before registration.

9.8.2 Average Atlas

An average (or groupwise) atlas is designed to represent the average anatomy of a population. The main idea is that average anatomy should require less deformation than a randomly selected

9 MR-Only Methodology

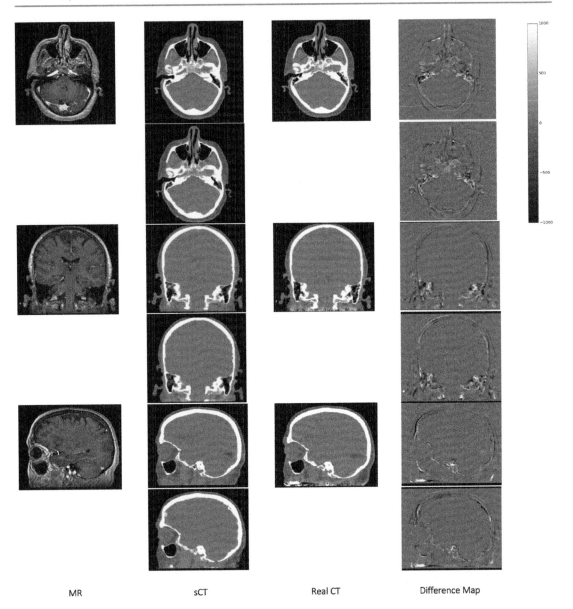

Fig. 9.10 Qualitative comparison of sCTs and real CT for subject #5 from (Han 2017). First column, MR; second column, sCTs (rows 1, 3 and 5 show the DCNN results, and rows 2, 4 and 6 show the atlas-based results); third column, real CT; fourth column, difference maps (rows 1, 3 and 5 correspond to the DCNN results, and rows 2, 4 and 6 correspond to the atlas-based results). The colour bar is associated with the difference maps. First and second rows, axial slices; third and fourth rows, coronal slices; fifth and sixth rows, sagittal slices. (Reprinted with permission from (Han 2017))

individual atlas when deformably registered to a target volume (Rohlfing et al. 2004). This method is commonly used for brain segmentation as it requires only a single registration, and it has been a common method for attenuation correction in PET-MRI of the brain.

An average atlas for sCT generation involves a training set of co-registered CT-MR volumes. The usual approach is groupwise registration: one *template* target MRI volume is identified from the training set (preferably one that is representative of the anatomical population of interest),

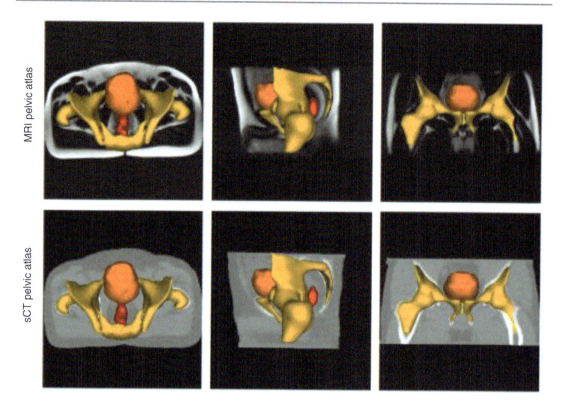

Fig. 9.11 Example MRI and sCT matching average atlases with average anatomical organs overlaid. This atlas can be deformably registered to a new MRI to generate an sCT volume

and all of the other MRIs in the atlas set are registered to that exemplar. Once all of the training sets are registered to the target, the resulting resampled moving MRI volumes are averaged to generate an initial average atlas. Then the MRI volumes in the training set are registered to the average atlas. This process is repeated (usually between three and five iterations). In practice the initial atlas is usually qualitatively blurry, and this blurriness decreases until convergence. Once this step is reached, the CT-MR volumes can be mapped to the average atlas using the same transformation matrices and deformation fields and the HU values averaged for each voxel. If manual contours are available, these can also be mapped into the atlas space and averaged. An example average pelvic atlas from (Dowling et al. 2012) is shown below. To convert a new MRI into an sCT volume, the average MRI atlas is registered (usually using rigid, affine and nonrigid registration) to the target MRI, and the average CT-MR volume is then propagated to the target MRI. Contours can also be propagated if auto-contouring is required (Fig. 9.11).

9.8.3 Multi-atlas Fusion

Methods based on multiple atlases generally provide better results than either average or single-atlas methods due to uncorrelated error cancellation and the power of consensus from multiple registered images (Mehranian et al. 2016). This approach is also the most computationally demanding, as it requires pairwise registration of all MR images in the atlas set to the target image. Once these registrations are completed, the co-registered CT-MR volumes can be propagated to the target MRI, and a fusion method is applied to generate an sCT volume.

One of the earliest papers using this approach, for MRI-based attenuation correction in the

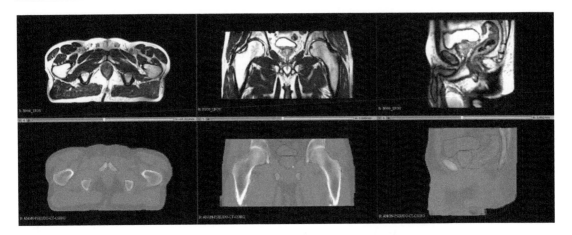

Fig. 9.12 Example MRI (top) and automatically contoured sCT using method from (Dowling et al. 2015)

brain, was published by Hofmann et al. (2008), who performed pairwise registration to initialise a patch-based search. A comparison of different atlas-based sCT generation methods for paediatric brain tumour patients was conducted by Uh et al. (2014) who found that multiple atlases outperformed the single-atlas Scheme.

A number of recent papers have focused on the use of this method for the pelvis. Dowling et al. (2015) applied this approach with the addition of a local-weighted voting method to generate a local similarity weighting between patches on each co-registered MR. These weightings were then applied to the propagated CT-MR volumes to generate both sCT output and automatic contours (Dowling et al. 2015) (Fig. 9.12). Siversson et al. (2015) use a similar pairwise registration approach; however, they perform an initial weighted voting method for segmenting the main organs of interest in the male pelvis and then use these structures to initialise a nonrigid pairwise registration step prior to a weighted fusion step. This method has received CE mark approval and has been commercialised (as MriPlanner from Spectronic Medical). In a slightly different approach, Arabi et al. (2018) used the multi-atlas-based segmentation to identify the pelvic bones from MRI, and these were then used to help optimise a locally weighted atlas fusion step. Unlike the previous pelvic papers which relied on a single MRI, Burgos et al. (2017) included both a T1-weighted and T2-weighted in an iterative multi-atlas propagation framework. Three of these approaches were compared with the same pelvic dataset in a 2018 paper (Arabi et al. 2018) with similar (high quality) output results.

9.8.4 Patch-Based Methods

Patch-based methods overlap with image registration methods (covered in Chap. 2) and are usually run after pairwise registration. The motivation is to refine the atlas-based prediction using pattern recognition on multiple 2D or 3D patches after the nonrigid registration. This may help when inter-patient anatomical variation is too high for global (rigid or affine) registration methods or where there are a limited number of co-registered CT-MR volumes for the atlas. A potential additional advantage is that patch-based approaches do not assume explicit one-to-one correspondence between images. One limitation of many existing patch-based methods is their computational complexity, which can limit the size of search windows centred at the target voxel (meaning there is a reliance to have a good initial registration of the atlas set to the target image).

A good example of this approach was provided by Andreasen et al. (2016) who were able to generate sCT of the male pelvis with similar HU MAE as multi-atlas fusion approaches using only nine training examples. In this paper, affine registration was used to align the atlas MRIs to the target MRI, and the CT-MRs were propagated using these transformations. After this step a 3D patch (7 × 7 × 5 voxels) centred at each voxel in the test image was extracted, and a search was performed within a local area of 13 × 13 × 11 (voxels centred at the same voxel). Finally the eight most similar patches were identified (using the square root of the sum of squared difference) and assigned a similarity weighting that was then used to generate a weighted contribution from the propagated CT-MR volumes.

Improved results for the prostate were later reported by Largent et al. (2019)) through the use of an original non-local mean patch-based method and by expanding the type of features used for patch similarity to include spatial, textural and texture information. A related patch-based approach was used for sCT brain generation by Huynh et al. (2016)) who used pairwise rigid registration followed by a structured random forest classification of each MRI patch to determine the most similar CT patch for sCT generation. They also use multi-scale features for their patches, and the resulting sCT volumes were highly accurate.

9.8.5 Summary

To date multi-atlas and patch-based sCT generation methods have exhibited good accuracy for both the pelvis and brain. However, this may change in the near future for two reasons: MRI sequences (UTE and ZTE) are being developed which show promise in accurately extracting bone signal and as deep learning approaches improve.

Advantages of atlas and patch-based approaches are that they use a priori geometric information and can apply registration regularisation to maintain realistic anatomical deformation. They are also more robust than other methods to intensity differences between images and have a demonstrated ability to generalise across MRI models and vendors (Wyatt et al. 2017). They are also able to incorporate automatic contouring (and automatic QA based on these contours) and usually require only a single MR sequence to be acquired.

Disadvantages of the approach are that they can be slow (especially for multi-atlas and patch approaches), there may be a greater influence from registration error and abnormal anatomy outside atlas set can cause problems. In addition, target volumes with a larger field of view than the training set can lead to missing data on the generated sCT (Fig. 9.1).

9.9 Clinical Translation

MRI-only-based RT planning has been implemented in few clinics and is in use as part of routine clinical protocols. In this chapter, the MRI-only-based RTP refers to an external RT planning protocol in which all the pretreatment tasks of RT are conducted by relying only on MRI without applying any other imaging modalities. Four clinics worldwide apply the protocol for their patients in routine workflow (Table 9.1).

Table 9.1 Clinics currently applying MRI-only RTP

Clinic	Site	Patients	Since	sCT method	Success rate (i.e. no need to apply CT), %
HUCH, Helsinki[a] (Korhonen et al. 2014; Koivula et al. 2017; Tenhunen et al. 2018)	Prostate	~400	2012	In-house	~92
TUCH, Turku[b]	Prostate	~300	2017	Commercial	~93
UMICH, Ann Arbor[c] (Hsu et al. 2013)	Brain	~100	2015	In-house	~95
UMC, Utrecht[d]	Prostate	~10	2018	Commercial	n/a

[a]Personal correspondence with Tiina Seppälä, Helsinki University Central Hospital, Helsinki, Finland (9/2018)
[b]Personal correspondence with Jani Keyriläinen, Turku University Hospital, Turku, Finland (9/2018)
[c]Personal correspondence with James Balter, University of Michigan, Ann Arbor, MI, US (9/2018)
[d]Personal correspondence with Nico van den Berg, University Medical Center Utrecht, The Netherlands (9/2018)

Table 9.2 Clinics applying MRI-only RTP together with QA scout CT[a] or full CT[b,c] (or other)

Clinic	Site	Patients	Since	sCT method	Success rate (i.e. CT was not mandatory), %
MSK, New York[a] (Tyagi et al. (2017a))	Prostate	~600	2016	Commercial	~95
SUS, Lund[b] (Persson et al. 2017)	Prostate	~40	2018	Commercial	~97
CMH, Newcastle[c] (Dowling et al. 2015)	Prostate	~20	2018	In-house	~100

[a]Personal correspondence with Neelam Tyagi, Memorial Sloan Kettering Cancer Center, NY, US (10/2018)
[b]Personal correspondence with Emilia Persson, Skåne University Hospital, Lund, Sweden (9/2018)
[c]Personal correspondence with Peter Greer, Calvary Mater Hospital, Newcastle, Australia (9/2018)

It is likely that external MRI-only-based RTP has been applied occasionally already during the last two decades in urgent patient cases while the CT simulator has been broken. Helsinki (HUCH) was the first clinic implementing MRI-only RTP workflow into the routine clinical protocols in 2012 (Korhonen et al. 2014; Koivula et al. 2017; Tenhunen et al. 2018). The clinic has relied on MRI-only RTP for over 400 prostate cancer patients (Tenhunen et al. 2018). The workflow has been successful for 92% of the patients. For 8% of the patients, also CT was applied, mainly due to uncertainties in gold marker visualisation (Tenhunen et al. 2018). Other excluding reasons were obesity (body contour reaching out of FOV) and image artefacts (mainly due to hip prosthesis).

Turku (TUCH) also is applying MRI-only RTP for prostate cancer patients. The clinic has treated over 300 patients since the beginning of 2017. The workflow has been carried out successfully for 93% of the patients. The failure reasons include problems with sCT construction (mainly due to metal in body), gold marker recognition uncertainties and patient obesity.

Ann Arbor (UMICH) started treating patients with brain metastasis by MRI-only protocol in 2015. Most of these roughly 100 patients have been treated by whole brain treatment. The workflow has been carried out successfully for nearly all these patients with few exceptions caused by patient claustrophobia or immobilisation issues, in which cases CT was applied.

Recently also Utrecht (UMC) has started treating prostate patients with MRI-only. Additionally, few clinics are relying mainly on MRI and applying other imaging modalities only for QA purposes of the MRI-based protocol (Table 9.2). These clinics are primarily implementing the workflow for prostate cancer patients. For example, New York (MSK) has relied mainly on MRI since 2016, and uses CT scouts for confirming gold marker identification. The CT is applied only for cases in which sCT reconstruction fails (e.g. due to patient size, femur angulation, blurry MR images, bony metastases or failure to determine the outer body contour) or if there are uncertainties in gold marker position on the MRI. Additionally, the clinics in Sweden (Lund) and Australia (Newcastle and Liverpool) are performing MRI-based RTP by applying CT only for backup and QA purposes (Dowling et al. 2015; Persson et al. 2017). The experiences are promising, and it is likely that these clinics will start MRI-only RTP shortly. There are also many other clinics that are aiming to apply MRI-only RTP protocol in the future and thus currently conducting, for example, sCT studies.

9.10 Is There a Future for CT?

A small number of clinics worldwide have shown that it is feasible to conduct MRI-only RTP, and implemented it into the routine clinical workflow. The experiences have shown that MRI-only RTP can be conducted successfully for over 90% of prostate patients (Tyagi et al. 2017a; Dowling et al. 2015; Tenhunen et al. 2018; Persson et al. 2017). The experiences are also encouraging for the brain (Hsu et al. 2013). However, it is important to underline that the clinics have been unable to use the workflow for all patients, even within the target group. The contraindications include such uncertainties as sCT construction, gold marker identification, image artefacts, metal objects in body and patient obesity. It is likely that technological and methodological development can overcome most of these issues.

While considering whether MRI-only RTP is suitable for the clinics, it is essential to consider also other factors than the accuracy compared to MRI + CT process. The potential benefits of MRI-only RTP include avoiding image co-registration (MRI + CT), saving hospital resources and saving patient exposure to ionising radiation applied in CT. The latter benefit can be questioned due to minimal imaging dose with high-quality optimised CT scanners. The imaging doses are negligible compared to dose in RT. Excluding one imaging modality (in this case CT) can reduce costs in a clinic. The calculated value for imaging can vary: the clinic in Helsinki evaluated that MRI-only RTP reduces costs by approximately 200€ per patient (this is the cost of CT simulation in such a public hospital) (Korhonen et al. 2016b). However, if the sCT construction is slow and requires additional resources (such as image reconstruction and QA), the process could potentially be as resource-intensive as applying CT. A clinic considering MRI-only RTP should evaluate the usefulness of the entire process. The potential benefits of MRI-only RTP could be replaced by additional drawbacks if the workflow is not robust, reliable, accurate, rapid and resource-saving. It is also essential to keep in mind that all the patients cannot be imaged by MRI and that CT includes valuable information in many patient groups. Also CT as an imaging modality is under constant development.

The sCT methods have focused mainly on the pelvis and the brain. Recent studies have shown also the possibility to construct high-quality sCTs also for other sites in the body (Korhonen et al. 2016a; Freedman et al. 2018; Wang et al. 2017). There are also sCT studies for attenuation correction of PET-MRI that aim for the whole body. These methods could be beneficial also for RTP. Additionally, the development of MRI simulators increases possibilities for the use of MRI-only RTP, for example, due to 4D imaging possibilities. The increase of MRI-Linacs will most likely boost research for MRI-only RTP. Currently, online adaptive planning with MRI-Linac is conducted by relying on simulation CT co-registered with the online MR image. It is worth also mentioning that MRI-only RTP is a standard protocol in other fields of RT apart from external beam RT. MRI-only RTP is increasingly applied for brachytherapy planning. It has been applied also for gamma knife and for Boron Neutron Capture Therapy (BNCT). The use of MRI-only for external RTP will most likely increase, but CT will still play a key role in the future as it's geometrically accurate, includes well-known calibration to electron density, is easy to reproduce and is relatively cheap, and there is an RT community with a lot of experience.

9.11 Summary

A variety of methods have been described for the generation of sCT from MRI. There are now effective solutions for the brain and prostate (with two FDA-approved systems), and they appear to have converged on similar levels of accuracy (Edmund and Nyholm 2017; Arabi et al. 2018). Almost all methods have some reliance on image registration for training. The sCT generation speed possible with deep learning is a significant advantage, and this method has achieved rapid impact in the field.

At this time there are still a number of outstanding issues and opportunities for further research in the field. These include:

- Increasing the generalizability of methods (to address different magnet strengths, scanner models, different centres).
- Improving the speed of acquisition (single vs. multiple sequences).
- Improving the speed of conversion (particularly multi-atlas/patches).
- Increasing robustness (such as abnormal anatomy, artefacts).

- Guaranteeing reliability (for example, with internal quality assurance).
- Accurate identification of cortical bone (UTE and ZTE sequences may help).
- Automatic gold seed fiducial detection (for the prostate (Gustafsson et al. 2017; Ghose et al. 2016)).
- There is a need for standardised reporting metrics.
- Determining how many training cases is required to adequately represent the population of interest.
- There is a need for open-source benchmark data to enable the objective comparison of sCT generation methods.

Acknowledgements Lauri Koivula (Department of Radiation Oncology, Cancer Center, Helsinki University Hospital, Helsinki, Finland). Xiao Han (Elekta Inc., Maryland Heights, MO, USA). Neelam Tyagi (Memorial Sloan Kettering Cancer Center, New York, USA). Filipa Guerreiro and Bas Raaymakers (Department of Radiotherapy, University Medical Center Utrecht, The Netherlands).

References

Andreasen D, Van Leemput K, Edmund JM. A patch-based pseudo-CT approach for MRI-only radiotherapy in the pelvis. Med Phys. 2016;43(8):4742–52. https://doi.org/10.1118/1.4958676.

Arabi H, Dowling JA, Burgos N, et al. Comparative study of algorithms for synthetic CT generation from MRI: consequences for MRI-guided radiation planning in the pelvic region. Med Phys. 2018;45(11):5218–33. https://doi.org/10.1002/mp.13187.

Bankman IN. Handbook of medical image processing and analysis. Amsterdam: Elsevier; 2009.

Brock KK. Image processing in radiation therapy. London: Taylor & Francis; 2014.

Brock KK, Dawson LA. Point: Principles of magnetic resonance imaging integration in a computed tomography-based radiotherapy workflow. Semin Radiat Oncol. 2014;24(3):169–74. https://doi.org/10.1016/j.semradonc.2014.02.006.

Burgos N, Guerreiro F, McClelland J, et al. Iterative framework for the joint segmentation and CT synthesis of MR images: application to MRI-only radiotherapy treatment planning. Phys Med Biol. 2017;62(11):4237–53. https://doi.org/10.1088/1361-6560/aa66bf.

Chandra S, Dowling J, Shen K, et al. Patient specific prostate segmentation in 3D magnetic resonance images. IEEE Trans Med Imaging. 2012;31:1955–64.

Chen L, Nguyen T-B, Jones E, et al. Magnetic resonance-based treatment planning for prostate intensity-modulated radiotherapy: creation of digitally reconstructed radiographs. Int J Radiat Oncol Biol Phys. 2007;68(3):903–11.

Cootes TFF, Taylor CJJ, Cooper DHH, Graham J, et al. Active shape models\their training and application. Comput Vis Image Underst. 1995;61(1):38–59. https://doi.org/10.1006/cviu.1995.1004.

Dice LR. Measures of the amount of ecologic association between species. Ecology. 1945;26(3):297–302.

Dowling JA, Lambert J, Parker J, et al. An atlas-based electron density mapping method for magnetic resonance imaging (MRI)-alone treatment planning and adaptive MRI-based prostate radiation therapy. Int J Radiat Oncol Biol Phys. 2012;83(1):e5–11.

Dowling JA, Sun J, Pichler P, et al. Automatic substitute computed tomography generation and contouring for magnetic resonance imaging (MRI)-alone external beam radiation therapy from standard MRI sequences. Int J Radiat Oncol Biol Phys. 2015;93(5):1144–53. https://doi.org/10.1016/j.ijrobp.2015.08.045.

Edmund JM, Nyholm T. A review of substitute CT generation for MRI-only radiation therapy. Radiat Oncol. 2017;12(1):28. https://doi.org/10.1186/s13014-016-0747-y.

Edmund JM, Kjer HM, Van Leemput K, Hansen RH, Al AJ, Andreasen D. A voxel-based investigation for MRI-only radiotherapy of the brain using ultra short echo times. Phys Med Biol. 2014;59(23):7501–19. https://doi.org/10.1088/0031-9155/59/23/7501.

Freedman J, Bainbridge H, Wetscherek A, et al. PO-0959: dosimetric evaluation of midposition pseudo-ct for MR-only lung radiotherapy treatment planning. Radiother Oncol. 2018;127:S526–7. https://doi.org/10.1016/S0167-8140(18)31269-6.

Ghose S, Mitra J, Rivest-Hénault D, et al. MRI-alone radiation therapy planning for prostate cancer: automatic fiducial marker detection. Med Phys. 2016;43(5):2218–28. https://doi.org/10.1118/1.4944871.

Ghose S, Dowling JA, Rai R, Liney GP. Substitute CT generation from a single ultra short time echo MRI sequence: preliminary study. Phys Med Biol. 2017a;62(8):2950–60. https://doi.org/10.1088/1361-6560/aa508a.

Ghose S, Greer PB, Sun J, et al. Regression and statistical shape model based substitute CT generation for MRI alone external beam radiation therapy from standard clinical MRI sequences. Phys Med Biol. 2017b;62:8566–80. https://doi.org/10.1088/1361-6560/aa9104.

Glide-Hurst CK, Wen N, Hearshen D, et al. Initial clinical experience with a radiation oncology dedicated open 1.0T MR-simulation. J Appl Clin Med Phys. 2015;16(2):5201. https://doi.org/10.1120/jacmp.v16i2.5201.

Greer PB, Dowling JA, Lambert JA, et al. A magnetic resonance imaging-based workflow for planning radiation therapy for prostate cancer. Med J Aust. 2011;194(4):S24–7.

Gustafsson C, Korhonen J, Persson E, Gunnlaugsson A, Nyholm T, Olsson LE. Registration free automatic identification of gold fiducial markers in MRI target delineation images for prostate radiotherapy. Med Phys. 2017;44(11):5563–74. https://doi.org/10.1002/mp.12516.

Han X. MR-based synthetic CT generation using a deep convolutional neural network method. Med Phys. 2017;44(4):1408–19. https://doi.org/10.1002/mp.12155.

Herman MG, Balter JM, Jaffray DA, et al. Clinical use of electronic portal imaging: report of AAPM radiation therapy committee task group 58. Med Phys. 2001;28(5):712–37. https://doi.org/10.1118/1.1368128.

Hofmann M, Steinke F, Scheel V, et al. MRI-based attenuation correction for PET/MRI: a novel approach combining pattern recognition and atlas registration. J Nucl Med. 2008;49(11):1875–83. https://doi.org/10.2967/jnumed.107.049353.

Hsu S-H, Cao Y, Huang K, Feng M, Balter JM. Investigation of a method for generating synthetic CT models from MRI scans of the head and neck for radiation therapy. Phys Med Biol. 2013;58(23):8419–35. https://doi.org/10.1088/0031-9155/58/23/8419.

Huynh T, Gao Y, Kang J, et al. Estimating CT image from MRI data using structured random forest and auto-context model. IEEE Trans Med Imaging. 2016;35(1):174–83. https://doi.org/10.1109/TMI.2015.2461533.

Ibanez L, Schroeder W. The ITK software guide 2.4. New York, NY: Kitware, Inc; 2005.

Johansson A, Karlsson M, Nyholm T. CT substitute derived from MRI sequences with ultrashort echo time. Med Phys. 2011;38(5):2708–14.. http://link.aip.org/link/MPHYA6/v38/i5/p2708/s1&Agg=doi

Johansson A, Karlsson M, Yu J, Asklund T, Nyholm T. Voxel-wise uncertainty in CT substitute derived from MRI. Med Phys. 2012;39(6):3283–90. https://doi.org/10.1118/1.4711807.

Johansson A, Garpebring A, Karlsson M, Asklund T, Nyholm T. Improved quality of computed tomography substitute derived from magnetic resonance (MR) data by incorporation of spatial information--potential application for MR-only radiotherapy and attenuation correction in positron emission tomography. Acta Oncol. 2013;52(7):1369–73. https://doi.org/10.3109/0284186X.2013.819119.

Johnstone E, Wyatt JJ, Henry AM, et al. Systematic review of synthetic computed tomography generation methodologies for use in magnetic resonance imaging–only radiation therapy. Int J Radiat Oncol. 2018;100(1):199–217. https://doi.org/10.1016/j.ijrobp.2017.08.043.

Karlsson M, Karlsson MG, Nyholm T, Amies C, Zackrisson B. Dedicated magnetic resonance imaging in the radiotherapy clinic. Int J Radiat Oncol Biol Phys. 2009;74(2):644–51.

Kerkmeijer LGW, Maspero M, Meijer GJ, van der Voort van Zyp JRN, de Boer HCJ, van den Berg CAT. Magnetic resonance imaging only workflow for radiotherapy simulation and planning in prostate cancer. Clin Oncol. 2018;30(11):692–701. https://doi.org/10.1016/J.CLON.2018.08.009.

Khan FM. Treatment planning in radiation oncology. 2nd ed. Philadelphia, PA: Lippincott Williams & Wilkins; 2007.

Kim J, Glide-Hurst C, Doemer A, Wen N, Movsas B, Chetty IJ. Implementation of a novel algorithm for generating synthetic CT images from magnetic resonance imaging data sets for prostate cancer radiation therapy. Int J Radiat Oncol Biol Phys. 2015;91(1):39–47. https://doi.org/10.1016/j.ijrobp.2014.09.015.

Koivula L, Kapanen M, Seppälä T, et al. Intensity-based dual model method for generation of synthetic CT images from standard T2-weighted MR images – generalized technique for four different MR scanners. Radiother Oncol. 2017;125(3):411–9. https://doi.org/10.1016/j.radonc.2017.10.011.

Korhonen J, Kapanen M, Keyriläinen J, Seppälä T, Tenhunen M. A dual model HU conversion from MRI intensity values within and outside of bone segment for MRI-based radiotherapy treatment planning of prostate cancer. Med Phys. 2014;41(1):011704. https://doi.org/10.1118/1.4842575.

Korhonen J, Koivula L, Seppälä T, Kapanen M, Tenhunen M. PO-0912: MRI-only based RT: adopting HU conversion technique for pseudo-CT construction in various body parts. Radiother Oncol. 2016a;119:S440. https://doi.org/10.1016/S0167-8140(16)32162-4.

Korhonen J, Visapää H, Seppälä T, Kapanen M, Saarilahti K, Tenhunen M. Clinical experiences of treating prostate cancer patients with magnetic resonance imaging–only based radiation therapy treatment planning workflow. Int J Radiat Oncol. 2016b;96(2):S225. https://doi.org/10.1016/j.ijrobp.2016.06.558.

Ladefoged CN, Law I, Anazodo U, et al. A multi-centre evaluation of eleven clinically feasible brain PET/MRI attenuation correction techniques using a large cohort of patients. NeuroImage. 2017;147:346–59. https://doi.org/10.1016/j.neuroimage.2016.12.010.

Lagendijk JJW, Raaymakers BW, Van den Berg CAT, Moerland MA, Philippens ME, van Vulpen M. MR guidance in radiotherapy. Phys Med Biol. 2014;59(21):R349–69. https://doi.org/10.1088/0031-9155/59/21/R349.

Lambert J, Greer PPB, Menk FFFF, et al. MRI-guided prostate radiation therapy planning: Investigation of dosimetric accuracy of MRI-based dose planning. Radiother Oncol. 2011;3:330–4. https://doi.org/10.1016/j.radonc.2011.01.012.

Largent A, Barateau A, Nunes J-C, et al. Pseudo-CT generation for MRI-only radiotherapy treatment planning: comparison between patch-based, atlas-based, and bulk density methods. Int J Radiat Oncol Biol Phys. 2019;103(2):479–90.

Lee YK, Bollet M, Charles-Edwards G, et al. Radiotherapy treatment planning of prostate cancer using magnetic resonance imaging alone. Radiother Oncol. 2003;66(2):203–16.

Litjens G, Kooi T, Bejnordi BE, et al. A survey on deep learning in medical image analysis. Med Image Anal. 2017;42:60–88. https://doi.org/10.1016/j.media.2017.07.005.

Lu C, Chelikani S, Jaffray DA, Milosevic MF, Staib LH, Duncan JS. Simultaneous nonrigid registration, segmentation, and tumor detection in MRI guided cervical cancer radiation therapy. IEEE Trans Med Imaging. 2012;31(6):1213–27. https://doi.org/10.1109/TMI.2012.2186976.

Marshall HR, Patrick J, Laidley D, et al. Description and assessment of a registration-based approach to include bones for attenuation correction of whole-body PET/MRI. Med Phys. 2013;40(8):082509. https://doi.org/10.1118/1.4816301.

Maspero M, Savenije MHF, Dinkla AM, et al. Dose evaluation of fast synthetic-CT generation using a generative adversarial network for general pelvis MR-only radiotherapy. Phys Med Biol. 2018;63(18):185001. https://doi.org/10.1088/1361-6560/aada6d.

Mehranian A, Arabi H, Zaidi H. Vision 20/20: magnetic resonance imaging-guided attenuation correction in PET/MRI: Challenges, solutions, and opportunities. Med Phys. 2016;43(3):1130–55. https://doi.org/10.1118/1.4941014.

Meyer P, Noblet V, Mazzara C, Lallement A. Survey on deep learning for radiotherapy. Comput Biol Med. 2018;98:126–46. https://doi.org/10.1016/j.compbiomed.2018.05.018.

Nyul LG, Udupa JK, Xuan Zhang X. New variants of a method of MRI scale standardization. IEEE Trans Med Imaging. 2000;19(2):143–50. https://doi.org/10.1109/42.836373.

Owrangi AM, Greer PB, Glide-Hurst CK. MRI-only treatment planning: benefits and challenges. Phys Med Biol. 2018;63(5):05TR01. https://doi.org/10.1088/1361-6560/aaaca4.

Persson E, Gustafsson C, Nordström F, et al. MR-OPERA: a multicenter/multivendor validation of magnetic resonance imaging-only prostate treatment planning using synthetic computed tomography images. Int J Radiat Oncol Biol Phys. 2017;99(3):692–700. https://doi.org/10.1016/j.ijrobp.2017.06.006.

Rivest-Hénault D, Greer P, Fripp J, Dowling J. Structure-guided nonrigid registration of CT-MR pelvis scans with large deformations in MR-based image guided radiation therapy. LNCS. 2014;8361:65–73. https://doi.org/10.1007/978-3-319-05666-1_9.

Rohlfing T, Brandt R, Maurer CR, Menzel R. Bee brains, B-splines and computational democracy: generating an average shape atlas. In: Brandt R, editor. Proceedings IEEE MMBIA. Kauai, HA: MMBIA; 2001. p. 187–94. https://doi.org/10.1109/MMBIA.2001.991733.

Rohlfing T, Brandt R, Menzel R, Maurer CR. Evaluation of atlas selection strategies for atlas-based image segmentation with application to confocal microscopy images of bee brains. NeuroImage. 2004;21(4):1428–42.

Siversson C, Nordström F, Nilsson T, et al. Technical note: MRI only prostate radiotherapy planning using the statistical decomposition algorithm. Med Phys. 2015;42(10):6090–7. https://doi.org/10.1118/1.4931417.

Stanescu T, Jans H-S, Pervez N, Stavrev P, Fallone BG. A study on the magnetic resonance imaging (MRI)-based radiation treatment planning of intracranial lesions. Phys Med Biol. 2008;53(13):3579–93. https://doi.org/10.1088/0031-9155/53/13/013.

Tenhunen M, Korhonen J, Kapanen M, et al. MRI-only based radiation therapy of prostate cancer: workflow and early clinical experience. Acta Oncol (Madr). 2018;57:1–6. https://doi.org/10.1080/0284186X.2018.1445284.

Toennies KD. Guide to medical image analysis: methods and algorithms. London: Springer; 2012. https://doi.org/10.1007/978-1-4471-2751-2.

Tustison NJ, Avants BB, Cook PA, et al. N4ITK: improved N3 bias correction. Med Imaging IEEE Trans. 2010;29(6):1310–20. https://doi.org/10.1109/TMI.2010.2046908.

Tyagi N, Fontenla S, Zhang J, et al. Dosimetric and workflow evaluation of first commercial synthetic CT software for clinical use in pelvis. Phys Med Biol. 2017a;62(8):2961–75. https://doi.org/10.1088/1361-6560/aa5452.

Tyagi N, Fontenla S, Zelefsky M, et al. Clinical workflow for MR-only simulation and planning in prostate. Radiat Oncol. 2017b;12(1):119. https://doi.org/10.1186/s13014-017-0854-4.

Uh J, Merchant TE, Li Y, Li X, Hua C. MRI-based treatment planning with pseudo CT generated through atlas registration. Med Phys. 2014;41(5):051711. https://doi.org/10.1118/1.4873315.

Wang C, Chao M, Lee L, Xing L. MRI-based treatment planning with electron density information mapped from CT images: a preliminary study. Technol Cancer Res Treat. 2008;7(5):341–8. http://www.ncbi.nlm.nih.gov/pubmed/18783283. Accessed 17 Feb 2011.

Wang H, Chandarana H, Block KT, Vahle T, Fenchel M, Das IJ. Dosimetric evaluation of synthetic CT for magnetic resonance-only based radiotherapy planning of lung cancer. Radiat Oncol. 2017;12(1):108. https://doi.org/10.1186/s13014-017-0845-5.

Weistrand O, Svensson S. The ANACONDA algorithm for deformable image registration in radiotherapy. Med Phys. 2014;42(1):40–53. https://doi.org/10.1118/1.4894702.

Wyatt JJ, Dowling JA, Kelly CG, et al. Investigating the generalisation of an atlas-based synthetic-CT algorithm to another centre and MR scanner for prostate MR-only radiotherapy. Phys Med Biol. 2017;62(24):N548–60. https://doi.org/10.1088/1361-6560/aa9676.

Xiang L, Wang Q, Nie D, et al. Deep embedding convolutional neural network for synthesizing CT image from T1-weighted MR image. Med Image Anal. 2018;47:31–44. https://doi.org/10.1016/j.media.2018.03.011.

Part IV

MRI for Guidance

MRI Linac Systems

Brendan Whelan, Brad Oborn, Gary Liney, and Paul Keall

10.1 Introduction

Radiotherapy is a cornerstone of modern cancer treatment, being indicated for 48% of all cancer patients across almost the entire spectrum of disease sites and stages (Barton et al. 2014). However, current state-of-the-art radiotherapy faces a constraint: it cannot adapt to the complex changes in patients' anatomy and physiology caused by the functioning musculoskeletal (Erridge et al. 2003), circulatory (Seppenwoolde et al. 2002), respiratory (Keall et al. 2006) and other human systems as well as of the treatment itself (e.g. tumour regression). As a result, radiation beams can be off-target, missing the tumour and striking healthy tissue. This results in reduced therapeutic efficacy and increased toxicity.

To solve this problem, a new generation of radiotherapy machines is being developed with magnetic resonance imaging (MRI) replacing X-rays as the image guidance strategy. These integrated MRI-linear accelerators (MRI-Linacs) combine exquisite soft tissue and physiologic imaging with targeted cancer treatment. MRI-Linacs will enable treatment to be adapted to the patient's changing anatomy and physiology in real time, so the radiation always targets the tumour—and the most aggressive and resistant volumes within the tumour—rather than healthy organs.

Major advances in radiotherapy in the last two decades have come from improvements in imaging of tumours and normal tissues. These advances include image-guided radiotherapy (Zelefsky et al. 2012), intensity-modulated radiotherapy (IMRT) (Pignol et al. 2008; Donovan et al. 2007; Nutting et al. 2011), 4D CT combined with IMRT (Liao et al. 2010), stereotactic body radiotherapy (Palma et al. 2010) and improved dose calculation (Latifi et al. 2014). Clinically, they have resulted in higher tumour doses, better cancer control and fewer side effects.

MRI is the best imaging tool available for radiotherapy guidance. MRI-Linacs allow exquisite imaging of complex tumour and normal tissue, far exceeding the image quality of X-ray guidance, the current standard of care. MRI-Linacs also challenge the current paradigm that the tumour is treated as a uniform whole rather than as a dynamic, heterogeneous and evolving complex of tumour cells in an ever-changing

B. Whelan · P. Keall
ACRF Image X Institute, University of Sydney, Sydney, NSW, Australia
e-mail: paul.keall@sydney.edu.au

B. Oborn
Centre for Medical Radiation Physics, University of Wollongong, Wollongong, NSW, Australia

Illawarra Cancer Care Centre, Wollongong Hospital, Wollongong, NSW, Australia

G. Liney (✉)
Ingham Institute of Applied Medical Research, Liverpool, NSW, Australia
e-mail: gary.liney@sswahs.nsw.gov.au

© Springer Nature Switzerland AG 2019
G. Liney, U. van der Heide (eds.), *MRI for Radiotherapy*,
https://doi.org/10.1007/978-3-030-14442-5_10

microenvironment. The physiologic imaging capabilities of the MRI could enable a virtual whole tumour biopsy prior to and during each treatment, enabling real-time adaptive physiological targeting as a unique way to treat cancer. The daily physiological images acquired also offer the opportunity to monitor treatment efficacy and enable rapid changes of treatment plans to improve therapy. The increased accuracy can also change how radiation is delivered, enabling higher dose, shorter course treatments that benefit patients and the health system. MRI offers a broad range of physiological imaging capabilities, for example, R2* imaging is correlated with hypoxia (Chopra et al. 2009), diffusion-weighted imaging with cellularity (Gibbs et al. 2009), blood oxygen level-dependent (BOLD) contrast imaging with neural activity (Ogawa et al. 1990) and dynamic contrast-enhanced (DCE) imaging with proliferation, vascular permeability and relative extravascular volume (Turnbull et al. 1999).

In this chapter we describe the current MRI-Linac systems and, based on the technology trajectory, predict how these systems may evolve in the future.

10.2 MRI-Linac Integration Challenges

The major engineering challenge in designing integrated MRI-linac systems is the mutual electromagnetic interference from/to the two major subsystems. As shall be seen below, the most challenging aspect is mutual coupling caused by the permanent B0 field of the MRI scanner. As such, the challenges differ depending on the relative orientation of the MRI scanner and linear accelerator. Two possible configurations exist as shown in Fig. 10.1. In the perpendicular configuration, the B0 field is orientated perpendicular to the treatment beam, whilst in the in-line configuration, they are parallel. Two separate designs based on the perpendicular configuration have been used to treat patients. Two designs based on the in-line configuration exist and remain in the development phase.

10.2.1 Impact of MRI Scanner on Linear Accelerator, Dose Transport and Dosimetry

10.2.1.1 Impact on Accelerating Structures

Radiotherapy treats cancer by irradiating it with a high-energy beam of radiation, most commonly X-rays. The device most commonly utilised to produce a treatment beam in X-ray radiotherapy is the linear accelerator or linac. A schematic of a simple accelerating structure is shown in Fig. 10.2. The accelerating structure can be split into two components: the electron gun injects a steady-state electron beam into the accelerating waveguide. Each accelerating cavity contains an oscillating electromagnetic field such that an electron injected into the first cavity at the correct time will be continually accelerated as it passes through each cavity. In MRI-Linac therapy, the electrons are accelerated to approximately 6 MeV. To produce X-rays, this electron beam is collided with a heavy metal target to produce an MV X-ray bremsstrahlung spectrum. A detailed explanation regarding accelerator physics is beyond the scope of this book but has been described in many excellent references (Karzmark et al. 1993).

When a linear accelerator is operated in proximity to an MRI scanner, the fringe magnetic field produces a force on the electrons according to the Lorentz equation, in which $\bar{F}$ is the force on an individual electron, $\bar{v}$ is the electron velocity, $\bar{B}$ is the magnetic field and q is the electron charge:

$$\bar{F}_{\text{magnetic}} = q\left(\bar{E} + \bar{v} \times \bar{B}\right) \quad (10.1)$$

As can be seen from Eq. (10.1), the force produced on an electron is dependent on both the magnitude and direction of a magnetic field relative to the velocity direction. The magnetic force is zero in the instance that the magnetic field and velocity vectors are parallel and is maximal when the magnetic field and velocity vectors are perpendicular. Magnetic forces can cause an electron beam to bend, focus, or defocus—all of

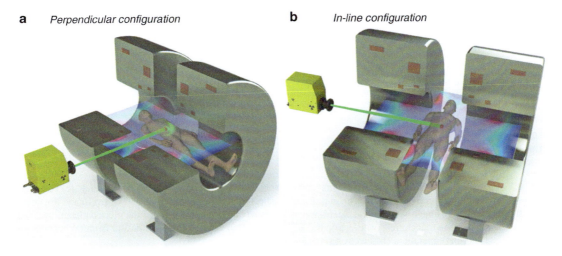

Fig. 10.1 MRI-Linac systems can be constructed in two possible configurations: (**a**) perpendicular, where the radiation beam is orthogonal to the magnetic field, or (**b**) in-line, where the radiation beam is parallel to the magnetic field. These schematics are loosely based on the Australian MRI-Linac system (Keall et al. 2014). Figure adapted from Paganelli et al. (2018)

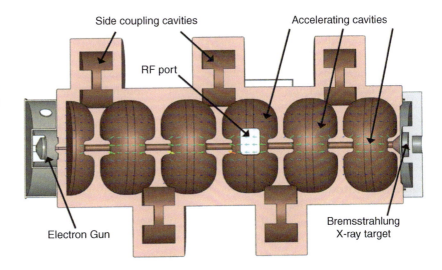

Fig. 10.2 A cut plane view of a basic side-coupled linac suitable for producing a therapeutic 6MV X-ray beam. A snapshot of the electric field distribution in the accelerating cavities is overlayed. This is the basic accelerator design currently being used in all MRI-Linac systems

which are deleterious to correct linear accelerator operation.

The effects of both in-line and perpendicular magnetic fields on linear accelerator operation have previously been studied via computational simulations. For the perpendicular case, total beam loss occurs at approximately 14 Gauss (G) and 45% at 6 G, whilst beam loss can begin as low as 2 G (Constantin et al. 2011; St Aubin et al. 2010a). This means that to produce a treatment beam for the perpendicular orientation, the linac must be operated in a near-zero field environment. This can be achieved by modifying the magnet and/or magnetically shielding the linac (Overweg et al. 2009; Whelan et al. 2018)—however, MRI magnet design (and redesign) is not a trivial task, and magnetic shielding causes distortion in the scanner. For the in-line case, maximum beam loss is approximately 80% at a field of 600 G (St Aubin et al. 2010a). It has also been shown that current loss due to in-line magnetic fields occurs nearly entirely in the electron gun as opposed to the linac

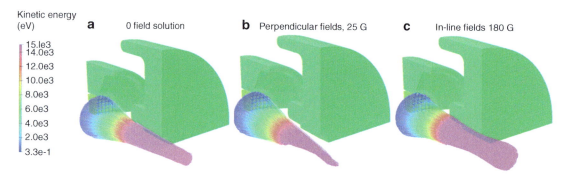

Fig. 10.3 The simulated effect of external magnetic fields on electron trajectories within an electron gun. Each image shows a cut-away image of a clinical electron gun geometry and the electron trajectories. (**a**) Electron trajectories at 0 field (normal operation), (**b**) electron trajectories at 25 G perpendicular fields and (**c**) electron trajectories in in-line fields of 180 G. In (**b**) and (**c**), beam loss results from collisions of the electron beam with the anode. Reproduced with permission from (Whelan et al. 2016b)

(St Aubin et al. 2010a; Whelan et al. 2016a). An example of the effects of perpendicular and in-line magnetic fields on the beam within an electron gun is shown in Fig. 10.3. In-line fields can also cause focusing or defocusing of an electron beam as described by Busch's theorem (Kumar 2009). It has been shown that this can result in substantial variations in the spatial intensity of the radiation beam impinging on the X-ray target (Whelan et al. 2016a). The major design ramification of this is a change in the thermal fatigue cycle of the target (Wang et al. 2017); however, to date this has not been explored in the literature.

10.2.1.2 Impact on Motors and Encoders

The multileaf collimator (MLC) is a crucial part of the treatment beam apparatus used to dynamically shape and modulate the photon treatment beam such that a complex dose distribution can be delivered to the patient. The MLC consists of a number of radiation blocking leaves which move independently of each other. Each leaf is attached to a stepper motor and encoder assembly. The purpose of the encoder is to verify that each stepper motor has taken the correct number of steps and hence the leaf is at the correct position. In conventional systems, optical and magnetic encoders are typically used—however, the function of this magnetic encoder is compromised when it is placed in an external magnetic field. Motor performance in magnetic fields has been assessed using independent optical encoders. It was found that depending on the specific motor used, performance began to degrade from 450 Gauss (Yun et al. 2010). Therefore, to operate a conventional MLC in an MRI-Linac system, the MLC must be redesigned or located far enough from the MRI scanner that the field is less than 0.05 T, magnetic shielding utilised or the component redesigned to function in magnetic fields. Another potential effect is increased motor burnout due to magnetic force on the motors—however, to date this effect has not been reported in the scientific literature.

10.2.1.3 Impact of Magnetic Fields on RF Power Flow

Magnetic fields can impact on the flow of RF power down a travelling waveguide via the Faraday effect. The Faraday effect refers to the rotation of polarised light propagating in a dielectric medium via magnetic fields (Ingersoll and Liebenberg 1954, 1956). Since the travelling waveguides only support certain modes, rotation of this distribution can lead to decreasing RF power flow. As yet, there are no reports in the literature quantifying this effect in MRI-Linac systems, although it has been noted as a potential concern in conference abstracts (Low et al. 2016).

10.2.1.4 Impact on Dose Transport

The dose in MRI-Linac systems is delivered by photons, which have no charge and hence are not affected by magnetic fields. However, a beam of photons deposit dose in matter via free radicals—largely electrons—which are subject to the Lorentz force defined by Eq. (10.1). When the patient is placed in a strong magnetic field, the trajectories of the electrons are altered—in zero field, the electrons undertake a 'random walk' from their point of creation, whereas in magnetic fields, the direction they take is biased. The exact behaviour again depends on the relative orientation of the radiation beam and the magnetic field. When the beam and the magnetic field lines are in (roughly) the same direction, the effect is to reduce lateral scattering. This is not necessarily a bad thing, since it allows for dose to be more focused along the photon beam. In fact, the theoretical benefits of strong in-line fields on dose transport within the patient had been studied in some detail well before the advent of MRI-Linacs for both electron beams (Shih 1975; Weinhous et al. 1985; Whitmire et al. 1977) and photon beams (Bielajew 1993; Chen et al. 2005). Recent developments towards MRI-guided radiotherapy have prompted further quantification of these effects for scenarios which align with potential MRI-Linac systems. This includes the reporting of small positive dose changes in general patient dosimetry (Kirkby et al. 2008) and furthermore positive dose enhancement effects in lung dosimetry (Kirkby et al. 2010; Oborn et al. 2016, 2017). The latter involves a narrowing of penumbral widths as the magnetic field encourages minimal lateral spread of secondary electrons when produced by the photon beam. In general, it seems that the presence of in-line magnetic fields has a positive impact on dose distributions around the treatment volume; however, the same mechanism that enhances the dose to tumours also acts to focus dose to the patient surface. Based on the results of Monte Carlo simulations, these effects can cause skin dose increases of up to 1000% (Oborn et al. 2012, 2014). However, these hotspots can be greatly reduced using electron purging devices and optimisation of the magnetic fringe field (Oborn et al. 2014). An alternative option is to add an absorbing layer between the beam and the patient, e.g. 2 cm of solid water, to absorb the electron-generated hotspots. This pragmatic approach would bring the surface dose to approximately 100%.

In contrast, when the magnetic fields are perpendicular to the beam direction, increased skin dose is not a problem as most contaminant electrons are swept away before reaching the patient (Oborn et al. 2009, 2010). However, in this configuration other issues emerge—the dose distribution inside the patient begins to become skewed, and at tissue-air interfaces (e.g. lung), hotspots can appear due to the much storied 'electron return effect', which has been shown to result in dose differences of up to 30–40% (Raaijmakers et al. 2004, 2005, 2007a, b, c, 2008). It has also been shown that there are various ways to compensate for this effect—for instance, by using an opposed beam to compensate for the effect, including the impact of the magnetic fields in the inverse plan optimisation, or by utilising a low-field MRI magnet (Bol et al. 2012, 2015; Mutic and Dempsey 2014). One question which remains somewhat open is the efficacy of these approaches in the presence of organ motion (remembering the fact that the target geometry may move is one of the main motivators for developing an MRI-Linac in the first place). Whilst some early promising work on this has been undertaken (Bol et al. 2012; Kontaxis et al. 2015, 2017), further quantification of these effects in the presence of motion is needed.

10.2.1.5 Impact of Magnetic Fields on Dosimetry

In addition to the magnetic field affecting radiation transport in human tissue for cancer treatment, charged particle transport will also be affected in dosimetry devices. This change is particularly important for ionisation chambers since (1) they are used for reference dosimetry measurements and (2) because the charge is measured from electrons moving in an air volume which has a density three orders of magnitude below that of water (and the majority of human tissue) and therefore the impact of magnetic fields on dose transport is magnified. Smit et al. (2013) reported a 5% effect in a 1.5 T MRI-Linac. Further studies on ion chambers in magnetic fields include (Smit et al. 2013; Meijsing et al. 2009; O'Brien et al. 2016; Reynolds et al. 2013; Spindeldreier et al. 2017).

There are also various experimental and Monte Carlo-based studies on solid-state detectors such as diodes and array detectors which also report various dosimetry calibration issues (Gargett et al. 2015, 2018; Reynolds et al. 2014, 2015). For ex vivo-style dosimetry, EPIDs have also been used in MRI-Linacs with good success as the detector lies in a relatively weak magnetic field (Raaymakers et al. 2011). MRI-Linac dosimetry with a variety of different detectors remains an important area of research and development of dosimetry standards.

10.2.2 Impact of Linear Accelerator on MRI Scanner

10.2.2.1 Impact of Externally Generated Magnetic Fields on the MRI Scanner

MRI requires an extremely homogenous field within the region being imaged to operate. Any magnetic fields generated near the MRI scanner degrade this field, compromising the geometric accuracy and image quality of images returned by the scanner. There are two ways in which external magnetic fields could be generated within the imaging volume of the MRI scanner by a linear accelerator. The first is the same way in which the MRI scanner itself generates a magnetic field—through current carrying wires. Although there are many currents in a linac, it turns out these are nowhere near strong enough to impact on normal imaging performance. The second way is the more familiar example of magnetism—magnetic materials. When magnetic materials are placed in a magnetic field (such as exists in an MRI scanner), they become magnetised and as such generate their own magnetic field. A linac tends to use a lot of ferromagnetic materials—for instance, bending magnets, MLC motors, ion pumps, magnetrons, ferrite recirculators, etc. (Karzmark et al. 1993). The impact of most of these components has yet to be studied or quantified in any detail within the scientific literature; however, since most of them are small and can be moved quite far away from the accelerator, it is broadly assumed that impact of these components is negligible. In any case, the magnetic field is optimised at installation through the process of passive shimming and/or use of additional superconducting shim coils to account for adjacent equipment. The most concerning component is the MLC, since it is the closest component to the magnet, it contains the largest mass of metal, and it doesn't remain stationary post magnet installation. As such, this is one of the few components which has been studied in detail (Kolling et al. 2013). The results of this study showed that a standard MLC would have minimal impact on the imaging field, provided it was operated more than ~1 metre from the centre of the magnet. However, if the equipment is moved, for example, on a rotating gantry or to change the SID, the field may need to be corrected for dynamically using electromagnet coils; this is achieved with the gradient coils (for 'first-order' correction) or using extra sets of coils for higher-order shimming (Liney et al. 2016).

Based on this information, it might seem that the impact of the linear accelerator on the MRI operation can be easily managed—but there's a catch. The easiest way to minimise the impact of the MRI fields on the linear accelerator is to magnetically shield the sensitive components. Shielding can be either passive (using magnetic materials to reduce the field in a volume of interest) or active (using current loops). However magnetic shielding by definition distorts magnetic fields! This is where a lot of the difficulty and compromise in MRI-Linac design stems from. Improved linac performance via magnetic shielding must be carefully balanced against potential degradation in the magnetic field of the MRI scanner. Magnetic shielding is discussed below.

10.2.2.2 Impact of RF Noise on the MRI Scanner

MRI scanners produce images by the measuring the RF signal of protons in the body. As such, MRI scanners are very sensitive to RF noise. A linear accelerator emits a wide spectrum of RF noise, which, if not accounted for, could interfere with the functionality of the MRI systems. The RF noise spectrum from three clinical linacs has been measured and found to be comparable in power and frequency to that measured in MRI, as such there is the potential of image artefacts occurring if correct shielding is not used (Lamey et al. 2010a). However, multiple studies and experimental results have demonstrated that it is possible to decouple the RF signals from the two devices to the extent that simultaneous operation is not affected (Lamey et al. 2010b; Fallone et al. 2009; Lagendijk et al. 2014). In addition to the study on RF noise from linacs above, the noise from MLC's and modulators has been quantified. It was shown that it is straightforward to shield the RF noise from the MLC (Lamey et al. 2010a) and that the largest source of RF noise from the linac was the magnetron. As such, it was recommended that the magnetron be stored in a different RF cage to the MRI scanner (Lamey et al. 2010b). In summary, whilst RF decoupling is an important design consideration, it is the magnetic decoupling which poses the greatest design challenges for MRI-Linac integration. This is because unlike magnetic shielding, RF shielding does not fundamentally interfere with the operation of an MRI magnet.

10.2.2.3 Interaction Between the Radiation Beam and Imaging Coil

In diagnostic MRI a closely fitting radio-frequency coil is used to receive the signal and minimise noise from outside anatomy. On an MRI-Linac this coil could conceivably be placed in the path of the radiation beam leading to several undesirable effects. These include attenuation of the beam and an increase in skin dose from contaminating electrons. A third effect referred to as 'radiation induced current' arises from electron disequilibrium in the conducting materials leading to artefacts and a reduction in signal-to-noise ratio (Burke et al. 2012). An alternative solution is to consider radiotranslucent materials (Hoogcarspel et al. 2018) or even open coil designs that maintain good image quality with a simultaneous radiation beam (Liney et al. 2018a).

10.2.3 Integration Strategies

Sections 10.2.1 and 10.2.2 provided an overview of the many interference effects that occur between MRI and linac systems. Here, we summarise the three major strategies one may use to overcome these interference issues. It should be noted that each of these strategies is independent, that is, an optimal design may use some combination of all three approaches.

10.2.3.1 Bespoke Magnet Design

The largest challenges in integrating an MRI scanner and a linear accelerator together stem from magnetostatic interference. This interference can be minimised by minimising the field magnitude in the locations in which linac components that have magnetostatic sensitivity or ferromagnetic components are placed. The most elegant means of achieving this is to incorporate this low-field region requirement into the initial magnet design. The fringe field distribution can be altered using superconducting shielding coils, ferromagnetic materials, or a combination of both. The Elekta MRI-Linac utilises a magnet design in which the conventional active shielding coils have been modified to create a toroidal low-field region in which the linear accelerator is placed (Overweg et al. 2009; Lagendijk et al. 2014). The Alberta group has presented a framework in which ferromagnetic materials are included in the magnet optimisation process and used to lower the fringe field (Tadic and Fallone 2012; Tari et al. 2017). A similar concept has been utilised in their MRI-Linac prototype; a steel 'yoke' is used to minimise the fringe field at the location of the linac (Fallone 2014). A potential issue with this approach is the temperature dependence of the magnetisation curves ferromagnetic materials, which can affect the homogeneity of the imaging volume of the scanner. As such, temperature control is an important consideration in magnet designs utilising a large amount of ferromagnetic material (Webb and Van de Moortele 2016).

The other MRI-Linac parameter which strongly influences magnet design is the choice of relative orientation of the linac and magnet. The impact of the B0 field on the linear accelerator can be minimised if the linac is orientated in-line with the B0 field (St Aubin et al. 2010a; Whelan et al. 2016a)—a configuration being pursued by the Alberta and Sydney groups (Keall et al. 2014; Fallone 2014). However, this requires that the patient is unconventionally positioned between the two poles of the magnet, which in turn requires some form of 'split bore' design. Creating a MRI magnet with a split between the two poles large enough to fit a person into carries its own unique set of challenges in terms of both magnet and gradient design (Liu et al. 2013). However, the Australian system has demonstrated how an open design incorporating both integrated gradient and RF coils can still provide sufficient image quality in both supine and vertical positions (Liney et al. 2018a). On the other hand, a more conventional closed bore (or small split bore) design necessitates that the linac is placed perpendicular to B0, which increases the effect of the B0 field on accelerator operation (St Aubin et al. 2010b).

The major challenge in utilising bespoke magnet design as an MRI-Linac integration strategy is the difficult and time-consuming nature of magnet design (Webb and Van de Moortele 2016). As such, although the most elegant means to minimise magnetostatic interference in MRI-Linac systems is bespoke magnet design, in many cases it may be more efficient to begin with an existing design and work to 'retrofit' it to the need at hand. The other challenge with bespoke magnet design is that if other system specifications are changed, the magnet may also need to be redesigned. As an example, the current Elekta MRI-Linac has a source to isocentre distance (SID) of ~1.5 m. If a future design aimed to utilise a more conventional SID of 1 m, the magnet optimisation process would have to be repeated.

10.2.3.2 Magnetic Shielding

Magnetic shielding refers to use of either ferromagnetic materials or current loops to produce a low-field region. Although this broad definition could be applied to the magnet optimisation strategies described in Sect. 10.2.3.1, the focus on this section is on magnet shielding that is introduced post magnet optimisation. The major advantage of this approach is that it can be implemented independently of magnet design, meaning the expertise required is substantially reduced. Of course, the major disadvantage is that any magnetic shielding not included in the original magnet design will perturb the imaging volume of the MRI scanner. As such, the presence of magnet shielding materials must be compensated for using some form of shimming (Webb and Van de Moortele 2016).

At present, all MRI-Linac designs utilise at least some passive shielding. Active shielding approaches have been explored in the literature (Santos et al. 2012); however, to the best of our knowledge, they are not currently in use on any system. This is largely due to convenience: active shielding requires optimisation of the coil placement and current depth, an independent power source and (potentially) cooling systems to cool the coils. In contrast, a well-designed passive shield will work in a wide variety of magnetic field strengths with no power or source or cooling requirements. A qualitative understanding of passive magnetic shielding can be achieved by considering the shield as a magnetic circuit, which describes a shield as a low reluctance path for magnetic flux. The formula for the ratio of the field inside and outside a spherical magnetic shell is given by Eq. 10.2:

$$K_{\text{sphere}} \quad \frac{2t\mu_r}{3R}+1 \quad (10.2)$$

This formula illustrates the important aspects of a good magnetic shield: high magnetic permeability and adequate thickness. It is important to note that the permeability of shielding materials

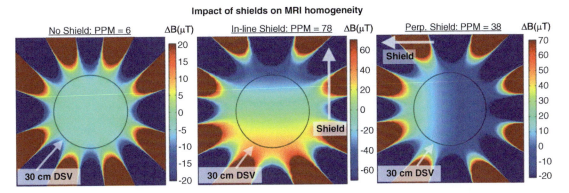

Fig. 10.4 The impact of passive shields on in-line and perpendicular MRI-Linac configuration

is a non-linear function of the applied field, which limits the applicability of analytic equations such as Eq. (10.2) for real-world simulations. As such, some form of computational electrodynamics is typically used. Computational electrodynamics is also necessary to assess the impact of a shield on the B0 field of the MRI scanner.

The use of passive magnetic shielding in MRI-Linac systems has been explored in some detail (Whelan et al. 2018; Santos et al. 2012; St Aubin et al. 2010c). One of the most important conclusions one can draw from this literature is that a cylindrical magnetic shield is more effective in the perpendicular configuration and also tends to cause less distortion (Whelan et al. 2018). This partly compensates for the increased effect of the magnet on the linear accelerator in this configuration (Sect. 10.2.1.1). Examples of the impact of passive shields on in-line and perpendicular MRI-Linac configurations are shown in Fig. 10.4.

10.2.3.3 Redesign of Individual Components

The final approach one may use to ensure MRI compatibility of a given component is to redesign that component. Ideally, a component would be reengineered to remove magnetic sensitivity altogether. For example, the magnetic encoders often used for MLC lead positioning verification have been demonstrated to have magnetic field sensitivity (Yun et al. 2010). In the Elekta Unity system, a novel optical system is used (Woodings et al. 2018). The possibility of redesigning accelerator structures to enable operation in certain magnetic fields has also been explored (Constantin et al. 2011; Whelan et al. 2016a); in this instance, it appears that there is potential to design an accelerator to operate correctly in certain fields, but not to remove the magnetic field sensitivity altogether.

In general, there are two drawbacks to redesigning components from the ground up to ensure MRI compatibility. Firstly, this process is time-consuming, requires considerable expertise and is expensive. In many cases it may be more straightforward to simply shield the components in question. Secondly, in instances where only partial MRI compatibility is achieved, changes in other system parameters such as SID or magnet strength/fringe field can void this limited compatibility.

10.3 Existing MRI-Linac Systems

At the time of writing, there are two commercial MRI-Linacs, the Elekta Unity and ViewRay MRIdian and two University-based systems, the University of Alberta MRI-Linac being commercialised by MagnetTx as the Aurora and the Australian MRI-Linac. These systems are shown in Fig. 10.5 with a comparison of different features given in Table 10.1. The systems are similar in some respects, for example, there are none with high energy of 10 MV or higher, though they differ in the field strength, beam-MRI-field orientation and source-isocentre distance. A more

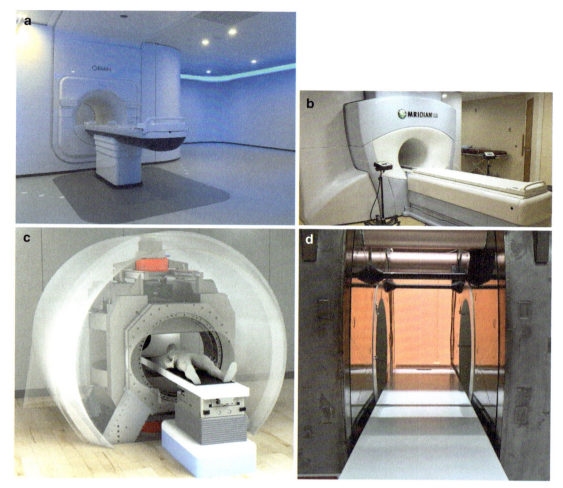

Fig. 10.5 Images of the existing systems. (**a**) Elekta Unity (courtesy Uulke van der Heide, Netherlands Cancer Institute), (**b**) ViewRay MRIdian (courtesy Carri Glide-Hurst, Henry Ford Hospital System), (**c**) MagnetTx Aurora (courtesy Gino Fallone, University of Alberta) and (**d**) Australian MRI-Linac (courtesy Gary Liney, Ingham Institute)

Table 10.1 Specifications of the existing systems

System	Radiation type	Field strength	Magnet type	Orientation	Source-isocentre distance	First patient Tx
Elekta Unity	7 MV FFF	1.5 T	Closed superconducting	Perpendicular	1.47 m	May 2017
ViewRay MRIdian	6 MV or ^{60}Co FFF	0.35 T	Split superconducting	Perpendicular	0.9 m	February 2014 (^{60}Co), July 2017 (Linac)
MagnetTx Aurora	6 MV	0.5 T	High temperature superconducting with steel yoke	In-line	1.4 m	Has not yet occurred
Australian MRI-Linac	4 & 6 MV FFF	1.0 T	Open superconducting	In-line with perpendicular option	1.8 m	Has not yet occurred

FFF flattening filter free, *MV* megavoltage, *Tx* treatment detailed comparison of the different systems is given in (Liney et al. 2018b).

2017 was a milestone year for integrated MRI-linear accelerators (MRI-Linacs). The first MRI-Linac patient treatments were performed in Utrecht (Raaymakers et al. 2017), and ViewRay successfully transitioned its MRIdian system from a cobalt radioisotope to a linac source, with the first patients treated at Henry Ford Hospital.[1] Adaptive radiotherapy, a long-standing challenge for traditional linacs, has become mainstream on ViewRay's integrated radiotherapy systems (Acharya et al. 2016). The early clinical findings for pancreas cancer (Rudra et al. 2017) have raised tremendous interest in the community and, if validated via clinical trials, will completely transform patterns of care for many cancer patients.

10.4 Future MRI-Guided Systems

Some future predictions do not need a crystal ball. The number of MRI-Linacs will grow, and with the large market opportunity, we will see some innovative new MRI-Linac designs with different features and strengths than those available today. A clinical MRI-guided particle therapy treatment room will be built (see chapter 13).

In parallel with this development, amazing new tools will be built to improve anatomic imaging, functional imaging, spatiotemporal resolution and tumour and normal tissue differentiation. We will use these tools to increase the efficacy of current treatments to improve local control and reduce toxicity and explore workflow increases and cost reductions within radiotherapy. However, a thought-provoking question is *With this new technology, what new opportunities for therapy are created?* Can we use MRI-Linacs for cardiac disease or other non-oncologic conditions? A five-patient *New England Journal of Medicine* paper showed profound benefits of radiotherapy for ventricular tachycardia (Cuculich et al. 2017). MRI-Linacs are uniquely positioned to non-invasively image the heart to maximise the therapeutic benefit of such procedures and also to treat more technically challenging sites, such as atrial fibrillation (Ipsen et al. 2014). The potential sub-mm accuracy of MRI-Linacs will enable us to rethink our anatomy and normal tissue sparing, such as sparing small neurovascular bundles linked with erectile dysfunction during prostate cancer radiotherapy (Lee et al. 2016). And of course no conversation of the future of cancer treatment can occur without mentioning immunotherapy, where the focused, tailored treatments offered by MRI-Linacs will provide the ideal immunostimulation environment with which to leverage adjuvant pharmacologic therapeutics.

10.5 Summary

In summary, MRI-Linac systems are changing the face of cancer radiotherapy. They arm clinicians with a new tool to visualise the target and normal tissues in real time and adapt the radiation beam to maximise tumour control and reduce side effects. They offer the potential of physiologic targeting to focus radiation dose where it is needed most, to the most resistant and aggressive regions of the tumour and the regions with the highest metastatic potential. MRI-Linac systems are the first to routinely offer online adaptive radiotherapy to facilitate reduced dose to critical structures that change position with respect to the tumour target on a day-to-day basis. MRI-Linacs have been installed in many of the leading cancer centres in the world. The future is exciting as to the growth of MRI-Linac systems, what new systems will emerge and how the current systems will evolve with time. Ultimately the question is how they will directly impact the duration and quality of life of cancer patients and indirectly their families and society.

---

[1] https://www.henryford.com/news/2017/07/viewray-firstpatient

References

Acharya S, Fischer-Valuck BW, Kashani R, et al. Online magnetic resonance image guided adaptive radiation therapy: first clinical applications. Int J Radiat Oncol Biol Phys. 2016;94:394–403.

Barton MB, Jacob S, Shafiq J, et al. Estimating the demand for radiotherapy from the evidence: a review of changes from 2003 to 2012. Radiother Oncol. 2014;112:140–4.

Bielajew AF. The effect of strong longitudinal magnetic fields on dose deposition from electron and photon beams. Med Phys. 1993;20:1171–9.

Bol G, Hissoiny S, Lagendijk J, et al. Fast online Monte Carlo-based IMRT planning for the MRI linear accelerator. Phys Med Biol. 2012;57:1375.

Bol GH, Lagendijk JJ, Raaymakers BW. Compensating for the impact of non-stationary spherical air cavities on IMRT dose delivery in transverse magnetic fields. Phys Med Biol. 2015;60:755–68.

Burke B, Wachowicz K, Fallone B, et al. Effect of radiation induced current on the quality of MR images in an integrated linac-MR system. Med Phys. 2012;39:6139–47.

Chen Y, Bielajew AF, Litzenberg DW, et al. Magnetic confinement of electron and photon radiotherapy dose: a Monte Carlo simulation with a nonuniform longitudinal magnetic field. Med Phys. 2005;32:3810–8.

Chopra S, Foltz WD, Milosevic MF, et al. Comparing oxygen-sensitive MRI (BOLD R2*) with oxygen electrode measurements: a pilot study in men with prostate cancer. Int J Radiat Biol. 2009;85:805–13.

Constantin DE, Fahrig R, Keall PJ. A study of the effect of in-line and perpendicular magnetic fields on beam characteristics of electron guns in medical linear accelerators. Med Phys. 2011;38:4174–85.

Cuculich PS, Schill MR, Kashani R, et al. Noninvasive cardiac radiation for ablation of ventricular tachycardia. N Engl J Med. 2017;377:2325–36.

Donovan E, Bleakley N, Denholm E, et al. Randomised trial of standard 2D radiotherapy (RT) versus intensity modulated radiotherapy (IMRT) in patients prescribed breast radiotherapy. Radiother Oncol. 2007;82:254–64.

Erridge SC, Seppenwoolde Y, Muller SH, et al. Portal imaging to assess set-up errors, tumor motion and tumor shrinkage during conformal radiotherapy of non-small cell lung cancer. Radiother Oncol. 2003;66:75–85.

Fallone BG. The rotating biplanar linac–magnetic resonance imaging system. Semin Radiat Oncol. 2014;24:200–2.

Fallone BG, Murray B, Rathee S, et al. First MR images obtained during megavoltage photon irradiation from a prototype integrated linac-MR system. Med Phys. 2009;36:2084–8.

Gargett M, Oborn B, Metcalfe P, et al. Monte Carlo simulation of the dose response of a novel 2D silicon diode array for use in hybrid MRI-LINAC systems. Med Phys. 2015;42:856–65.

Gargett MA, Oborn B, Alnaghy SJ, et al. A high resolution 2d array detector system for small-field MRI-Linac applications. Biomed Phys Eng Express. 2018;4:035041.

Gibbs P, Liney GP, Pickles MD, et al. Correlation of ADC and T2 measurements with cell density in prostate cancer at 3.0 Tesla. Investig Radiol. 2009;44:572–6.

Hoogcarspel SJ, Zijlema SE, Tijssen RH, et al. Characterization of the first RF coil dedicated to 1.5 T MR guided radiotherapy. Phys Med Biol. 2018;63:025014.

Ingersoll L, Liebenberg D. The Faraday effect in gases and vapors. I. J Opt Soc Am. 1954;44:566–71.

Ingersoll L, Liebenberg D. Faraday effect in gases and vapors. II. J Opt Soc Am. 1956;46:538–42.

Ipsen S, Blanck O, Oborn B, et al. Radiotherapy beyond cancer: target localization in real-time MRI and treatment planning for cardiac radiosurgery. Med Phys. 2014;41:120702.

Karzmark C, Nunan CS, Tanabe E. Medical electron accelerators. New York City, NY: McGraw-Hill; 1993.

Keall PJ, Mageras GS, Balter JM, et al. The management of respiratory motion in radiation oncology report of AAPM Task Group 76. Med Phys. 2006;33:3874–900.

Keall PJ, Barton M, Crozier S. The Australian magnetic resonance imaging–linac program. Semin Radiat Oncol. 2014;24:203–6.

Kirkby C, Stanescu T, Rathee S, et al. Patient dosimetry for hybrid MRI-radiotherapy systems. Med Phys. 2008;35:1019–27.

Kirkby C, Murray B, Rathee S, et al. Lung dosimetry in a linac-MRI radiotherapy unit with a longitudinal magnetic field. Med Phys. 2010;37:4722–32.

Kolling S, Oborn B, Keall P. Impact of the MLC on the MRI field distortion of a prototype MRI-linac. Med Phys. 2013;40:12705.

Kontaxis C, Bol G, Lagendijk J, et al. A new methodology for inter-and intrafraction plan adaptation for the MR-linac. Phys Med Biol. 2015;60:7485.

Kontaxis C, Bol G, Stemkens B, et al. Towards fast online intrafraction replanning for free-breathing stereotactic body radiation therapy with the MR-linac. Phys Med Biol. 2017;62:7233.

Kumar V. Understanding the focusing of charged particle beams in a solenoid magnetic field. Am J Phys. 2009;77:737–41.

Lagendijk JJ, Raaymakers BW, van Vulpen M. The magnetic resonance imaging–linac system. Semin Radiat Oncol. 2014;24:207–9.

Lamey M, Burke B, Blosser E, et al. Radio frequency shielding for a linac-MRI system. Phys Med Biol. 2010a;55:995–1006.

Lamey M, Rathee S, Johnson L, et al. Radio frequency noise from the modulator of a linac. IEEE Trans Electromagn Compat. 2010b;52:530–6.

Latifi K, Oliver J, Baker R, et al. Study of 201 non-small cell lung cancer patients given stereotactic ablative radiation therapy shows local control dependence on dose calculation algorithm. Int J Radiat Oncol Biol Phys. 2014;88:1108–13.

Lee JY, Spratt DE, Liss AL, et al. Vessel-sparing radiation and functional anatomy-based preservation for erectile function after prostate radiotherapy. Lancet Oncol. 2016;17:e198–208.

Liao ZX, Komaki RR, Thames HD Jr, et al. Influence of technologic advances on outcomes in patients with unresectable, locally advanced non-small-cell lung cancer receiving concomitant chemoradiotherapy. Int J Radiat Oncol Biol Phys. 2010;76:775–81.

Liney GP, Dong B, Begg J, et al. Technical note: experimental results from a prototype high-field inline MRI-linac. Med Phys. 2016;43:5188–94.

Liney GP, Dong B, Weber E, et al. Imaging performance of a dedicated radiation transparent RF coil on a 1.0 Tesla inline MRI-linac. Phys Med Biol. 2018a;63:135005.

Liney G, Whelan B, Oborn B, et al. MRI-linear accelerator radiotherapy systems. Clin Oncol. 2018b;30:686–91.

Liu L, Sanchez-Lopez H, Liu F, et al. Flanged-edge transverse gradient coil design for a hybrid LINAC–MRI system. J Magn Reson. 2013;226:70–8.

Low D, Mutic S, Shvartsman S, et al. TU-H-BRA-02: the physics of magnetic field isolation in a novel compact linear accelerator based MRI-guided radiation therapy system. Med Phys. 2016;43:3768.

Meijsing I, Raaymakers BW, Raaijmakers AJ, et al. Dosimetry for the MRI accelerator: the impact of a magnetic field on the response of a Farmer NE2571 ionization chamber. Phys Med Biol. 2009;54:2993–3002.

Mutic S, Dempsey JF. The ViewRay system: Magnetic resonance-guided and controlled radiotherapy. Semin Radiat Oncol. 2014;24:196–9.

Nutting CM, Morden JP, Harrington KJ, et al. Parotid-sparing intensity modulated versus conventional radiotherapy in head and neck cancer (PARSPORT): a phase 3 multicentre randomised controlled trial. Lancet Oncol. 2011;12:127–36.

Oborn BM, Metcalfe PE, Butson MJ, et al. High resolution entry and exit Monte Carlo dose calculations from a linear accelerator 6 MV beam under the influence of transverse magnetic fields. Med Phys. 2009;36:3549–59.

Oborn BM, Metcalfe PE, Butson MJ, et al. Monte Carlo characterization of skin doses in 6 MV transverse field MRI-LINAC systems: effect of field size, surface orientation, magnetic field strength, and exit bolus. Med Phys. 2010;37:5208–17.

Oborn B, Metcalfe PE, Butson M, et al. Electron contamination modeling and skin dose in 6 MV longitudinal field MRIgRT: Impact of the MRI and MRI fringe field. Med Phys. 2012;39:874–90.

Oborn B, Kolling S, Metcalfe PE, et al. Electron contamination modeling and reduction in a 1 T open bore inline MRI-linac system. Med Phys. 2014;41:051708.

Oborn BM, Ge Y, Hardcastle N, et al. Dose enhancement in radiotherapy of small lung tumors using inline magnetic fields: a Monte Carlo based planning study. Med Phys. 2016;43:368.

Oborn BM, Gargett MA, Causer TJ, et al. Experimental verification of dose enhancement effects in a lung phantom from inline magnetic fields. Radiother Oncol. 2017;125:433–8.

O'Brien DJ, Roberts DA, Ibbott GS, et al. Reference dosimetry in magnetic fields: formalism and ionization chamber correction factors. Med Phys. 2016;43:4915.

Ogawa S, Lee T-M, Kay AR, et al. Brain magnetic resonance imaging with contrast dependent on blood oxygenation. Proc Natl Acad Sci U S A. 1990;87:9868–72.

Overweg J, Raaymakers B, Lagendijk J, et al. System for MRI guided radiotherapy. Proc Int Soc Magn Reson Med. 2009;2009:593.

Paganelli C, Whelan BM, Peroni M, et al. MRI-guidance for motion management in external beam radiotherapy: current status and future challenges. Phys Med Biol. 2018;63:22TR03.

Palma D, Visser O, Lagerwaard FJ, et al. Impact of introducing stereotactic lung radiotherapy for elderly patients with stage I non-small-cell lung cancer: a population-based time-trend analysis. J Clin Oncol. 2010;28:5153–9.

Pignol J-P, Olivotto I, Rakovitch E, et al. A multicenter randomized trial of breast intensity-modulated radiation therapy to reduce acute radiation dermatitis. J Clin Oncol. 2008;26:2085–92.

Raaijmakers AJ, Raaymakers BW, Lagendijk JJ. Integrating a MRI scanner with a 6 MV radiotherapy accelerator: dose increase at tissue-air interfaces in a lateral magnetic field due to returning electrons. Phys Med Biol. 2005;50:1363–76.

Raaijmakers AJ, Hardemark B, Raaymakers BW, et al. Dose optimization for the MRI-accelerator: IMRT in the presence of a magnetic field. Phys Med Biol. 2007a;52:7045–54.

Raaijmakers AJ, Raaymakers BW, Lagendijk JJ. Experimental verification of magnetic field dose effects for the MRI-accelerator. Phys Med Biol. 2007b;52:4283–91.

Raaijmakers AJ, Raaymakers BW, van der Meer S, et al. Integrating a MRI scanner with a 6 MV radiotherapy accelerator: impact of the surface orientation on the entrance and exit dose due to the transverse magnetic field. Phys Med Biol. 2007c;52:929–39.

Raaijmakers AJ, Raaymakers BW, Lagendijk JJ. Magnetic-field-induced dose effects in MR-guided radiotherapy systems: dependence on the magnetic field strength. Phys Med Biol. 2008;53:909–23.

Raaymakers BW, Raaijmakers AJ, Kotte AN, et al. Integrating a MRI scanner with a 6 MV radiotherapy accelerator: dose deposition in a transverse magnetic field. Phys Med Biol. 2004;49:4109–18.

Raaymakers BW, de Boer JC, Knox C, et al. Integrated megavoltage portal imaging with a 1.5 T MRI linac. Phys Med Biol. 2011;56:N207–14.

Raaymakers BW, Jurgenliemk-Schulz IM, Bol GH, et al. First patients treated with a 1.5 T MRI-Linac: clinical proof of concept of a high-precision, high-field MRI guided radiotherapy treatment. Phys Med Biol. 2017;62:L41–50.

Reynolds M, Fallone BG, Rathee S. Dose response of selected ion chambers in applied homogeneous transverse and longitudinal magnetic fields. Med Phys. 2013;40:042102.

Reynolds M, Fallone BG, Rathee S. Dose response of selected solid state detectors in applied homogeneous transverse and longitudinal magnetic fields. Med Phys. 2014;41:092103.

Reynolds M, Fallone BG, Rathee S. Technical note: response measurement for select radiation detectors in magnetic fields. Med Phys. 2015;42:2837–40.

Rudra S, Jiang N, Rosenberg SA, et al. High dose adaptive MRI guided radiation therapy improves overall survival of inoperable pancreatic cancer. Int J Radiat Oncol Biol Phys. 2017;99:E184.

Santos D, St Aubin J, Fallone B, et al. Magnetic shielding investigation for a 6 MV in-line linac within the parallel configuration of a linac-MR system. Med Phys. 2012;39:788–97.

Seppenwoolde Y, Shirato H, Kitamura K, et al. Precise and real-time measurement of 3D tumor motion in lung due to breathing and heartbeat, measured during radiotherapy. Int J Radiat Oncol Biol Phys. 2002;53:822–34.

Shih CC. High energy electron radiotherapy in a magnetic field. Med Phys. 1975;2:9–13.

Smit K, Van Asselen B, Kok J, et al. Towards reference dosimetry for the MR-linac: magnetic field correction of the ionization chamber reading. Phys Med Biol. 2013;58:5945.

Spindeldreier CK, Schrenk O, Bakenecker A, et al. Radiation dosimetry in magnetic fields with Farmer-type ionization chambers: determination of magnetic field correction factors for different magnetic field strengths and field orientations. Phys Med Biol. 2017;62:6708–28.

St Aubin J, Santos DM, Steciw S, et al. Effect of longitudinal magnetic fields on a simulated in-line 6 MV linac. Med Phys. 2010a;37:4916–23.

St Aubin J, Steciw S, Fallone B. Effect of transverse magnetic fields on a simulated in-line 6 MV linac. Phys Med Biol. 2010b;55:4861.

St Aubin J, Steciw S, Fallone BG. Magnetic decoupling of the linac in a low field biplanar linac-MR system. Med Phys. 2010c;37:4755–61.

Tadic T, Fallone BG. Design and optimization of superconducting MRI magnet systems with magnetic materials. IEEE Trans Appl Supercond. 2012;22:4400107.

Tari SY, Wachowicz K, Fallone BG. A non-axial superconducting magnet design for optimized patient access and minimal SAD for use in a Linac-MR hybrid: proof of concept. Phys Med Biol. 2017;62:N147.

Turnbull LW, Buckley DL, Turnbull LS, et al. Differentiation of prostatic carcinoma and benign prostatic hyperplasia: correlation between dynamic Gd-DTPA-enhanced MR imaging and histopathology. J Magn Reson Imaging. 1999;9:311–6.

Wang J, Trovati S, Borchard PM, et al. Thermal limits on MV x-ray production by bremsstrahlung targets in the context of novel linear accelerators. Med Phys. 2017;44:6610–20.

Webb A, Van de Moortele P. The technological future of 7 T MRI hardware. NMR Biomed. 2016;29:1305–15.

Weinhous MS, Nath R, Schulz RJ. Enhancement of electron beam dose distributions by longitudinal magnetic fields: Monte Carlo simulations and magnet system optimization. Med Phys. 1985;12:598–603.

Whelan B, Gierman S, Holloway L, et al. A novel electron accelerator for MRI-linac radiotherapy. Med Phys. 2016a;43:1285–94.

Whelan B, Holloway L, Constantin D, et al. Performance of a clinical gridded electron gun in magnetic fields: implications for MRI-linac therapy. Med Phys. 2016b;43:5903.

Whelan B, Kolling S, Oborn BM, et al. Passive magnetic shielding in MRI-Linac systems. Phys Med Biol. 2018;63:075008.

Whitmire DP, Bernard DL, Peterson MD, et al. Magnetic enhancement of electron dose distribution in a phantom. Med Phys. 1977;4:127–31.

Woodings SJ, Bluemink J, de Vries J, et al. Beam characterisation of the 1.5 T MRI-linac. Phys Med Biol. 2018;63:085015.

Yun J, St Aubin J, Rathee S, et al. Brushed permanent magnet DC MLC motor operation in an external magnetic field. Med Phys. 2010;37:2131–4.

Zelefsky MJ, Kollmeier M, Cox B, et al. Improved clinical outcomes with high-dose image guided radiotherapy compared with non-IGRT for the treatment of clinically localized prostate cancer. Int J Radiat Oncol Biol Phys. 2012;84:125–9.

11. MRI at the Time of External Beam Treatment

Michael Roach and Carri K. Glide-Hurst

11.1 Overview: MR for Onboard IGRT (MR-IGRT) Treatment Guidance

Magnetic resonance image-guided radiation therapy (MR-IGRT) offers simultaneous tracking of the target during treatment delivery while taking advantage of the excellent soft tissue contrast of MRI. Even at low magnetic field strengths (i.e., 0.35 T), visualization of tissues and most critical structures has been shown to be superior to cone beam CT (CBCT) (Noel et al. 2015) for many disease sites, particularly in the abdomen and pelvis. By eliminating radiation exposure, daily monitoring of intrafractional motion and treatment plan adjustments based on changes in anatomy can be made in near real time (Acharya et al. 2016a). Historically, MR-IGRT was unavailable due to the challenges of decoupling the radiation delivery device from the influence of a magnetic field and vice versa, but these technical limitations have been recently overcome. The world's first clinical MR-IGRT machine utilized cobalt-60 for treatment delivery with a low-field 0.35 T magnet (Mutic and Dempsey 2014), but now devices with linear accelerators for treatment delivery and higher strength magnets for IGRT are available (Lagendijk et al. 2014; Keall et al. 2014). Complete descriptions of the MR-IGRT devices that have been developed can be found in Chap. 10. This chapter will provide the clinical context, including highlighting clinical workflows and specific case examples and revealing the major advantages of MR-IGRT for gating and adaptive radiation therapy (ART).

11.2 MR-Co-60 in Clinical Practice

The first MR-IGRT system was installed at Washington University in St. Louis. Between January 2014 and June 2016, the program treated a total of 316 patients (Fischer-Valuck et al. 2017). The most frequent disease sites were abdomen, 88 patients (28%); breast, 82 patients (26%), pelvis, 68 patients (21%); and thorax, 61 patients (19%). Patients were selected for treatment with the MR-IGRT system as opposed to conventional linear accelerator-based treatment based primarily upon improved soft tissue imaging, 168 patients (53%); cine gating, 81 patients (26%); or online adaptation, 67 patients (21%), with most being selected for a combination of these factors. Seventy-six patients (24%) were treated with three-dimensional conformal RT, 146 (46%) with intensity-modulated radiation

M. Roach (✉)
Department of Radiation Oncology, Washington University in Saint Louis, St. Louis, MO, USA
e-mail: roachm@wustl.edu

C. K. Glide-Hurst
Department of Radiation Oncology, Henry Ford Cancer Institute, Detroit, MI, USA
e-mail: CHURST2@hfhs.org

therapy (IMRT), and 94 (30%) with stereotactic body radiation therapy (SBRT). Overall, high patient compliance was observed with only nine patients (3%) unable to tolerate the simulation due to claustrophobia and/or pain in the treatment position. An average of eight patients/day were treated (range: 0–15), with significant variation based on treatment complexity. During these initial 2.5 years, the machine was offline for 39 business days (6%) for scheduled cobalt-60 source changes, software upgrades, and machine maintenance. While the MR-Co-60 clinical experience has laid the groundwork for the initial clinical experience with MR-IGRT, the lower-energy and broader penumbra as compared to a six MV beam has moved the evolution of the technology toward higher beam energies.

11.3 MR-Linac in Clinical Practice

The integration of a modified six MV Elekta (Stockholm, Sweden) linear accelerator and 1.5 T Philips (Best, Netherlands) Achieva MRI system was first developed at the University Medical Center-Utrecht in the Netherlands, and the system has been installed in several institutions (Raaymakers et al. 2009). The system was first used to treat patients in May 2017 at the University Medical Center-Utrecht. Four patients with lumbar spine bone metastases were treated with 8 Gy in a single fraction with a three or five beam step-and-shoot IMRT plan. Plans were created while the patient was on the treatment table. Pretreatment CT was deformably registered to the online MRI for treatment planning (Raaymakers et al. 2017). This treatment procedure averaged 41 min (range: 33–44) and was well tolerated by patients. The international MRI-Linear Accelerator Consortium has been formed to facilitate evidence-based introduction of this technology, and it plans to form a central data registry program for future reports on how this technology is utilized clinically (Kerkmeijer et al. 2016).

The MRIdian Linac system (ViewRay, Mountain View, CA) has been in clinical operation since July 2017 at Henry Ford Health System and has since been installed at several other institutions. The system is equipped with a double-stack, double-focus multi-leaf collimator (MLC), to achieve 2 mm spatial resolution (half the MLC leaf width), thereby enabling more precise RT using six MV flattening filter free at a higher dose rate (~600 MU/min) than its Co-60 predecessor. During the first year of clinical operation, 127 patients were treated (89% IMRT, 11% 3D conformal), with ~57% treated with hypofractionated dosing schemes. Sixty percent of the disease sites treated were located in the abdominal and thorax regions (abdominal metastases, liver, lung, and pancreas) requiring gated treatments delivered at either end-inhalation or end-exhalation breath holds based on patient compliance.

Recently, a dosimetric comparison was conducted for pancreatic cancer SBRT between the tri-cobalt MR-IGRT and MRIdian Linac systems, revealing that while similar target coverage could be obtained, the dose to the nearby organs at risk were higher for the tri-cobalt system (Ramey et al. 2018). In this study, the MRIdian Linac system performed similarly to a conventional linac for planning target volume (PTV) coverage and OAR constraints. Given the higher dose rate and sharper penumbra for the MR-linac, advanced planning strategies including the treatment of small brain metastases in an MR-guided stereotactic radiosurgery (MRgSRS) setting have also been explored (Wen et al. 2018).

11.4 Clinical Workflows

Patients must be screened for contraindications to determine eligibility for MR-IGRT following standard guidelines such as those from the American College of Radiology (Safety et al. 2013). Initial screening is commonly performed by nursing staff prior to consult, by the physician during the patient history interview, and/or by treatment therapists prior to treatment. Prior to each fraction, patients are queried for any medical procedures since they were last seen and for any metal on their person.

The following workflow pertains to MR-IGRT conducted for ViewRay systems, which may differ from the Elekta Unity clinical workflows that are emerging. To guide any necessary CT simulation (CT-SIM) and emulate patient setup during MR-IGRT, MRI "dummy" surface phased array receiver coils, with attenuation properties similar to that of the actual MR receiver surface coils, are often built into or around immobilization devices as shown in Fig. 11.1. This ensures a high signal-to-noise ratio while also maintaining setup conditions between MR-IGRT, MRI simulation (MR-SIM) on the MR-IGRT system, and CT-SIM. With the benefits of real-time tracking and monitoring, some institutions have reduced their immobilization device use in MR-IGRT settings. Patient clearance in the MRI bore may also be of concern given the typical MRI bore size (~70 cm) as compared to the wide bore CT-SIM (~85 cm).

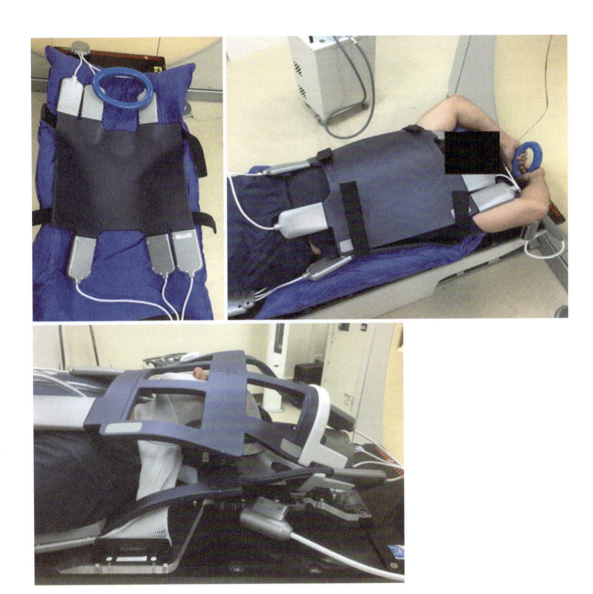

Fig. 11.1 Example of radiofrequency receiver coils built into immobilization devices for high signal-to-noise ratio as used on a low-field MR-linear accelerator. The coils shown are the two-part phase array coil with 12-elements (torso, top row) and 10-elements (head and neck, bottom row)

11.4.1 Multimodality (CT/MR Combined) and Single-Modality (MR-Primary) Treatment Planning

In the standard multimodality workflow, the standard CT-SIM is used for dose calculation and treatment planning with daily MR-IGRT images co-registered to the CT-SIM dataset. Advantages of this workflow include that the CT-SIM dataset is known for its spatial integrity and accuracy for dose calculations, while disadvantages include that then the reference dataset for daily treatment requires a multimodality image registration with the lower contrast resolution of CT. In the MR-primary workflow, a synthetic CT (either derived from electron densities from the CT dataset or via bulk density overrides) must be used for dose calculation as the MR does not contain electron density information. The ViewRay Treatment Planning System enables the generation of an electron density map using the CT that has been rigidly or deformably registered to the MRI dataset to facilitate dose calculation (Henke et al. 2018; Bohoudi et al. 2017a). One disadvantage of the MR-primary planning approach is that attention must be paid to transient regions of air or changes in organ at risk filling differences (i.e., rectum, bladder, stomach, etc.) between the acquisitions to ensure a robust electron density map is used. However, daily IGRT using single-modality registration (MR-MR) is generally more straightforward than multimodality (MR-CT) for determining the couch shifts. It should be noted that the MRI bore limits shifts much more than conventional linear accelerators.

11.4.2 MR-Based Gating

Following AAPM Task Group Report 76 guidelines, when tumor excursion is >5 mm in any direction, motion management is employed (Keall et al. 2006). Using the currently available low-field MR-linac and MR-Co (McPartlin et al. 2016) technologies, cine images can be acquired in the sagittal plane for one or three slices with acquisition frame rates of four and two frames/second, respectively, using a balanced steady-state free precession sequence (BSSFP, 5–10 mm slice thickness, 3.5 × 3.5 mm^2 in-plane spatial resolution). It is customary to acquire this data through the target volume with sufficient contrast from surrounding structures to facilitate MR-based gating. Two gating parameters are typically selected: boundary expansion, which can be isotropic or anisotropic and defines the gating window, and the % region of interest (%ROI), which defines the percentage of the tracked volume that can extend outside boundary while allowing beam to remain on. Many institutions are incorporating audio or visual feedback to improve the duty cycle and treatment efficiency. While end-exhalation provides the most reproducible portion of the respiratory cycle, patient compliance may be challenging for repeated breath holds, particularly for hypofractionated cases.

Implementing MR-IGRT for real-time tumor tracking and gating offers distinct advantages including the elimination of the invasive procedure required for fiducial placement and avoiding issues with subsequent marker migration that can lead to pneumonias, fistulas, and inaccurate treatment (Matsuo et al. 2014). Direct tumor tracking is preferable to respiratory surrogates such as patient surface anatomy for correlation with internal motion (Malinowski et al. 2012). MRI allows for this direct tracking while avoiding additional exposure to the ionizing radiation used in fluoroscopy. Gating is currently being performed routinely with many MR-IGRT systems (Green et al. 2012), and similar tracking has been reported for MRI-linacs (Yun et al. 2013).

11.5 MR-Based Adaptive Radiation Therapy (ART)

Typically, conventional radiation therapy uses a single dataset of a patient's anatomy taken at the time of simulation. Additional datasets can be acquired at the time of treatment with 2D kV or MV images, with cone beam CT, or with MRI, but the use of these datasets is usually limited to rigid matching with the anatomy on the original planning dataset in order to make small shifts in patient alignment to improve treatment precision. Geometric deformations in internal anatomy cannot be easily accounted for with this process, however, and the initial treatment plan that was optimized to sculpt dose around targets and away from normal tissue may become suboptimal.

Adaptive radiation therapy (ART) is a methodology that adjusts patient treatment according to physical or functional changes of both the target and organs at risk (OARs). This offers potential for dose escalation to the target and may improve treatment tolerance by better sparing OARs. ART relies on in-room treatment image guidance, accurate image registration, recontouring of target and OARs, plan evaluation and reoptimization, dose calculation, and quality assurance (QA) (Lim-Reinders et al. 2017). This can be done either offline or online. In offline adaptation, a new dataset is acquired, the patient is taken off the simulation or treatment table, and a new treatment plan is generated over hours or days. In online adaptation, a new plan is generated while the patient is on the treatment table in their treatment position. Though online adaptation offers potential improvements in treatment accuracy, it can be challenging to complete both plan adaptation, QA, and plan delivery quickly enough that the patient can tolerate remaining still in their treatment position.

11.5.1 Online Adaptation

The following workflow description is that of the first published online adaptive MR-IGRT treatments as summarized in Fig. 11.2. It should be stressed that online adaptation is highly reliant on the quality of the daily MRI taken for both patient alignment and radiation therapy replanning. Before the delivery of each adaptive fraction, immobilized patients undergo volumetric MRI in their treatment position. Next, to facilitate dose calculation, both the electron density map and the contours from either the planning scan or the most recently used plan are transferred via deformable image registration to the daily MRI scan. After review of the image registration, many institutions perform a rigid copy of their original target volumes as they were developed using adjunct imaging at time of initial planning, and in hypofractionated settings, minimal change

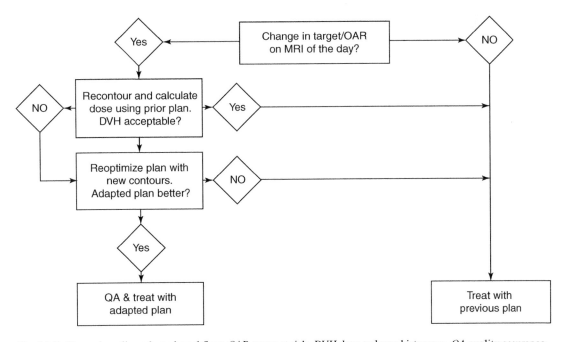

Fig. 11.2 Example online adapted workflow. *OAR* organ at risk, *DVH* dose-volume histogram, *QA* quality assurance

is expected in the target volume (Henke et al. 2018; Bohoudi et al. 2017a). Currently, recontouring is the most resource intense and rate-limiting step of the process. The electron density map is also reviewed by a physicist, and manual corrections may be made to ensure high-fidelity dose calculation accuracy.

After contour and electron density corrections, a dose prediction is performed using either the initial treatment plan or the most recently used plan. If the target coverage is below prespecified physician defined acceptable thresholds or if OAR doses exceed constraints, online reoptimization is performed. One current limitation is that the plan is projected as if that day's anatomy existed for all fractions when a dose-volume histogram (DVH) is created. As violation of OAR constraints is most likely to occur in close proximity to the target, recontouring is often performed in a region of interest limited to 3–5 cm around the PTV to improve efficiency (Bohoudi et al. 2017a). Next, a side-by-side comparison of the reoptimized plan's isodose distribution and DVH with that of the prior plan is performed (Fig. 11.3). Further reoptimization can be done by changing optimization calculation parameters and/or with plan normalization. The physician then selects the plan to be used after a final review of isodose lines and DVH.

If the adapted plan is selected for treatment, rapid online QA is performed. In a conventional workflow, initial plans often undergo measurement-based QA; however online ART with the patient on the table requires reliance on computer-based QA. The reoptimized plan, the electron density map, and the Digital Imaging

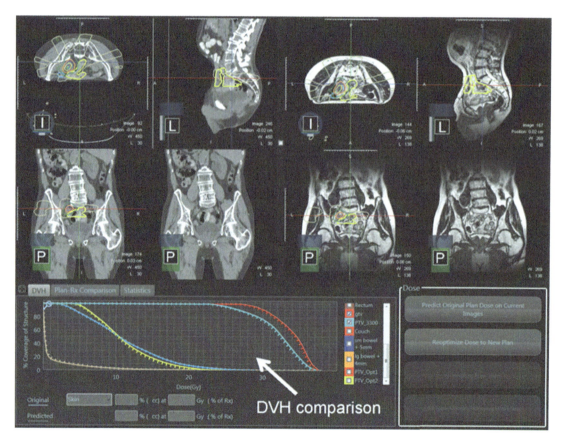

Fig. 11.3 Comparison of original plan (four upper left CT images) on the original CT simulation scan, and the original plan's beams when calculated on the first day's MRI scan on ViewRay. The lower half of the panel shows a dose-volume histogram (DVH) showing the percent of structures receiving a certain dose

and Communications in Medicine (DICOM) dose and structure files can be used either online or via an external workstation to perform a secondary Monte Carlo dose calculation and comparison via three-dimensional gamma analysis with 2–3% and 2–3 mm gamma criteria over the entire treatment volume (Sun et al. 2012). Plan parameter comparisons can be performed between beam angles, segment number, beam-on time, fluence patterns, and changes/gaps in structure volumes between the prior and new plans to ensure agreement and discrepancies can be flagged for physics review (Rangaraj et al. 2013; Li et al. 2015).

Given the resource-intense nature of the online ART process, particularly for time required for physicists to perform plan adjustments and QA and for physicians to recontour, the median online ART that was first reported with MR-IGRT was 26 min including time required for recontouring, reoptimization, and QA with only 2% of treatments requiring >40 min. It should be noted that this was time that was in addition to usual setup and treatment delivery time. Efforts to improve efficiency include having dosimetrists or specially trained therapists delineate appropriate structures rather than physicians, improving contour propagation quality on the vendor side, and having dedicated physician/physicist staffing at the ART procedures to avoid delays due to availability. From a patient care perspective, some patients will require anxiolytics and pain medication to get through these longer treatments.

The currently available online ART workflow has limitations. Current technology with MRI IGRT cannot reproducibly identify point volumes of deformable OARs like the bowel for accurate calculations of cumulative dose. The isotoxicity approach described above is conservative by projecting the same treatment over that day's anatomy for the entire treatment course. While this approach ensures that no point volume of OAR will exceed dose constraints, this approach may limit PTV coverage and further dose escalation. This workflow also does not account for intrafraction OAR motion. Plan adaptation based on intrafraction imaging feedback has been proposed but is far from clinical implementation (Glitzner et al. 2016; Kontaxis et al. 2015).

11.5.2 Tumor Response Adaptation

As described in Chap. 6, in addition to adapting treatment based upon interfraction anatomic changes, treatment target volumes and dose can be adapted based upon tumor response (Kishan and Lee 2016). Diffusion-weighted imaging (DWI) has been shown to predict response to radiation therapy sooner than gross tumor volume changes on CT and metabolic changes on fluorodeoxyglucose-positron emission tomography (FDG-PET) (Malayeri et al. 2011; Tsien et al. 2014). While treatment response assessment is typically performed by tracking changes in the tumor's apparent diffusion coefficient (ADC) from baseline using higher field strengths, University of California Los Angeles has successfully developed a spin echo-based diffusion sequence at 0.35 T and found good ADC measurement agreement with 1.5 T or higher MRIs (Yang et al. 2016). Here, a single-shot echo-planar imaging k-space sampling scheme (maximum gradient amplitude of 18 mT/m and gradient slew rate of 200 mT/(m/ms)) was implemented immediately after treatment, while the patient was still in the treatment position. Results for several sarcoma and head and neck carcinoma cases (2–5 fractions per patient) were promising, yielding relatively constant ADC values in reference regions (i.e., brainstem) while tumor ADC maps changed during treatment and with more heterogeneity within larger tumors.

A similar feasibility study was conducted for response assessment to neoadjuvant therapy in three patients with rectal cancer also treated on ViewRay (Shaverdian et al. 2017). Patients in this study received 50.4–54 Gy in 1.8 Gy daily fractions with concurrent oral capecitabine for locally advanced rectal adenocarcinoma. Changes in ADC were correlated to pathological responses after total mesorectal excisions by a single pathologist blinded to all imaging and clinical data. The authors proposed DWI as a noninvasive modality that could assess response to treatment, with higher posttreatment ADC values predicting a pathologic complete response. While further investigation is needed, functional imaging taken at the end of treatment could potentially be used to spare patients the morbidity of surgery, particularly for low rectal tumors where a permanent colostomy must be created.

Serial DWI data obtained via MR-IGRT may thus provide an additional biomarker that could be used to tailor doses based on tumor response. Explorations in other disease sites and with 1.5 T MR-linacs offer potential for a paradigm shift in the future of IGRT and plan adaptation as described more extensively in Chap. 6.

11.6 MRI at the Time of Thorax Treatment

Lung cancer remains the most common type of cancer worldwide, with non-small cell lung cancer (NSCLC) making up the majority of cases with ~20% of cases diagnosed in early stages before the cancer has spread to regional lymph nodes. The increasing adoption of low-dose CT-based screening in high-risk patient populations with significant tobacco smoking histories is expected to increase the numbers of cases caught in early stages (Team 2011; Moyer 2014). Historically, medically inoperable lung cancer patients were treated with conventionally fractionated radiation therapy. In the past decade, however, SBRT has emerged as the standard of care for the medically inoperable early stage NSCLC patients, showing improved local control in both randomized (Nyman et al. 2016) and population-based comparisons (Koshy et al. 2015). SBRT is also being adopted for early stage small cell lung cancer (Shioyama et al. 2015; Verma et al. 2017) and lung oligometastases (Navarria et al. 2015). Instead of delivering radiation in small doses over several weeks, SBRT delivers very high doses extremely precisely to targets over a course that is only 1–2 weeks in duration. Improvements in tumor staging, target delineation, treatment planning, patient immobilization, respiratory motion management, and image guidance allow for the reproducible and safe delivery of these large fraction sizes to tumors with narrow margins. Narrow treatment margins and sharp drop-off of dose help minimize injury to surrounding OARs including the spinal cord, brachial plexus, trachea, proximal bronchial tree, esophagus, heart, great vessels, chest wall, and, in some lower lobe tumors, abdominal organs like the stomach, bowel, and liver (Ritter et al. 2011).

Given the high doses per fraction that are used in SBRT, precise patient positioning is needed. However as opposed to many advanced robotic treatment couches with 6 degrees of freedom that are used in treatment machines that specialize in SBRT, the restricted bore size on MRI treatment machines limits corrections largely to the superior-inferior direction. To correct for large shifts in other directions or rotations, online adaptation may be utilized using the initial treatment plan (Ates et al. 2016). Real-time tracking and gating is particularly advantageous for tumors in the lower lobes of the lung where respiratory motion is greatest (Fig. 11.4). While clinical evidence is still being established, with MR guidance and gated delivery, local control is expected to be similar to X-ray-based alignment, with a potential for a decrease in toxicity due to decreased treatment volumes when compared to internal target volume approaches that treat the entirety of the tumor's trajectory during respiration.

With more advanced stage lung tumors such as those invading central structures or with regional spread to mediastinal lymph nodes, using MR-IGRT for daily pretreatment alignment may allow for a potential reduction in the setup component of CTV-PTV margin when compared to CBCT (Bainbridge et al. 2017). The combination of real-time tracking and online adaptation has been proposed to allow for safer dose escalation in more advanced lung cancers with better OAR sparing, particularly within the central thorax near the proximal bronchial tree, esophagus, and heart (Henke et al. 2016). An early retrospective study of patients receiving hypofractionated radiation therapy alone for more advanced central malignancies showed that after 1 week of treatment at fraction 6, patients demonstrated significant on-treatment MRI-defined GTV

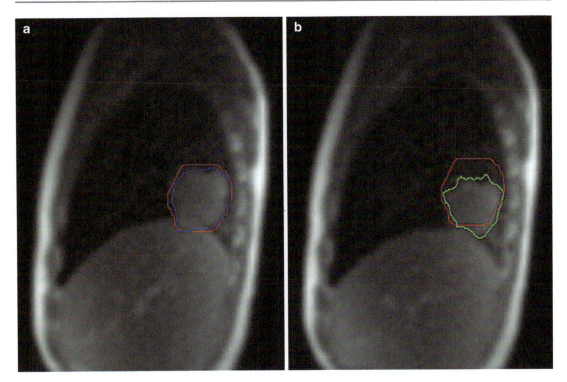

Fig. 11.4 Demonstration of gating in the lung without fiducials on ViewRay. In all panels, the red line is the gating boundary, a static 3 mm expansion on the gross tumor volume. The blue and green lines are the deformable gating target contour that is tracked in real time. In panel **a**, the lung target is largely within bounds and the beam is on. In panel **b**, it is out of bounds and the beam is off

reduction, with a median reduction of 27%. Application of the initial plan at fraction 6 resulted in violations of OAR constraints in approximately half of the patients. Adaptive planning was shown to be able to reverse all of these OAR violations. In 40% of fractions corrected for OAR constraint violations, PTV coverage was able to be increased concomitantly. Prospective clinical trials of this combination of MR for both alignment and adaptation are being planned at several institutions with MRI IGRT.

11.7 MRI at the Time of Abdomen Treatment

11.7.1 Pancreas

Although surgical resection offers the only chance of cure for pancreatic cancer, just 20% of patients have resectable, nonmetastatic disease at diagnosis. The remainder of patients with exocrine pancreatic cancer present roughly equally between those with distant metastases and those with locally advanced but unresectable disease. Typically in these locally advanced cases, the primary tumor is wrapped around or is invading blood vessels like the celiac axis or superior mesenteric artery that cannot be reconstructed and cannot be sacrificed without irreversibly damaging the stomach and bowel. Management of such patients is controversial as local control benefits are often obscured by high rates of distant progression within the abdomen or thorax (Hammel et al. 2016). At present, median patient survival with either chemotherapy or chemoradiation therapy is just 15 months. Phase II studies suggest a downstaging benefit to neoadjuvant chemotherapy and radiation therapy, with a greater rate of achieving a complete resection compared to historical controls. As resection offers curative potential, successful downstaging from neoadjuvant chemoradiation therapy has the potential to improve long-term overall survival in patients with unresectable disease at diagnosis.

Unfortunately, pancreatic tumors are located in close proximity to the stomach, duodenum, and bowel, all of which are sensitive parallel structures that have historically limited dose escalation with radiation. These gastrointestinal organs also deform daily and are not easily visualized with CBCT. While fiducials can be placed in the primary tumor to allow for tracking, the movement from stomach filling and peristalsis of the bowel cannot be so easily tracked with X-ray-based IGRT. MRI-guided radiation therapy and MRI-based ART have the potential to overcome these challenges using gating and adaptation based on OAR location, with promising early clinical results. Thirty-six patients with locally advanced or borderline resectable pancreatic cancer were treated with MRI-guided radiation from October 2014 to September 2016 at three institutions. Doses ranged from conventionally fractionated radiation of 50–60 Gy in 25–30 fractions and SBRT to 30–36 Gy in five fractions to higher ablative doses with either 50–67.5 Gy in 15 fractions or SBRT to 40–50 Gy in five fractions. These higher ablative doses had a biologically effective dose (BED) ≥ 70 Gy based on an alpha/beta of 10 for the tumor. With a median follow-up of 7 months, those treated with the higher ablative doses had significantly improved overall survival (OS). Those who received lower BED had a median survival of just 7 months, while those who received higher BED had not yet reached median survival. On multivariate analysis, BED ≥70 Gy remained predictive of improved OS even after controlling for the tumor marker CA 19–9 at diagnosis and the use of induction chemotherapy. Two-thirds of treatments were adapted online in the high-dose group, while <5% were in the low-dose group (Rudra et al. 2017). Given these results, a prospective multi-institutional trial of stereotactic MRI-guided adapted therapy (SMART) is planned.

The approach was considered isotoxic (Zindler et al. 2016) in contrast to conventional radiation, where the PTV is typically covered by >95% of the prescription dose according to International Committee on Radiation Units and Measurements (ICRU) guidelines (ICRU83 2010). These clinicians limited daily PTV coverage by OAR tolerance with "hard" OAR constraints that were lower than the prescription dose. These "hard" constraints included OAR hotspots, with <0.5 cc of each OAR allowed to exceed a dose constraint that was approximately 70% of the PTV prescription dose for both the 15 and 5 fraction regimens. However, rather than aiming for relatively homogenous PTV coverage by 95–107% of the prescription dose like with conventional radiation, heterogeneous hotspots were allowed within the PTV away from the OARs. This created a steep dose gradient at the OAR rim while simultaneously allowing for dose escalation to the PTV. Dose accumulation to deformable OARs was not performed due to challenges previously described.

11.7.2 Liver

Primary liver cancer is the third most common cause of cancer death worldwide. The liver is also one of the most common sites of secondary metastases, particularly from gastrointestinal primaries. While surgery is considered the main curative treatment option, complete resection or liver transplant is feasible in only a minority of patients. Nonsurgical local treatment options for both primary and secondary liver malignancies include radiofrequency ablation, microwave ablation, cryoablation, alcohol injection, transarterial chemoembolization, yttrium-90 microspheres, and external beam radiation therapy.

An increasing number of retrospective and prospective series have explored the efficacy and safety of SBRT for local control of both liver primaries and metastases (Murray and Dawson 2017). To date, local control has been excellent and ranges from 75% to 100% at 1 year. Of note, SBRT is often done in Child-Pugh class A patients with preserved liver function, though there are more limited reports of using SBRT in the more compromised Child-Pugh class B patients. Grade 3 or greater toxicity has been reported in up to a third of patients, with increasing rates in the Child-Pugh class B patients. Death from liver failure after SBRT has been seen in up to 13% of patients. Ongoing research is looking into optimizing planning based on pretreatment functional imaging of the liver in order to spare healthier segments to reduce toxicity.

Localization for liver SBRT is critical. This has almost always been done after placement of a fiducial, usually by interventional radiology (Mahadevan et al. 2018). However, like with lung SBRT, the use of MRI at the time of treatment can spare the patient this invasive procedure. Some tumors are readily visible on MRI without contrast. If not, one approach is the daily use of gadolinium-ethooxybenzyl-deithylenetri-amine pentaacetic acid (Gadolinium-EOB-DPTA, Eovist). This intravenous contrast agent is selectively taken up by hepatocytes and increases the signal intensity of normal liver parenchyma on T1-weighted MRI (Ringe et al. 2010; Cruite et al. 2010). Liver tumors will appear hypointense on delayed phase contrast scans with this agent. These hypodense lesions can then be tracked to facilitate respiratory gating (Fig. 11.5) (Rosenberg et al. 2015). Patients with chronic, severe kidney disease or acute kidney injury are at risk for nephrogenic systemic fibrosis with this contrast agent though, and it is thus best avoided in such patients. If the lesion is not well seen with the use of this daily contrast,

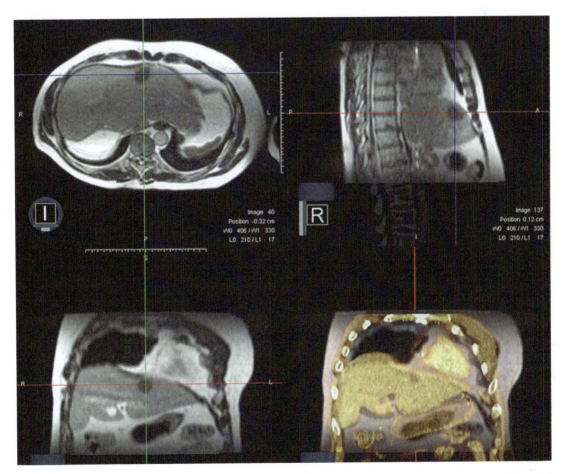

Fig. 11.5 Stereotactic body radiation therapy in five fractions was planned to a liver target on ViewRay. Eovist contrast was given prior to each fraction highlighting normal liver parenchyma. The target is hypodense and is easily tracked for gating. Clockwise from upper left: axial simulation, sagittal simulation, coronal overlay of setup MRI (gold) and simulation MRI (gray), and coronal simulation

the entire liver contour or a surrogate landmark can be used as a gating structure, though attention needs to be paid to potential deformations occurring during the respiratory cycle.

11.7.3 Abdominal Metastases

The peritoneum, para-aortic lymph nodes, and especially the adrenal gland, are common locations for metastatic spread of cancer within the abdomen. For patients with a limited metastatic disease burden (oligometastatic) or with limited progressing sites (oligoprogressive), SBRT has been investigated as an addition to systemic therapy to increase local control and progression-free survival. Much like with primary pancreatic cancer, both intrafraction respiratory motion and interfraction physiologic organ motion make SBRT to metastases within the abdomen challenging. The first prospective phase I trial using SMART showed that this approach was both clinically deliverable and safe, allowing PTV dose escalation and simultaneous OAR sparing compared to nonadaptive abdominal SBRT (Henke et al. 2018) (Fig. 11.6).

In this phase I study of SMART, 20 patients were split evenly between those with oligometastatic or unresectable primary liver cancer and those with non-liver abdominal malignancies. Initial plans

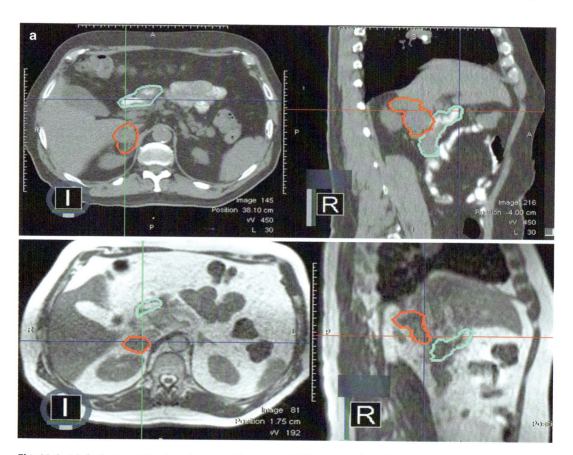

Fig. 11.6 (a) Online/on-table adaptation of a right adrenal target (red) on ViewRay. The top two panels are axial and sagittal slices of the simulation CT scan where nearby duodenum (cyan) is nearby. The bottom panels show that on the set-up MRI for the first day of treatment, the duodenum has shifted further away from the target, potentially allowing for better dose coverage of the target. (b) Online adaptation of a right adrenal target (blue color wash) on ViewRay. On the top panels, the original plan is shown where high dose coverage (orange and red) is limited due to target proximity to the duodenum (cyan). On the bottom panels, the plan has been adapted to increase coverage of the target

11 MRI at the Time of External Beam Treatment

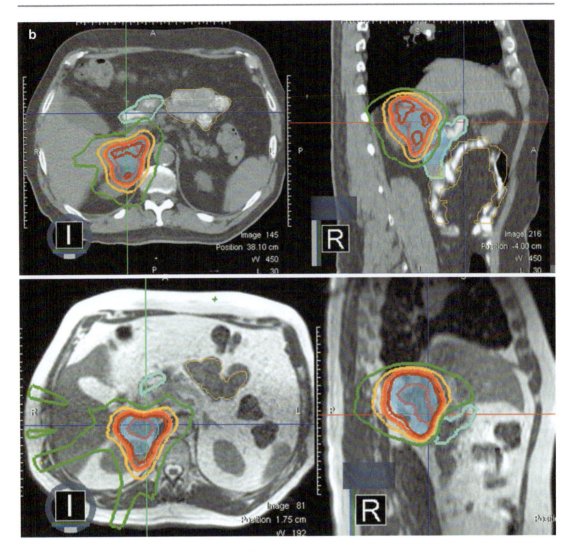

Fig. 11.6 (continued)

prescribed 50 Gy in five fractions of 10 Gy each to the PTV, though escalation/condensing to 60 Gy in four fractions of 15 Gy each was allowed if OAR constraints could be met. OAR constraints took priority over PTV coverage. Either the initial plan or prior fraction's plan (whichever was more recent) was loaded and contours were then manually edited as needed. If there was a violation in an OAR maximum dose constraint or an opportunity for PTV coverage improvement, a new adaptive plan was generated. Online adaptive plans were used in 81 of 97 fractions. Adaptation was done due to OAR constraint violations in 61 of 97 plans and for opportunities for PTV dose escalation in 20 of 97. PTV coverage increased in 64 of 97 fractions. Median on-table time was 79 min. Zero grade 3 or greater acute (<6 month) treatment toxicities were found, despite the high ablative doses used. Hopefully these promising results will be replicated and reported soon by other institutions adopting SMART.

11.8 MRI at the Time of Breast Treatment

Prospective randomized controlled trials and meta-analyses have established that breast conservation therapy, consisting of partial mastectomy and adjuvant radiation therapy, offers equivalent disease control in women with early-stage breast cancer as compared to mastectomy. Breast conserving therapy offers significantly superior disease control when compared to partial mastectomy alone. For ductal carcinoma in situ, adjuvant radiation therapy increases local control. Typically, adjuvant breast irradiation includes whole-breast irradiation over 3–5 weeks, often followed by a boost to the surgical cavity. Accelerated partial breast irradiation (APBI), consisting of twice-daily treatments over 5 days or shorter schedules, was developed to improve compliance with adjuvant radiation therapy. Common treatment options for APBI include interstitial techniques, intracavitary applicators, single intraoperative treatments, and external beam radiation, each technique having its advantages and disadvantages.

MR-guided RT is well suited for either boosting of the partial mastectomy surgical cavity after whole breast treatment or for APBI. In addition to aiding alignment when compared to conventional X-ray-based IGRT approaches such as CBCT, MR-guided RT allows for gating and for smaller PTV margins (Fig. 11.7). One prospective registry study of 30 women with early-stage breast cancer receiving external beam APBI halved the conventional 2 cm margin from cavity to PTV (CTV + 1 cm = PTV). Of note, the CTV excluded the chest wall, pectoral muscles, and 5 mm from skin. Instead with MRI IGRT, the surgical cavity was expanded to 1 cm for CTV with no further PTV expansion (Acharya et al. 2016c). The dose prescribed was 38.5 Gy in 3.85 Gy twice-daily fractions separated by at least 6 hours delivered on 5 consecutive weekdays. Target dose constraints were 95% of the PTV to receive 95% of prescription dose and 98% of PTV to receive 90% of prescription.

On this study, a volumetric MRI with 1.5 × 1.5 × 3 mm resolution was acquired for each fraction's setup with alignment to the cavity contour. Cine images from a single sagittal plane through the surgical cavity were then acquired daily (four frames per second, BSSFP sequence, 7 mm slice thickness, 3.5 × 3.5 mm^2 spatial resolution). The calculated margin required for at least 90% of the cavity to be contained for 90% of the treatment time was 0.7 mm. The fifth to the 95th percentile intrafractional cavity motion was

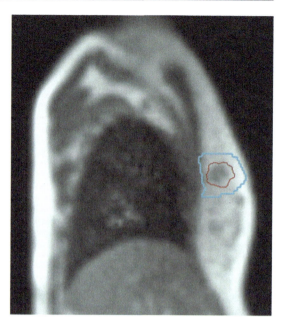

Fig. 11.7 Accelerated partial breast irradiation in ten total fractions delivered twice a day on ViewRay. The red line is the outline of the surgical cavity which is tracked continuously during treatment and respiration. The blue line is a 1 cm expansion for CTV, subtracted off the chest wall and 5 mm from skin

<3 mm in anterior-posterior and superior-inferior directions with excellent agreement between the planned and delivered V95 dose (<1% difference). Preliminary results suggest good to excellent cosmetic outcomes. Clinical trials using similar cavity alignment and tracking strategies are ongoing using once a day APBI and even single fraction treatments with long-term cosmetic and disease outcomes pending.

11.9 MRI at the Time of Pelvic Treatment

11.9.1 Prostate

Prostate cancer is the most commonly diagnosed malignancy in men, and its treatment with surveillance alone, surgery, and radiation therapy is rapidly evolving. Radiation therapy for prostate cancer has moved from 3D techniques to conventionally fractionated dose-escalated IMRT to hypofractionated IMRT and, most recently, SBRT. Regardless of the dose and fractionation selected for treatment, IGRT is often used given the prostate's location between the bladder and rectum. These two organs can not only be damaged by RT but also can shift the internal location of the prostate based on their respective day-to-day filling. Given this, localization for prostate RT is most often done through implanted fiducial markers, electromagnetic beacons, or volumetric imaging with CBCT, rather than relying on external skin markings and 2D MV/kV matching to bone. MRI is currently used mainly at the time of screening/diagnosis and at the time of simulation as described in earlier chapters but shows promise for use in both alignment and adaptation during treatment (Pathmanathan et al. 2018).

MR-IGRT offers strengths in this setting for assessing and tracking prostate, rectum, and bladder motion in real time, while incorporating MRI for treatment planning improves autocontouring (Klein et al. 2008; Pasquier et al. 2007). As shown in Fig. 11.8, the prostate, seminal vesicles, and nearby organs can be clearly demarcated using

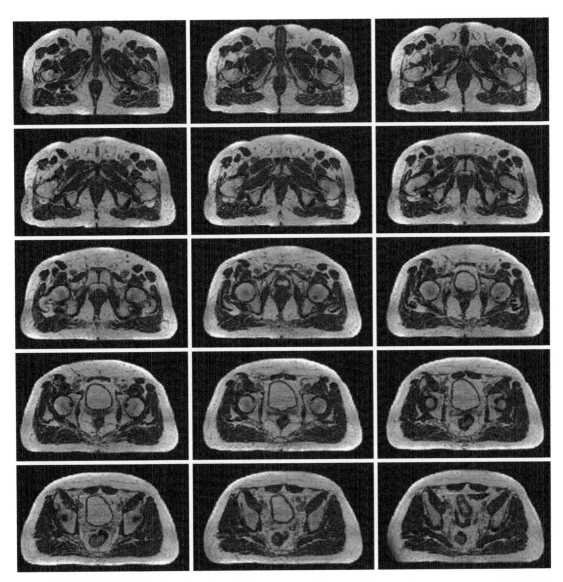

Fig. 11.8 Example of prostate cancer patient acquisition on a 0.35 T MR-linac with a field of view of 45 × 30 × 36 cm (1.5 mm isotropic voxels) acquired in ~3 min, often used for treatment planning. Scans with shorter acquisition times (~20 s) can be used for daily image-guided radiation therapy at the expense of a coarser slice thickness (3 mm)

the clinical balanced steady-state free precession sequence, offering advantages for daily prostate and seminal vesicle localization. Conventionally fractionated radiation has been shown to cause the prostate to first swell and then constrict over weeks (King et al. 2011), or with SBRT, swelling has often been observed (Gunnlaugsson et al. 2014). Online adaptations taking advantage of this allow not only for adaptation due to change in prostate size as well as deformation of the bladder and rectum but also for adaptation based on independent movements of other potential targets like the seminal vesicles and pelvic lymph nodes in higher-risk disease and of other potential OARs like the urethra. Online adaptation can be based upon a library of plans or with dynamic recalculation. Gating can also be done to account for patient movement and changes in bladder and rectum filling during treatment (Bohoudi et al. 2017b). It has been proposed that using MR-IGRT, CTV to PTV margins may be safely reduced to ≤ 3 mm (McPartlin et al. 2016).

In addition to localization, MRI can also theoretically be used as an indication of treatment response and a tool to adapt to this. There have been preliminary reports of using diffusion for this purpose on small samples of patients undergoing radiation receiving one to two MRI scans during treatment as well as scans following treatment completion (Park et al. 2012; Liu et al. 2014; Decker et al. 2014). There is the suggestion that the greatest changes in diffusion are seen in patients with the best outcomes. However, all of these diffusion studies during treatment were performed with 3 T diagnostic MRIs, and available MR-IGRT machines are currently limited to 0.35 or 1.5 T. In theory, daily treatment could be adapted to these tumor load changes with "dose painting by numbers" based upon voxel-specific functional MRI characteristics as recently described in a study that correlated MRI characteristics of prostates that were then surgically removed (van Schie et al. 2017). Current practice with daily MRI-guided therapy, however, is largely limited to alignment alone (McDonald et al. 2013), particularly for SBRT and postoperative/salvage. Practical considerations when treating the prostate with MR-IGRT include the management of bladder/rectal filling, which may be limiting for longer procedures that incorporate online ART.

11.9.2 Bladder

For operable patients with a bladder cancer that has invaded into the organ's muscular layer, the current standard treatment is either a radical cystectomy or a bladder preservation approach. For bladder preservation, patients first undergo a maximal debulking with transurethral bladder tumor (TURBT) local resection, followed by concurrent chemotherapy and radiation therapy with the aim to eliminate any residual disease after TURBT but to also avoid the need for an ileal conduit or urostomy. For medically inoperable patients, concurrent chemotherapy and radiation therapy are used together as an alternate definitive treatment. Outcomes with radiation alone have historically been inferior to surgical outcomes, but adverse patient selection is often cited as one potential explanation.

Other potential explanations for radiation's inferior outcomes with bladder cancer treatment are the dose and volumes used. With conventional techniques, large amounts of small bowel can be irradiated which can result in both acute and late toxicity. Many treatment schemes rely on a "cone down" approach with shrinking volumes. A typical scheme radiates the pelvic nodes at risk in addition to the bladder and then focuses on the whole bladder and then on just the region of the tumor. This "cone down" can be either done sequentially or with a simultaneous integrated boost technique. Regardless of the scheme, strict bladder filling or voiding protocols are needed with patients in order to minimize interfraction setup variability.

Adaptive radiation therapy can help account for this interfraction variability. To date, this has often been done with a daily cone beam and a "library" of plans (McDonald et al. 2013; Vestergaard et al. 2014; Foroudi et al. 2014; Meijer et al. 2012; Tuomikoski et al. 2011; Murthy et al. 2016). Most reports create three or more plans based on different volumes of bladder filling (e.g., small, medium, and large). Each day of treatment, therapists select the plan with the smallest PTV that will still provide appropriate coverage of the bladder and tumor boost. If no plan PTV covers the bladder adequately, the patient is removed from the treatment couch.

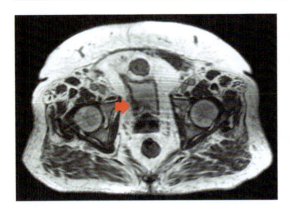

Fig. 11.9 Patient with a muscle invasive bladder cancer in the right posterior wall of the bladder as seen on a 0.35 T tri-cobalt system. 1.5 × 1.5 mm high resolution scan performed with patient free breathing, approximately 2 min acquisition time

Most studies of inter- and intrafraction anatomy changes in patients being treated for bladder cancer have been performed with implanted fiducial markers and with either orthogonal kV imaging or CT. MRI IGRT allows for better soft tissue visualization than either of these approaches (Fig. 11.9) and can also be combined with iodinated fiducials to even better demarcate tumor or tumor beds. One study of patients with muscle-invasive bladder cancer treated on a MR-IGRT system showed that in 28% of cases, the vector shift required for accurate alignment by soft tissue targets was greater than the PTV margin (Fischer-Valuck et al. 2016). In addition to initial alignment, the use of MRI IGRT has potential for its ability to potentially better spare normal tissues than a plan library and also for target shifting midtreatment due to steadily increasing bladder filling (Vestergaard et al. 2016).

11.10 Summary and Future Directions

For many cancers, external beam radiation therapy guided by MRI at the time of treatment enables radiation oncologists to more accurately target their therapy with improved soft tissue contrast and with respiratory gating without invasive fiducial placement. MRI at the time of treatment does so without adding any additional ionizing radiation exposure to the patient, allowing for safe, constant tracking of both malignant and normal targets. MRI at the time of treatment has made online adaptive radiation therapy feasible, allowing for better dose escalation to targets while simultaneously better sparing of normal tissues. Emerging applications for MR-based treatment include the use of radiation to treat cardiac arrhythmias such as ventricular tachycardia and atrial fibrillation (Cuculich et al. 2017; Ipsen et al. 2014). MR-based localization and gating are well suited to compensate for both the respiratory and cardiac motion that complicates these novel ablative treatments. In addition, recently an offline investigation was performed to characterize localization accuracy, treatment planning capabilities, and delivery accuracy of a low-field MR-linac for stereotactic radiosurgery in the brain (Wen et al. 2018). This work revealed that the accuracy and plan quality were comparable to other frameless stereotactic systems, thereby offering future potential for implementing MR-IGRT for benign and malignant brain diseases. Overall when fully realized, MRI at the time of treatment has the potential to change treatment intent based upon continuously acquired data, to allow for dose escalation when anatomy is in a favorable condition, and to use real-time imaging biomarkers to further optimize disease and patient outcomes (Pollard et al. 2017).

References

Acharya S, Fischer-Valuck BW, Kashani R, Parikh P, Yang D, Zhao T, Green O, Wooten O, Li HH, Hu Y, Rodriguez V, Olsen L, Robinson C, Michalski J, Mutic S, Olsen J. Online magnetic resonance image guided adaptive radiation therapy: first clinical applications. Int J Radiat Oncol Biol Phys. 2016a;94:394–403.

Acharya S, Fischer-Valuck BW, Mazur TR, Curcuru A, Sona K, Kashani R, Green O, Ochoa L, Mutic S, Zoberi I. Magnetic resonance image guided radiation therapy for external beam accelerated partial-breast irradiation: evaluation of delivered dose and intrafractional cavity motion. Int J Radiat Oncol Biol Phys. 2016c;96:785–92.

Ates O, Ahunbay EE, Moreau M, Li XA. A fast online adaptive replanning method for VMAT using flattening filter free beams. Med Phys. 2016;43:2756–64.

Bainbridge H, Salem A, Tijssen RHN, Dubec M, Wetscherek A, Van Es C, Belderbos J, Faivre-Finn C,

McDonald F. Magnetic resonance imaging in precision radiation therapy for lung cancer. Transl Lung Cancer Res. 2017;6:689–707.

Bohoudi O, Bruynzeel AME, Senan S, Cuijpers JP, Slotman BJ, Lagerwaard FJ, Palacios MA. Fast and robust online adaptive planning in stereotactic MR-guided adaptive radiation therapy (SMART) for pancreatic cancer. Radiother Oncol. 2017a;125:439–44.

Bohoudi O, Bruynzeel A, Senan S, Slotman B, Palacios M, Lagerwaard F. SP-0494: using a MRI-guided radiation therapy system for prostate cancer patients. Radiother Oncol. 2017b;123:S263.

Cruite I, Schroeder M, Merkle EM, Sirlin CB. Gadoxetate disodium-enhanced MRI of the liver: part 2, protocol optimization and lesion appearance in the cirrhotic liver. Am J Roentgenol. 2010;195:29–41.

Cuculich PS, Schill MR, Kashani R, Mutic S, Lang A, Cooper D, Faddis M, Gleva M, Noheria A, Smith TW, Hallahan D, Rudy Y, Robinson CG. Noninvasive cardiac radiation for ablation of ventricular tachycardia. N Engl J Med. 2017;377:2325–36.

Decker G, Mürtz P, Gieseke J, Träber F, Block W, Sprinkart AM, Leitzen C, Buchstab T, Lütter C, Schüller H. Intensity-modulated radiotherapy of the prostate: dynamic ADC monitoring by DWI at 3.0 T. Radiother Oncol. 2014;113:115–20.

Fischer-Valuck BW, Green OL, Mutic S, Gay H, Michalski JM. Vector analysis of bladder cancer patient setup utilizing a magnetic resonance image guided radiation therapy (MR-IGRT) system. Int J Radiat Oncol Biol Phys. 2016;96:E261.

Fischer-Valuck BW, Henke L, Green O, Kashani R, Acharya S, Bradley JD, Robinson CG, Thomas M, Zoberi I, Thorstad W. Two-and-a-half-year clinical experience with the world's first magnetic resonance image guided radiation therapy system. Adv Radiat Oncol. 2017;2:485–93.

Foroudi F, Pham D, Rolfo A, Bressel M, Tang CI, Tan A, Turner S, Hruby G, Williams S, Hayne D. The outcome of a multi-centre feasibility study of online adaptive radiotherapy for muscle-invasive bladder cancer TROG 10.01 BOLART. Radiother Oncol. 2014;111:316–20.

Glitzner M, Fast MF, de Senneville BD, Nill S, Oelfke U, Lagendijk J, Raaymakers B, Crijns S. Real-time auto-adaptive margin generation for MLC-tracked radiotherapy. Phys Med Biol. 2016;62:186.

Green OP, Goddu S, Mutic S. SU-E-T-352: commissioning and quality assurance of the first commercial hybrid MRI-IMRT system. Med Phys. 2012;39:–3785.

Gunnlaugsson A, Kjellén E, Hagberg O, Thellenberg-Karlsson C, Widmark A, Nilsson P. Change in prostate volume during extreme hypo-fractionation analysed with MRI. Radiat Oncol. 2014;9:22.

Hammel P, Huguet F, van Laethem J-L, Goldstein D, Glimelius B, Artru P, Borbath I, Bouché O, Shannon J, André T. Effect of chemoradiotherapy vs chemotherapy on survival in patients with locally advanced pancreatic cancer controlled after 4 months of gemcitabine with or without erlotinib: the LAP07 randomized clinical trial. JAMA. 2016;315:1844–53.

Henke L, Kashani R, Yang D, Zhao T, Green O, Olsen L, Rodriguez V, Wooten HO, Li HH, Hu Y. Simulated online adaptive magnetic resonance–guided stereotactic body radiation therapy for the treatment of oligometastatic disease of the abdomen and central thorax: characterization of potential advantages. Int J Radiat Oncol Biol Phys. 2016;96:1078–86.

Henke L, Kashani R, Robinson C, Curcuru A, DeWees T, Bradley J, Green O, Michalski J, Mutic S, Parikh P, Olsen J. Phase I trial of stereotactic MR-guided online adaptive radiation therapy (SMART) for the treatment of oligometastatic or unresectable primary malignancies of the abdomen. Radiother Oncol. 2018;126:519–26.

P.ICRU83. Recording and reporting intensity modulated photon beam therapy, IMRT (ICRU). 2010.

Ipsen S, Blanck O, Oborn B, Bode F, Liney G, Hunold P, Rades D, Schweikard A, Keall PJ. Radiotherapy beyond cancer: target localization in real-time MRI and treatment planning for cardiac radiosurgery. Med Phys. 2014;41:120702.

Keall PJ, Mageras GS, Balter JM, Emery RS, Forster KM, Jiang SB, Kapatoes JM, Low DA, Murphy MJ, Murray BR. The management of respiratory motion in radiation oncology report of AAPM Task Group 76. Med Phys. 2006;33:3874–900.

Keall PJ, Barton M, Crozier S, Australian MRI-Linac Program. The Australian magnetic resonance imaging-linac program. Semin Radiat Oncol. 2014;24:203–6.

Kerkmeijer LG, Fuller CD, Verkooijen HM, Verheij M, Choudhury A, Harrington KJ, Schultz C, Sahgal A, Frank SJ, Goldwein J. The MRI-linear accelerator consortium: evidence-based clinical introduction of an innovation in radiation oncology connecting researchers, methodology, data collection, quality assurance, and technical development. Front Oncol. 2016;6:215.

King BL, Butler WM, Merrick GS, Kurko BS, Reed JL, Murray BC, Wallner KE. Electromagnetic transponders indicate prostate size increase followed by decrease during the course of external beam radiation therapy. Int J Radiat Oncol Biol Phys. 2011;79:1350–7.

Klein S, Van Der Heide UA, Lips IM, Van Vulpen M, Staring M, Pluim JP. Automatic segmentation of the prostate in 3D MR images by atlas matching using localized mutual information. Med Phys. 2008;35:1407–17.

Kontaxis C, Bol G, Lagendijk J, Raaymakers B. A new methodology for inter-and intrafraction plan adaptation for the MR-linac. Phys Med Biol. 2015;60:7485.

Koshy M, Malik R, Mahmood U, Husain Z, Sher DJ. Stereotactic body radiotherapy and treatment at a high volume facility is associated with improved survival in patients with inoperable stage I non-small cell lung cancer. Radiother Oncol. 2015;114:148–54.

Lagendijk JJ, Raaymakers BW, Van Vulpen M. The magnetic resonance imaging-linac system. Semin Radiat Oncol. 2014;24:207–9.

Li HH, Rodriguez VL, Green OL, Hu Y, Kashani R, Wooten HO, Yang D, Mutic S. Patient-specific quality assurance for the delivery of 60co intensity modulated radiation therapy subject to a 0.35-T lateral magnetic field. Int J Radiat Oncol Biol Phys. 2015;91:65–72.

Lim-Reinders S, Keller BM, Al-Ward S, Sahgal A, Kim A. Online adaptive radiation therapy. Int J Radiat Oncol Biol Phys. 2017;99:994–1003.

Liu L, Wu N, Ouyang H, Dai J, Wang W. Diffusion-weighted MRI in early assessment of tumour response to radiotherapy in high-risk prostate cancer. Br J Radiol. 2014;87:20140359.

Mahadevan A, Blanck O, Lanciano R, Peddada A, Sundararaman S, D'Ambrosio D, Sharma S, Perry D, Kolker J, Davis J. Stereotactic body radiotherapy (SBRT) for liver metastasis–clinical outcomes from the international multi-institutional RSSearch® Patient Registry. Radiat Oncol. 2018;13:26.

Malayeri AA, El Khouli RH, Zaheer A, Jacobs MA, Corona-Villalobos CP, Kamel IR, Macura KJ. Principles and applications of diffusion-weighted imaging in cancer detection, staging, and treatment follow-up. Radiographics. 2011;31:1773–91.

Malinowski K, McAvoy TJ, George R, Dietrich S, D'Souza WD. Incidence of changes in respiration-induced tumor motion and its relationship with respiratory surrogates during individual treatment fractions. Int J Radiat Oncol Biol Phys. 2012;82:1665–73.

Matsuo Y, Ueki N, Takayama K, Nakamura M, Miyabe Y, Ishihara Y, Mukumoto N, Yano S, Tanabe H, Kaneko S. Evaluation of dynamic tumour tracking radiotherapy with real-time monitoring for lung tumours using a gimbal mounted linac. Radiother Oncol. 2014;112:360–4.

McDonald F, Lalondrelle S, Taylor H, Warren-Oseni K, Khoo V, McNair H, Harris V, Hafeez S, Hansen V, Thomas K. Clinical implementation of adaptive hypofractionated bladder radiotherapy for improvement in normal tissue irradiation. Clin Oncol. 2013;25:549–56.

McPartlin AJ, Li X, Kershaw LE, Heide U, Kerkmeijer L, Lawton C, Mahmood U, Pos F, van As N, van Herk M. MRI-guided prostate adaptive radiotherapy–a systematic review. Radiother Oncol. 2016;119:371–80.

Meijer GJ, van der Toorn P-P, Bal M, Schuring D, Weterings J, de Wildt M. High precision bladder cancer irradiation by integrating a library planning procedure of 6 prospectively generated SIB IMRT plans with image guidance using lipiodol markers. Radiother Oncol. 2012;105:174–9.

Moyer VA. Screening for lung cancer: US Preventive Services Task Force recommendation statement. Ann Intern Med. 2014;160:330–8.

Murray LJ, Dawson LA. Advances in stereotactic body radiation therapy for hepatocellular carcinoma. Semin Radiat Oncol. 2017;27:247–55.

Murthy V, Masodkar R, Kalyani N, Mahantshetty U, Bakshi G, Prakash G, Joshi A, Prabhash K, Ghonge S, Shrivastava S. Clinical outcomes with dose-escalated adaptive radiation therapy for urinary bladder cancer: a prospective study. Int J Radiat Oncol Biol Phys. 2016;94:60–6.

Mutic S, Dempsey JF. The ViewRay system: magnetic resonance-guided and controlled radiotherapy. Semin Radiat Oncol. 2014;24:196–9.

Navarria P, De Rose F, Ascolese AM. SBRT for lung oligometastases: who is the perfect candidate? Rep Pract Oncol Radiother. 2015;20:446–53.

Noel CE, Parikh PJ, Spencer CR, Green OL, Hu Y, Mutic S, Olsen JR. Comparison of onboard low-field magnetic resonance imaging versus onboard computed tomography for anatomy visualization in radiotherapy. Acta Oncol. 2015;54:1474–82.

Nyman J, Hallqvist A, Lund J-Å, Brustugun O-T, Bergman B, Bergström P, Friesland S, Lewensohn R, Holmberg E, Lax I. SPACE—a randomized study of SBRT vs conventional fractionated radiotherapy in medically inoperable stage I NSCLC. Radiother Oncol. 2016;121:1–8.

Park SY, Kim CK, Park BK, Park W, Park HC, Han DH, Kim B. Early changes in apparent diffusion coefficient from diffusion-weighted MR imaging during radiotherapy for prostate cancer. Int J Radiat Oncol Biol Phys. 2012;83:749–55.

Pasquier D, Lacornerie T, Vermandel M, Rousseau J, Lartigau E, Betrouni N. Automatic segmentation of pelvic structures from magnetic resonance images for prostate cancer radiotherapy. Int J Radiat Oncol Biol Phys. 2007;68:592–600.

Pathmanathan AU, van As NJ, Kerkmeijer LGW, Christodouleas J, Lawton CAF, Vesprini D, van der Heide UA, Frank SJ, Nill S, Oelfke U, van Herk M, Li XA, Mittauer K, Ritter M, Choudhury A, Tree AC. Magnetic resonance imaging-guided adaptive radiation therapy: a "game changer" for prostate treatment? Int J Radiat Oncol Biol Phys. 2018;100:361–73.

Pollard JM, Wen Z, Sadagopan R, Wang J, Ibbott GS. The future of image-guided radiotherapy will be MR guided. Br J Radiol. 2017;90:20160667.

Raaymakers BW, Lagendijk JJ, Overweg J, Kok JG, Raaijmakers AJ, Kerkhof EM, van der Put RW, Meijsing I, Crijns SP, Benedosso F, van Vulpen M, de Graaff CH, Allen J, Brown KJ. Integrating a 1.5 T MRI scanner with a 6 MV accelerator: proof of concept. Phys Med Biol. 2009;54:N229–37.

Raaymakers B, Jürgenliemk-Schulz I, Bol G, Glitzner M, Kotte A, van Asselen B, de Boer J, Bluemink J, Hackett S, Moerland M. First patients treated with a 1.5 T MRI-Linac: clinical proof of concept of a high-precision, high-field MRI guided radiotherapy treatment. Phys Med Biol. 2017;62:L41.

Ramey SJ, Padgett KR, Lamichhane N, Neboori HJ, Kwon D, Mellon EA, Brown K, Duffy M, Victoria J, Dogan N. Dosimetric analysis of stereotactic body radiation therapy for pancreatic cancer using MR-guided Tri-60Co unit, MR-guided LINAC, and conventional LINAC-based plans. Pract Radiat Oncol. 2018;8(5):e312–21.

Rangaraj D, Zhu M, Yang D, Palaniswaamy G, Yaddanapudi S, Wooten OH, Brame S, Mutic S. Catching errors with patient-specific pretreatment machine log file analysis. Pract Radiat Oncol. 2013;3:80–90.

Ringe KI, Husarik DB, Sirlin CB, Merkle EM. Gadoxetate disodium-enhanced MRI of the liver: part 1, protocol optimization and lesion appearance in the noncirrhotic liver. Am J Roentgenol. 2010;195:13–28.

Ritter T, Quint DJ, Senan S, Gaspar LE, Komaki RU, Hurkmans CW, Timmerman R, Bezjak A, Bradley JD, Movsas B. Consideration of dose limits for organs at risk of thoracic radiotherapy: atlas for lung, proximal bronchial tree, esophagus, spinal cord, ribs, and brachial plexus. Int J Radiat Oncol Biol Phys. 2011;81:1442–57.

Rosenberg S, Labby Z, Wojcieszynski A, Hullett C, Geurts M, Bayliss R, Hill P, Paliwal B, Bayouth J, Bassetti M. First reported real-time MRI guided liver stereotactic body radiation therapy treatments: experience and clinical implications. Int J Radiat Oncol Biol Phys. 2015;93:S19.

Rudra S, Jiang N, Rosenberg S, Olsen J, Parikh P, Bassetti M, Lee P. High dose adaptive MRI guided radiation therapy improves overall survival of inoperable pancreatic cancer. Int J Radiat Oncol Biol Phys. 2017;99:E184.

Safety EPOM, Kanal E, Barkovich AJ, Bell C, Borgstede JP, Bradley WG Jr, Froelich JW, Gimbel JR, Gosbee JW, Kuhni-Kaminski E. ACR guidance document on MR safe practices: 2013. J Magn Reson Imaging. 2013;37:501–30.

van Schie MA, Steenbergen P, Dinh CV, Ghobadi G, van Houdt PJ, Pos FJ, Heijmink SW, van der Poel HG, Renisch S, Vik T. Repeatability of dose painting by numbers treatment planning in prostate cancer radiotherapy based on multiparametric magnetic resonance imaging. Phys Med Biol. 2017;62:5575.

Shaverdian N, Yang Y, Hu P, Hart S, Sheng K, Lamb J, Cao M, Agazaryan N, Thomas D, Steinberg M. Feasibility evaluation of diffusion-weighted imaging using an integrated MRI-radiotherapy system for response assessment to neoadjuvant therapy in rectal cancer. Br J Radiol. 2017;90:20160739.

Shioyama Y, Nagata Y, Komiyama T, Takayama K, Shibamoto Y, Ueki N, Yamada K, Kozuka T, Kimura T, Matsuo Y. Multi-institutional retrospective study of stereotactic body radiation therapy for stage I small cell lung cancer: Japan Radiation Oncology Study Group (JROSG). Int J Radiat Oncol Biol Phys. 2015;93:S101.

Sun B, Rangaraj D, Boddu S, Goddu M, Yang D, Palaniswaamy G, Yaddanapudi S, Wooten O, Mutic S. Evaluation of the efficiency and effectiveness of independent dose calculation followed by machine log file analysis against conventional measurement based IMRT QA. J Appl Clin Med Phys. 2012;13:140–54.

Team NLSTR. Reduced lung-cancer mortality with low-dose computed tomographic screening. N Engl J Med. 2011;365:395–409.

Tsien C, Cao Y, Chenevert T. Clinical applications for diffusion MRI in radiotherapy. Semin Radiat Oncol. 2014;24:218–26.

Tuomikoski L, Collan J, Keyriläinen J, Visapää H, Saarilahti K, Tenhunen M. Adaptive radiotherapy in muscle invasive urinary bladder cancer—an effective method to reduce the irradiated bowel volume. Radiother Oncol. 2011;99:61–6.

Kishan AU, Lee P. MRI-guided radiotherapy: opening our eyes to the future. Integr Cancer Sci Ther. 2016;3(2):420–7. https://doi.org/10.15761/ICST.1000181.

Verma V, Simone CB, Allen PK, Gajjar SR, Shah C, Zhen W, Harkenrider MM, Hallemeier CL, Jabbour SK, Matthiesen CL. Multi-institutional experience of stereotactic ablative radiation therapy for stage I small cell lung cancer. Int J Radiat Oncol Biol Phys. 2017;97:362–71.

Vestergaard A, Muren LP, Lindberg H, Jakobsen KL, Petersen JB, Elstrøm UV, Agerbæk M, Høyer M. Normal tissue sparing in a phase II trial on daily adaptive plan selection in radiotherapy for urinary bladder cancer. Acta Oncol. 2014;53:997–1004.

Vestergaard A, Hafeez S, Muren LP, Nill S, Høyer M, Hansen VN, Grønborg C, Pedersen EM, Petersen JB, Huddart R. The potential of MRI-guided online adaptive re-optimisation in radiotherapy of urinary bladder cancer. Radiother Oncol. 2016;118:154–9.

Wen N, Kim J, Doemer A, Glide-Hurst C, Chetty IJ, Liu C, Laugeman E, XhaferIlari I, Kumarasiri A, Victoria J, Bellon M, Kalkanis S, Siddiqui MS, Movsas B. Evaluation of a magnetic resonance guided linear accelerator for stereotactic radiosurgery treatment. Radiother Oncol. 2018;127(3):460–6.

Yang Y, Cao M, Sheng K, Gao Y, Chen A, Kamrava M, Lee P, Agazaryan N, Lamb J, Thomas D. Longitudinal diffusion MRI for treatment response assessment: preliminary experience using an MRI-guided tri-cobalt 60 radiotherapy system. Med Phys. 2016;43:1369–73.

Yun J, Wachowicz K, Mackenzie M, Rathee S, Robinson D, Fallone B. First demonstration of intrafractional tumor-tracked irradiation using 2D phantom MR images on a prototype linac-MR. Med Phys. 2013;40:051718.

Zindler JD, Thomas CR, Hahn SM, Hoffmann AL, Troost EG, Lambin P. Increasing the therapeutic ratio of stereotactic ablative radiotherapy by individualized isotoxic dose prescription. J Natl Cancer Inst. 2016;108:djv305.

Part V

Future Direction

Will We Still Need Radiotherapy in 20 Years?

12

Michael B. Barton, Trang Pham, and Georgia Harris

"Prediction is very difficult, especially about the future"

Niels Bohr

12.1 Introduction

The International Agency for Research on Cancer (IARC) predicts that the number of new cases of cancer will increase to about 24 million by 2035 (Ferlay et al. 2013). Radiotherapy has been shown to be the treatment of choice for about half of all cancer patients (Delaney et al. 2005; Barton et al. 2014). If the current practices and distribution of cases continue, then about 12 million new cases of cancer will need radiotherapy by 2035. We estimate that if all those who needed radiotherapy received it, then radiotherapy would save one million lives per year and prevent 2.5 million locoregional recurrences (Atun et al. 2015).

MRI offers the potential for extending the capabilities of radiotherapy beyond its current indications. This chapter examines the demand for radiotherapy over the next 20 years and discusses two approaches that may increase the number of cases who benefit from radiotherapy.

MRI provides exquisite soft tissue imaging, but even more intriguingly, it promises insights into the physiological responses of tumours and normal tissues that may significantly alter the way cancer treatment is delivered. Tumour heterogeneity is a defining feature of malignancy. We explore the potential of functional MRI to predict response to radiotherapy and direct differential targeting of radiation dose within tumours.

The spatial resolution and sensitivity of MRI combined with better definition of radiotherapy beams open up the possibility of using radiotherapy to treat widespread metastases with the aim of long-term control or even cure.

12.1.1 The Demand for Radiotherapy

The proportion of cases for whom radiotherapy is the treatment of choice because of superior clinical outcome or favourable side-effect profile is known as the optimal radiotherapy utilisation (RTU) rate (Delaney et al. 2005). Values have been calculated for the population of cancer patients as a whole and for individual tumour types such as breast and lung cancer. These proportions can be applied to populations with different case mixes to individualise the RTU to different populations.

M. B. Barton (✉)
Faculty of Medicine, Ingham Institute for Applied Medical Research, South West Clinical School, UNSW Sydney, Sydney, NSW, Australia
e-mail: michael.barton@health.nsw.gov.au

T. Pham
Clinical Academic in Radiation Oncology, Faculty of Medicine, Ingham Institute for Applied Medical Research, South West Clinical School, UNSW Sydney, Sydney, NSW, Australia

G. Harris
Department of Radiation Oncology, Chris O'Brien Lifehouse, Camperdown, NSW, Australia

© Springer Nature Switzerland AG 2019
G. Liney, U. van der Heide (eds.), *MRI for Radiotherapy*,
https://doi.org/10.1007/978-3-030-14442-5_12

We have used this method to estimate the demand for radiotherapy in 184 countries covered by IARC in their publically available database of cancer incidence and mortality. IARC has performed projections of cancer incidence based on demographic changes to estimate the number of new cases of country by 27 tumour types for 2035. Non-melanomatous skin cancer was excluded because it is not routinely notified to central cancer registries. The global optimal RTU was 50%. RTU ranged from 32% (Mongolia) to 59% (Comoros) (Yap et al. 2016).

In 2012 IARC estimated that there were 14 million new cases of cancer globally (Ferlay et al. 2013). They predict that this number will almost double by 2035 to 24 million cases. About 12 million of these cases would benefit from radiotherapy. This is a conservative estimate because the stage at diagnosis was assumed to have the same distribution in every country. In reality patients in low- and middle-income countries are more likely to have advanced cancer at diagnosis, and radiotherapy will play a larger role in their management because they are less likely to be suitable for surgery (Barton et al. 2006).

The optimal number of radiotherapy fractions (attendances) needed can be calculated by using evidence-based guidelines to assign a number of fractions to each indication. Overall the optimal number of fractions was 19.4 per course for the case mix in Australia (Wong et al. 2016). Taking into account the differing case mix globally, we estimate that over 200 million fractions will be required by 2035 to meet the total demand (Atun et al. 2015). Nearly two thirds of radiotherapy capacity will be needed in low- and middle-income countries.

12.1.2 Benefits of Radiotherapy

It is also possible to estimate the survival and local control benefit for each radiotherapy indication. We have calculated that globally, radiotherapy adds 4% to cancer survival at 5 years and 10% to local control (Hanna et al. 2018). The benefit of radiotherapy is greater in LMIC because the proportion of cervix and head and neck cancers is greater in these countries (Table 12.1).

By combining the data on new cases of cancer from Globocan with information on demand for fractions and the potential benefit of radiotherapy, we can calculate that there are seven million patients who would benefit from radiotherapy in 2012 and that if radiotherapy was available to all who needed it, then nearly 600,000 lives would be saved, and local failure would be avoided in 1.4 million cases (Table 12.2) (Atun et al. 2015). By 2035 there would be 12 million new radiotherapy cases each year needing 220 million fractions. If all of these cases received radiotherapy, then nearly one million lives would be saved and 2.5 million local recurrences avoided.

Table 12.1 Population benefit from radiotherapy by income range (World Bank Country and Lending Groups 2018)

Income	Average GNI per person, USD	Local control, %	Survival, %
High	>12,236	10.1	3.2
Upper Middle	3956–12,235	8.6	3.9
Lower middle	1006–3955	13.4	6.2
Low	<1005	13.6	6.3
All		10.4	4.1

Table 12.2 Demand for radiotherapy and benefit

	New cancer cases	RT cases	Fractions	5-Year benefit Survival	5-Year benefit Local control
2012	14,090,149	7,057,329	129,567,566	579,628	1,462,358
2015	15,230,336	8,590,624	140,125,759	624,782	1,580,362
2020	17,141,369	7,624,309	157,793,271	698,752	1,776,757
2025	19,311,062	9,661,786	177,662,458	780,483	1,995,212
2030	21,680,805	10,832,809	199,204,428	868,285	2,230,085
2035	24,019,837	11,985,210	220,408,307	953,994	2,460,285

12.1.3 Cost Benefits of Providing Access to Radiotherapy

Of course it would require significant investment in personnel, equipment and facilities to achieve worldwide coverage of radiotherapy by 2035. Atun et al. (2015) have calculated that it would cost $184 billion dollars to scale up radiotherapy in low- and middle-income countries using the standard model of radiotherapy delivery: a two machine department, simulator and planning equipment. An efficiency model that assumed technological innovation would reduce costs to $97 billion. Scale-up of radiotherapy delivery in low- and middle-income countries alone would save 27 million life years and produce a net benefit of $278 billion over the period 2015–2035.

To meet global demand by 2035, there would be a need for an extra 13,500 new megavoltage machines, 43,000 radiation oncologists, 40,000 medical physicists and 131,000 radiation therapists (Atun et al. 2015).

12.2 New Roles for Radiotherapy

The projections for the demand of radiotherapy assume that the proportion of cases that would benefit from radiotherapy will remain stable. A review of the change in optimal utilisation rate over 10 years found that it decreased from 52% to 48% primarily due to epidemiological changes (Barton et al. 2014). It is possible that some indications will decrease such as cervix cancer although the impact of HPV vaccination is likely to take many years to manifest as vaccination programmes are just beginning in LMIC.

In the remainder of this chapter, we consider two examples where MRI and in particular MRI-guided treatment have the potential to increase the proportion of cancer patients who would benefit from radiotherapy and to increase the efficacy of radiotherapy.

12.2.1 Using MRI to Target Tumour Heterogeneity

Tumours are biologically heterogeneous in nature. The tumour microenvironment is characterised by heterogeneity in vasculature, oxygenation, cellularity and metabolism (Vaupel 2004; Hanahan and Weinberg 2011). Proper assessment and characterisation of this physiologic heterogeneity is key to developing new radiotherapy approaches to targeting heterogeneity and improving outcomes. Functional MRI enables information to be obtained about key biological characteristics of tumour: (1) vascularisation and oxygenation, (2) cellularity and proliferation and (3) metabolism. In addition, MRI has the ability to assess the entire tumour, allowing for characterisation of intratumour heterogeneity in function and aggressiveness. This information could be used for early radiotherapy response prediction and stratification of management based on therapeutic response (Fig. 12.1).

Techniques in radiation oncology have been refined to enable accurate delivery of radiotherapy based on tumour morphology obtained from anatomical imaging modalities such as computed tomography (CT). The advent of dose painting with IMRT and VMAT enables a non-homogeneous dose to be given, opening up the possibility that extra doses can be given to heterogeneous biological targets (Bernier et al. 2004). MRI now offers potential for extending capabilities of radiotherapy to target tumour heterogeneity. The clinical development of radiotherapy-dedicated MRI-simulators and MRI-guided treatment systems (MRI-Linac) enables functional imaging to be incorporated for better radiotherapy targeting of tumour biology. An MRI biomarker map of tumour heterogeneity can be obtained, opening up new opportunities to further refine radiotherapy targeting based on tumour function (Fig. 12.2). Furthermore, MRI has the advantage of 'virtual' whole-tumour sampling and can be repeated on multiple occasions without ionising radiation exposure, opening up the possibility for intra- and inter-fraction targeting of tumour heterogeneity.

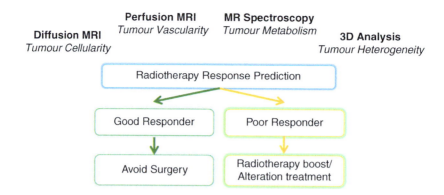

Fig. 12.1 Functional MRI for radiotherapy response prediction and stratification of management. Diffusion-weighted spectroscopy and dynamic contrast-enhanced MRI could provide biologic information predictive of radiotherapy response. Patients can be stratified according to therapeutic response. For example in rectal cancer, good responders to treatment may be able to avoid surgery with a 'wait and watch' approach following long-course chemoradiotherapy, thereby avoiding a permanent colostomy

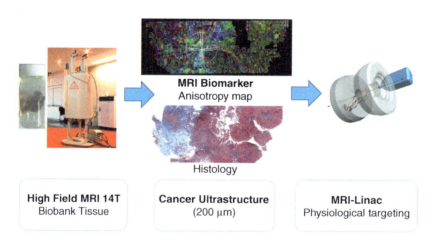

Fig. 12.2 MRI biomarker discovery and translational pipeline from ex vivo to clinical setting. High-field MRI examination of biobank tissue and correlation of MRI biomarker maps with histopathology allow for discovery of predictive MRI biomarkers. These MRI biomarkers could be translated to clinical field strengths for functional targeting on the MRI-linac

12.2.1.1 Dynamic Contrast-Enhanced MRI for Targeting Tumour Perfusion and Hypoxia

The tumour microenvironment is characterised by abnormal microcirculation with poor functionality of tumour vasculature (Vaupel 2004; Bernier et al. 2004). Newly formed tumour vasculature is immature, highly tortuous, dilated, leaky and poorly organised blood vessels resulting in unstable blood flow and regions of hypoxia. Tumour hypoxia is a well-established factor of radioresistance. Evidence has accumulated showing that patterns of hypoxia in tumours are highly heterogeneous, making it difficult to target with treatment. Tissue biopsy immunohistochemistry or direct methods of measuring hypoxia with oxygen electrodes are invasive and are unable to assess this heterogeneity. In addition, temporal heterogeneity in hypoxia exists, and repeated measurements would be required to assess this.

Information on spatial heterogeneity in tumour vascularisation and hypoxia can be obtained with dynamic contrast-enhanced (DCE) MRI. DCE-MRI is able to non-invasively assess characteristics of the tumour microvascular environment such as hypoxia and microvessel density that can influence radiosensitivity. Typically, the abnormal leaky tumour microvasculature results in a rapid wash-in and wash-out of contrast and a greater increase in signal intensity than in normal tissues. Regions of low perfusion, indicated by low signal intensity on DCE-MRI, may represent hypoxic regions in tumour, thereby presenting a potential target for radiotherapy boosting. Studies in patients with cervix cancer undergoing radiotherapy have shown correlation of DCE-MRI parameters with direct tumour oxygenation measurements (Cooper et al. 2000; Loncaster et al. 2002). Clinical DCE-MRI studies in rectal cancer have shown correlation of DCE-MRI parameters such as K_{ps} and K^{trans}, with factors of tumour angiogenesis, such as microvessel density, endothelial cell proliferation and VEGF (Zahra et al. 2007; de Lussanet et al. 2005; George et al. 2001; Zhang et al. 2008). DCE-MRI studies have also shown that higher K^{trans} pretreatment is predictive of good response to radiotherapy (Pham et al. 2017a; Intven et al. 2015).

12.2.1.2 Diffusion-Weighted MRI for Targeting Tumour Cellularity

Diffusion-weighted MRI assesses movement of water molecules through tissue and provides information about tumour cellularity and microarchitecture. Apparent diffusion coefficient (ADC) from diffusion-weighted imaging (DWI) measures water diffusion through tissue and shows an inverse relationship with tissue cellularity (Metcalfe et al. 2013). ADC values have been shown to correlate with tumour cellularity and grade in prostate (Gibbs et al. 2009) and CNS tumours (Sugahara et al. 1999; Higano et al. 2006).

Radiotherapy-induced cellular damage and necrosis occur early following commencement of treatment. Viable tumour cells restrict the diffusion of water through tissue resulting in a low ADC value, whereas necrotic tumour cells allow increased diffusion of water molecules resulting in a high ADC value. The ability of DWI to detect changes in tumour microstructure allows it to be used for prediction of radiotherapy response and differential targeting of radiation dose (e.g. boosting for poor responders) within tumours. Multiple studies have demonstrated the value of ADC in the early prediction of radiotherapy response. In general, studies in CNS, head and neck and rectal cancers have shown that low ADC pretreatment and greater percentage increase in ADC during treatment are predictive of good response to radiotherapy (Pham et al. 2017a; Barbaro et al. 2012; Lambrecht et al. 2012; Chen et al. 2014; Moffat et al. 2005). In contrast, a high ADC pretreatment is predictive poor response to radiotherapy, likely due to the presence of more radioresistant necrotic cells (van der Paardt et al. 2013; Dzik-Jurasz et al. 2002). The tumour heterogeneity in ADC has been assessed with a histogram method in a rectal cancer study and demonstrated that a higher relative fraction of high ADCs was predictive of poor response to radiotherapy; this was hypothesised to be due to the higher fraction of necrotic tumour cells (DeVries et al. 2003).

12.2.1.3 Magnetic Resonance Spectroscopy for Targeting Tumour Metabolism

Magnetic resonance spectroscopy (MRS) is an important tool for studying cancer metabolism. An activated choline pathway is typical of malignancy, and its discovery was mostly owing to the introduction of MRS in the study of cancer in the 1980s. Abnormal tumour metabolism is emerging as a hallmark of cancer and a possible therapeutic target (Hanahan and Weinberg 2011). The combination of malignant transformation, cellular proliferation and hypoxic tumour microenvironment is the cause of an increase in choline compounds in cancer. MRS is a non-invasive method of detecting an increase in choline-containing compounds. In addition, different cancers have unique metabolic 'fingerprints' as demonstrated in ex vivo studies (Griffin and Shockcor 2004).

Choline is currently the most studied metabolite in clinical studies and a potential novel therapeutic target. MRS studies in CNS, prostate, breast and rectal cancer have shown an increased level of choline in cancer and a reduction in choline levels in response to radiotherapy (Pham et al. 2017a; Kwock et al. 2006; Kim et al. 2012). In high-grade gliomas (WHO grade III and IV), response to therapy is heterogeneous, and early detection of poor response to therapy would allow patients to begin next-line treatment. Proton MRS has been shown to be able to differentiate between tumour, necrotic brain tissue and normal brain tissue through choline signal intensity (Kwock et al. 2006). Data from serial three-dimensional MRS allows for assessment of this heterogeneity in response to treatment and targeted biopsy to guide further treatment.

12.2.1.4 Quantifying Tumour Heterogeneity with Multi-parametric MRI Histogram Analysis

Tumours are physiologically heterogeneous in their response to treatment, and summary measures such as mean ADC or K^{trans} of a region of interest do not reflect tumour heterogeneity. Multi-parametric MRI combines whole-tumour anatomical and functional information in a single examination, and this can be repeated over the course of treatment. Multi-parametric MRI allows information on multiple biological parameters to be obtained, thereby providing a more comprehensive assessment of tumour biology; this can provide information on radiotherapy response and improve risk stratification for management (Pham et al. 2017b). Figure 12.3 shows images from multi-parametric MRI, combining information from T2-weighted, DWI and DCE-MRI.

Functional information on all tumour voxels can be visualised on a slice-by-slice map, enabling refined targeting or boosting of particular tumour regions that are biologically more aggressive, such as poorly perfused hypoxic regions. Histogram analysis techniques allow information on all tumour voxels to be captured for assessment of intratumour heterogeneity and its changes in response to treatment (Fig. 12.4 and 12.5). Quantitative information on tumour heterogeneity such as skewness, kurtosis and percentile distribution can be extracted from histograms. Overall trends from MRI histogram studies have shown that post-treatment, histograms demonstrate a shift of DWI ADC to the right with decreased kurtosis and skewness and a shift in DCE K^{trans} to the left with narrower and increased peak height (Just 2014).

12.2.2 Treatment of Metastases for Cure with Radiotherapy Alone

Most arguments for the contribution of radiotherapy to future cancer control consist of envisioning small increments in local and perhaps regional control. However, given the enormous burden of advanced metastatic disease globally and its associated morbidity and mortality, the possibility of achieving cure or survival prolongation for these patients has the potential for a huge impact at the population level.

Approximately a quarter of all cancer patients present with stage IV disease where the cancer has spread to distant organs, and most cancer patients who die do so from metastatic spread (Branch 2016). Survival of stage IV patients is the worst of all cancer patients and has barely improved over the last decade (Fig. 12.6).

These patients are generally classified as having incurable disease at the time of their cancer diagnosis, with some exceptions (including seminoma and haematological malignancies for example) where long-term remission may be achieved. Historically, once a solid tumour has developed the capacity to metastasise to distant sites, treatment has largely focussed on systemic therapy given with palliative intent and supportive care. In this setting, radiotherapy has traditionally been used for the palliation of focal symptoms. The exception is those patients with limited metastatic disease (usually defined as 1–5 metastases), in whom the use of ablative radiotherapy may prolong survival (Corbin et al. 2013; Tree et al. 2013; Lo et al. 2009, 2010a, b).

The term oligometastases was first coined by Hellman and Weichselbaum (1995) and describes the concept of an intermediary metastatic state in which cancer exists as a discrete number of metas-

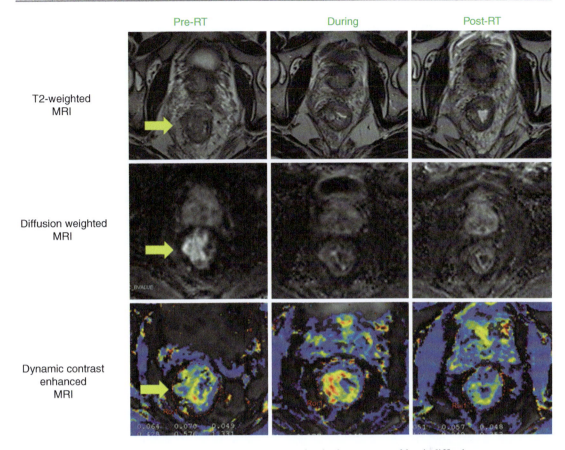

Fig. 12.3 Multi-parametric MRI for prediction and assessment of tumour response in a rectal cancer patient. Images at three time-points in a rectal cancer patient undergoing long-course chemoradiotherapy. This patient had a pathologic complete response (AJCC seventh edition tumour regression grade 0) to chemoradiotherapy. The anatomic images (top row) showed persistent thickening in the rectum making it difficult to assess response to therapy. The diffusion MR images (middle row) showed an early reduction in signal intensity at week 3, indicating early response to therapy. Perfusion MRI (bottom row) showed increase in perfusion during chemoradiotherapy and decreased perfusion post-chemoradiotherapy

tases at first before cells acquire the ability to metastasise more widely. It has been hypothesised that successful eradication of disease at an oligometastatic stage with more aggressive local treatments may improve survival outcomes and possibly result in cure in select cases (Khoo et al. 2018). There is a growing body of evidence to support this hypothesis, whereby long-term survival is possible following surgical resection of limited sites of metastatic disease (Fernandez et al. 2004; Pastorino et al. 1997). Furthermore, the use of stereotactic body radiotherapy (SBRT) to deliver ablative doses of radiotherapy to a variety of oligometastatic disease sites has been reported in a number of retrospective and prospective cohort studies to prolong overall survival and/or progression-free survival (Branch 2016; Corbin et al. 2013; Tree et al. 2013; Lo et al. 2009, 2010a). There are a number of randomised studies in progress which seek to evaluate the true benefit of adding local therapy to systemic therapy in patients with stage IV disease and also to ascertain which patients and primary tumour sites and histologies are most likely to benefit from such an approach. That said, there is little consensus on the total number or volume of metastases that constitute the oligometastatic state, which clearly exists on a continuum with advanced metastatic disease; an arbitrary number of 1–5 metastases has typically been used, whereby observational prospective

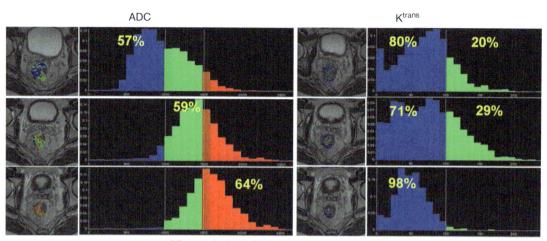

Fig. 12.4 Multi-parametric MRI-combined colour-coded maps and histogram analysis in a rectal cancer good responder to long-course chemoradiotherapy—histopathology tumour regression grade 0 (AJCC seventh edition TRG 0, pathologic complete response). Histogram analysis of ADC and K^{trans} was performed for three timepoints (top row pretreatment, middle row during treatment, bottom row post-treatment) on prototype software (Siemens OncoTreat). Colour-coded functional mapping of ADC and K^{trans} allows visualisation of changes in tumour cellularity (diffusion weighted) and perfusion (dynamic contrast enhanced) on a slice-by-slice basis. A shift in ADC histogram to the right and shift in K^{trans} histogram to the left can be seen in response to treatment

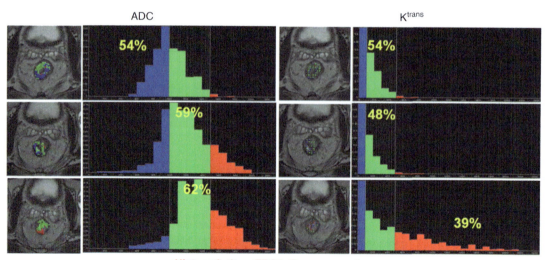

Fig. 12.5 Multi-parametric MRI-combined colour-coded maps and histogram analysis in a rectal cancer poor responder to long-course chemoradiotherapy—histopathology tumour regression grade 2 (AJCC seventh edition TRG 2, minimal response). The ADC histograms demonstrated a shift in ADC to moderate values during treatment. The K^{trans} histograms demonstrated a shift of K^{trans} voxels to the right following completion of treatment, suggesting residual perfusion and residual disease

studies have suggested improved outcomes with SBRT for those with fewer metastases (Salama et al. 2012), but there is little data regarding the use of SBRT for more widespread disease.

One of the tenets of radiation oncology practice is the concept of treating malignancy to a high or 'tumourcidal' dose but minimising normal tissue dose and volume to reduce the risk of

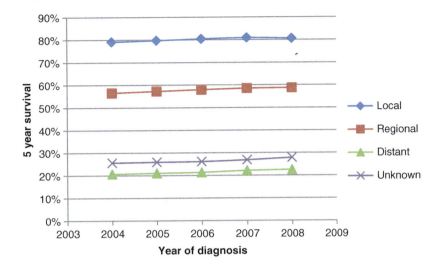

Fig. 12.6 Five-year survival by year of diagnosis and cancer stage (Branch 2016)

both acute and late morbidity. Over the past three decades, there have been dramatic improvements in sophisticated radiotherapy planning and delivery techniques which have made this more achievable (Moran et al. 2005). In line with this, Schulz and Kagan (2003) proposed the concept of the 'Infinitron', an idealised radiotherapy device which delivers dose only to cancer cells and no dose to adjacent normal tissues; this notion is particularly attractive in terms of the possible applicability to patients with advanced metastatic disease in whom eradication of all known cancer deposits may possibly result in cure or long-term survival.

The ability to treat metastases is obviously limited by our ability to detect tumour deposits and the sensitivity of current diagnostic and functional molecular imaging. Current diagnostic imaging resolution enables visualisation of deposits up to 3 mm in size (Forghani et al. 2015), which is thought to represent 3×10^8 cancer cells, at an early stage and size before they are likely to be symptomatic. Cancer deposits of this size or less are unlikely to cause harm directly unless occurring within a critical area (e.g. within the central nervous system) however may have potential to seed or spread to other areas or mutate to a more resistant tumour clone. Thus, eradicating even tiny cancer deposits with ablative radiotherapy might in theory prolong survival. In reality, at some stage selective irradiation of all visualised cancer deposits might result in an unacceptable whole body or organ at risk dose, at which point treatment would not be feasible.

With ongoing advancements in diagnostic imaging coupled with substantial improvements in radiotherapy delivery techniques (including the development of MRI simulators and MRI-guided treatment systems), it raises the question of how far along the continuum towards this idealised state we have come and what the technical and biological barriers to radiotherapy as a potential curative treatment tool for patients with advanced metastatic cancer might be. Currently, routine diagnostic surveillance imaging for patients with advanced metastatic disease is not widely recommended but rather reserved for symptomatic progression where a change in management may be indicated. The pursuit of a curative approach to management in patients with advanced metastatic disease would certainly be a paradigm shift in current oncological practice, whereby close clinical follow-up and regular surveillance imaging may be imperative with potentially huge implications on service delivery and resource utilisation in this patient cohort.

12.3 Conclusion

Radiotherapy for existing indications would benefit over seven million cancer patients worldwide, and this number will increase to 12 million by 2035, saving nearly one million lives each year and preventing 2.5 million cancer recurrences.

MRI guidance is likely to increase the number of patients who benefit for radiotherapy by opening up new indications such as previously uncontrollable metastatic disease and improve the efficacy of existing treatment by better targeting tumour heterogeneity.

References

Atun R, Jaffray D, Barton M, Baumann M, Vikram B, Bray F, et al.. Responding to the cancer crisis: expanding global access to radiotherapy: a Lancet Oncology Commission. European Cancer Congress; 2015.

Barbaro B, Vitale R, Valentini V, Illuminati S, Vecchio FM, Rizzo G, et al. Diffusion-weighted magnetic resonance imaging in monitoring rectal cancer response to neoadjuvant chemoradiotherapy. Int J Radiat Oncol Biol Phys. 2012;83(2):594–9.

Barton MB, Frommer M, Shafiq J. The role of radiotherapy in cancer control in low- and middle-income countries. Lancet Oncol. 2006;7(7):584–95.

Barton MB, Jacob S, Shafiq J, Wong K, Thompson SR, Hanna TP, et al. Estimating the demand for radiotherapy from the evidence: a review of changes from 2003 to 2012. Radiother Oncol. 2014;112(1):140–4.

Bernier J, Hall E, Giaccia A. Radiation oncology: a century of achievements. Nat Rev Cancer. 2004;4:737–47.

Branch SS. SEER*stat database: incidence – SEER 18 regs research data + Hurricane Katrina impacted Louisiana cases, Nov 2015 Sub (1973–2013 varying) – linked to county attributes – total U.S., 1969–2014 counties. Bethesda, MD: Surveillance Research Program, National Cancer Institute; 2016.

Chen Y, Liu X, Zheng D, Xu L, Hong L, Xu Y, et al. Diffusion-weighted magnetic resonance imaging for early response assessment of chemoradiotherapy in patients with nasopharyngeal carcinoma. Magn Reson Imaging. 2014;32(6):630–7.

Cooper RA, Carrington BM, Loncaster JA, Todd SM, Davidson SE, Logue JP, et al. Tumour oxygenation levels correlate with dynamic contrast-enhanced magnetic resonance imaging parameters in carcinoma of the cervix. Radiother Oncol. 2000;57(1):53–9.

Corbin KS, Hellman S, Weichselbaum RR. Extracranial oligometastases: a subset of metastases curable with stereotactic radiotherapy. J Clin Oncol. 2013;31(11):1384–90.

Delaney G, Jacob S, Featherstone C, Barton M. The role of radiotherapy in cancer treatment: estimating optimal utilization from a review of evidence-based clinical guidelines. Cancer. 2005;104(6):1129–37.

van der Paardt MP, Zagers MB, Beets-Tan RGH, Stoker J, Bipat S. Patients who undergo preoperative chemoradiotherapy for locally advanced rectal cancer restaged by using diagnostic MR imaging: a systematic review and meta-analysis. Radiology. 2013;269(1):101–12.

DeVries AF, Kremser C, Hein PA, Griebel J, Krezcy A, Öfner D, et al. Tumor microcirculation and diffusion predict therapy outcome for primary rectal carcinoma. Int J Radiat Oncol Biol Phys. 2003;56(4):958–65.

Dzik-Jurasz A, Domenig C, George M, Wolber J, Padhani A, Brown G, et al. Diffusion MRI for prediction of response of rectal cancer to chemoradiation. Lancet. 2002;360(9329):307–8.

Ferlay J, Soerjomataram I, Ervik M, Dikshit R, Eser S, Mathers C, et al. GLOBOCAN 2012 v1. 0, cancer incidence and mortality worldwide: IARC CancerBase no. 11. Lyon: International Agency for Research on Cancer; 2013.. http://globocaniarcfr

Fernandez FG, Drebin JA, Linehan DC, Dehdashti F, Siegel BA, Strasberg SM. Five-year survival after resection of hepatic metastases from colorectal cancer in patients screened by positron emission tomography with F-18 fluorodeoxyglucose (FDG-PET). Ann Surg. 2004;240(3):438.

Forghani R, Yu E, Levental M, Som PM, Curtin HD. Imaging evaluation of lymphadenopathy and patterns of lymph node spread in head and neck cancer. Expert Rev Anticancer Ther. 2015;15(2):207–24.

George M, Dzik-Jurasz A, Padhani A, Brown G, Tait D, Eccles S, et al. Non-invasive methods of assessing angiogenesis and their value in predicting response to treatment in colorectal cancer. Br J Surg. 2001;88(12):1628–36.

Gibbs P, Liney GP, Pickles MD, Zelhof B, Rodrigues G, Turnbull LW. Correlation of ADC and T2 measurements with cell density in prostate cancer at 3.0 Tesla. Investig Radiol. 2009;44(9):572–6.

Griffin JL, Shockcor JP. Metabolic profiles of cancer cells. Nat Rev Cancer. 2004;4(7):551–61.

Hanahan D, Weinberg RA. Hallmarks of cancer: the next generation. Cell. 2011;144(5):646–74.

Hanna TP, Shafiq J, Delaney GP, Vinod SK, Thompson SR, Barton MB. The population benefit of evidence-based radiotherapy: 5-year local control and overall survival benefits. Radiother Oncol. 2018;126(2):191–7.

Hellman S, Weichselbaum RR. Oligometastases. J Clin Oncol. 1995;13(1):8–10.

Higano S, Yun X, Kumabe T, Watanabe M, Mugikura S, Umetsu A, et al. Malignant astrocytic tumors: clinical importance of apparent diffusion coefficient in prediction of grade and prognosis. Radiology. 2006;241(3):839–46.

Intven M, Reerink O, Philippens ME. Dynamic contrast enhanced MR imaging for rectal cancer response assessment after neo-adjuvant chemoradiation. J Magn Reson Imaging. 2015;41(6):1646–53.

Just N. Improving tumour heterogeneity MRI assessment with histograms. Br J Cancer. 2014;111(12):2205–13.

Khoo V, Hawkins M, McDonald F, Ahmed M, Kirby A, Van As N, et al. CORE: a randomised trial of COventional care versus radioablation (stereotactic body radiotherapy) for extracranial oligometastases. Lung Cancer. 2018;115:S85–S6.

Kim MJ, Lee SJ, Lee JH, Kim SH, Chun HK, Kim SH, et al. Detection of rectal cancer and response to concurrent chemoradiotherapy by proton magnetic resonance spectroscopy. Magn Reson Imaging. 2012;30(6):848–53.

Kwock L, Smith JK, Castillo M, Ewend MG, Collichio F, Morris DE, et al. Clinical role of proton magnetic resonance spectroscopy in oncology: brain, breast, and prostate cancer. Lancet Oncol. 2006;7(10):859–68.

Lambrecht M, Vandecaveye V, De Keyzer F, Roels S, Penninckx F, Van Cutsem E, et al. Value of diffusion-weighted magnetic resonance imaging for prediction and early assessment of response to neoadjuvant radiochemotherapy in rectal cancer: preliminary results. Int J Radiat Oncol Biol Phys. 2012;82(2):863–70.

Lo SS, Fakiris AJ, Teh BS, Cardenes HR, Henderson MA, Forquer JA, et al. Stereotactic body radiation therapy for oligometastases. Expert Rev Anticancer Ther. 2009;9(5):621–35.

Lo SS, Fakiris AJ, Chang EL, Mayr NA, Wang JZ, Papiez L, et al. Stereotactic body radiation therapy: a novel treatment modality. Nat Rev Clin Oncol. 2010a;7(1):44.

Lo SS, Teh BS, Mayr NA, Olencki TE, Wang JZ, Grecula JC, et al. Stereotactic body radiation therapy for oligometastases. Discov Med. 2010b;10(52):247–54.

Loncaster JA, Carrington BM, Sykes JR, Jones AP, Todd SM, Cooper R, et al. Prediction of radiotherapy outcome using dynamic contrast enhanced MRI of carcinoma of the cervix. Int J Radiat Oncol Biol Phys. 2002;54(3):759–67.

de Lussanet QG, Backes WH, Griffioen AW, Padhani AR, Baeten CI, van Baardwijk A, et al. Dynamic contrast-enhanced magnetic resonance imaging of radiation therapy-induced microcirculation changes in rectal cancer. Int J Radiat Oncol Biol Phys. 2005;63(5):1309–15.

Metcalfe P, Liney G, Holloway L, Walker A, Barton M, Delaney G, et al. The potential for an enhanced role for MRI in radiation-therapy treatment planning. Technol Cancer Res Treat. 2013;12(5):429–46.

Moffat BA, Chenevert TL, Lawrence TS, Meyer CR, Johnson TD, Dong Q, et al. Functional diffusion map: a noninvasive MRI biomarker for early stratification of clinical brain tumor response. Proc Natl Acad Sci U S A. 2005;102(15):5524–9.

Moran JM, Elshaikh MA, Lawrence TS. Radiotherapy: what can be achieved by technical improvements in dose delivery? Lancet Oncol. 2005;6(1):51–8.

Pastorino U, Buyse M, Friedel G, Ginsberg RJ, Girard P, Goldstraw P, et al. Long-term results of lung metastasectomy: prognostic analyses based on 5206 cases. J Thorac Cardiovasc Surg. 1997;113(1):37–49.

Pham TT, Liney GP, Wong K, Barton MB. Functional MRI for quantitative treatment response prediction in locally advanced rectal cancer. Br J Radiol. 2017a;90(1072):20151078.

Pham TT, Liney G, Wong K, Rai R, Lee M, Moses D, et al. Study protocol: multi-parametric magnetic resonance imaging for therapeutic response prediction in rectal cancer. BMC Cancer. 2017b;17(1):465.

Salama JK, Hasselle MD, Chmura SJ, Malik R, Mehta N, Yenice KM, et al. Stereotactic body radiotherapy for multisite extracranial oligometastases. Cancer. 2012;118(11):2962–70.

Schulz R, Kagan AR. More precisely defined dose distributions are unlikely to affect cancer mortality. Med Phys. 2003;30(2):276.

Sugahara T, Korogi Y, Kochi M, Ikushima I, Shigematu Y, Hirai T, et al. Usefulness of diffusion-weighted MRI with echo-planar technique in the evaluation of cellularity in gliomas. J Magn Reson Imaging. 1999;9(1):53–60.

Tree AC, Khoo VS, Eeles RA, Ahmed M, Dearnaley DP, Hawkins MA, et al. Stereotactic body radiotherapy for oligometastases. Lancet Oncol. 2013;14(1):e28–37.

Vaupel P. Tumor microenvironmental physiology and its implications for radiation oncology. Semin Radiat Oncol. 2004;14(3):198–206.

Wong K, Delaney GP, Barton MB. Evidence-based optimal number of radiotherapy fractions for cancer: a useful tool to estimate radiotherapy demand. Radiother Oncol. 2016;119(1):145–9.

World Bank Country and Lending Groups [Internet]. The World Bank. 2018. https://datahelpdesk.worldbank.org/knowledgebase/articles/906519-world-bank-country-and-lending-groups. Accessed 5 Apr 2018.

Yap ML, Zubizarreta E, Bray F, Ferlay J, Barton M. Global access to radiotherapy services: have we made progress during the past decade? J Glob Oncol. 2016;207:JGO001545.

Zahra MA, Hollingsworth KG, Sala E, Lomas DJ, Tan LT. Dynamic contrast-enhanced MRI as a predictor of tumour response to radiotherapy. Lancet Oncol. 2007;8(1):63–74.

Zhang XM, Yu D, Zhang HL, Dai Y, Bi D, Liu Z, et al. 3D dynamic contrast-enhanced MRI of rectal carcinoma at 3T: correlation with microvascular density and vascular endothelial growth factor markers of tumor angiogenesis. J Magn Reson Imaging. 2008;27(6):1309–16.

Real-Time MRI-Guided Particle Therapy

13

Bradley M. Oborn

13.1 Rationale for MRI-Guided Particle Therapy (MRPT)

Particle-based cancer therapy has had a long and promising history that arguably dates back to the exciting work by Wilson in 1946 (Wilson 1946). In this work the potential use of a high-energy beam of protons for cancer therapy was described. At the time, Wilson proposed "It will be simple to collimate proton beams to less than 1.0 mm diameter or to expand them to cover any area uniformly". It seemed that this could be an ideal form of cancer treatment as dose could in principle be accurately tailored to cover a tumour volume precisely, with very minimal dose to surrounding tissues—somewhat an ideal method of external beam therapy using ionising radiation. Since this early exciting prediction, many practical elements of particle therapy, in particular with regard to pencil-beam scanning, have been discovered that in essence deteriorate the ideal dose distribution. These include the well-documented problems such as range uncertainty, penumbral widening near the Bragg peak, fragmentation dose tails, and nonideal accelerators and beamlines (i.e. polyenergetic pencil beams with angular divergence). These issues are then further compromised by patient setup errors and potential patient movement during treatment. In summary, particle therapy is more complex and not as robust as first predicted for many reasons. To overcome some of these issues, treatment methods have been altered through techniques such as including extended treatment margins (incorporate range uncertainty) and optimising plan robustness (accommodate patient anatomy changes or movement). At the end of the day, particle therapy does have superior dose distributions for many tumour sites, in particular the ability to spare healthy tissue more than x-ray therapy. There is evidence, and at least a suggestion, for a clinical benefit of proton therapy over x-ray therapy approaches for various challenging tumours such as paediatric central nervous system malignancies, large ocular melanomas, chordomas and hepatocellular carcinomas (Allen et al. 2012).

Interestingly, there does not appear to be any clinical gains for using particle (proton) therapy over the most accurate x-ray therapy methods for small-to-large motion tumours such as prostate (Yu et al. 2013) and lung (Liao et al. 2018). It is clear from the literature that more robust prospective clinical trials are needed to determine the appropriate clinical settings for particle therapy (Allen et al. 2012; Odei et al. 2016).

From a pure dosimetry viewpoint, a degraded or misaligned particle therapy dose distribution

B. M. Oborn (✉)
Centre for Medical Radiation Physics, University of Wollongong, Wollongong, NSW, Australia

Illawarra Cancer Care Centre,
Wollongong, NSW, Australia

may have stronger implications for patient toxicities as compared with x-ray beams. An analogy at this point could be "particle therapy beams offer the sharpest knife in radiotherapy, but the knife is wobbly".

If we consider that we have accurate and real-time MRI guidance at hand, then we can start to address these issues. The range of particle beams is heavily dependent on the material type and density being traversed. Patient anatomy is mostly soft tissue based, and MRI offers superior information on the distribution of soft tissues. Current planning methods use CT information which is geometrically accurate for patient outline and bony anatomy distribution. However, soft tissues are all close in Hounsfield unit (HU) or CT number (density), and so ultimately inaccuracies exist in how the materials are mapped into the dose planning stages. MR images, coupled with intelligent algorithms or manual contouring, will in principle enable greater anatomy delineation for planning purposes. The direct result envisaged in this case is that range uncertainty will be reduced from the current value of around 3.5% to a number that is perhaps 1%. It is worth noting that dual-energy CT scanning is also promising similar results (Han et al. 2016; Zhu and Penfold 2016; Taasti et al. 2016); however, the use of such ionising radiation for image guidance on a daily basis is simply not feasible. CT imaging including dual-energy CT will still likely play an important part in MRPT development as a reference tool, whilst MRI-based planning is advanced.

13.2 Existing Literature Related to MRPT

The first noted literature on MRI combined with particle therapy comes in the form of a patent awarded in 2004 (Bucholz and Miller 2004). Three other patents are noted from 2013 (John 2013), 2014 (Kruip 2014) and 2016 (Fallone et al. 2016). In each of these patents, the general concept of firing a proton or particle beam towards a patient in an MRI scanner is described and the modality to be used for real-time guidance.

In terms of scientific literature, the first work appears in 2008 by Raaymakers et al. (2008). In this work some basic Monte Carlo-based work was performed to ascertain the deflection that a therapeutic proton beam would undergo if subject to magnetic fields typical of a current clinical MRI-linac system (1.5 T). The encouraging result that the deflection of therapeutic proton beams is not too severe has perhaps encouraged a string of further studies on the various aspects of MRPT to date. The focus of several of these is that of MRI-only planning for proton and ion therapy, i.e. where MR images are used exclusively in the planning process. These include Koivula et al. (2016), Rank et al. (2013a, b) and Maspero et al. (2017). The remainder of the studies to date on MRPT concepts relate directly to real-time MRI-guided proton therapy. The various topics include beam delivery and deflections (Oborn et al. 2015; Wolf and Bortfeld 2012; Raaijmakers et al. 2008; Schellhammer and Hoffmann 2017) and dose planning inside magnetic fields (Hartman et al. 2015; Moteabbed et al. 2014; Kurz et al. 2017; Fuchs et al. 2017; PadillaCabal et al. 2018). Most recently, a research programme at OncoRay in Dresden (Germany) appears to have a functional proof-of-concept system where MR images of a phantom have been acquired with a clinical scanner, whilst proton beam delivery was occurring (Schellhammer et al. 2018; Hoffmann et al. 2018). Finally, we also note a recent "Future of Medical Physics"-themed article on real-time MRI-guided proton therapy (Oborn et al. 2017).

An important conclusion to draw from the current literature on MRPT development is that passively scattered beams will not be a feasible method for beam delivery. This is because these polyenergetic beams will be degraded, spatially, as they transport towards an MRI scanner (Oborn et al. 2015). This is not really an issue as the alternate option, pencil-beam scanning, is ideally suited for this modality. Each mostly monoenergetic pencil beam will be delivered to the patient with a known MRI fringe field map and be independent of the other pencil beams. Each particle within each pencil beam should therefore take a very similar path from the scanning magnets to the patient.

13.3 Workflow and Patient Selection in MRPT

The workflow and patient selection in MRPT would be similar to that of MRI-guided x-ray-based therapy. Particle therapy, through pencil-beam scanning, however, has some desirable advantages over x-rays. In the purest form, fractional doses that have been delivered slightly incorrectly can be easily patched up with rescanning (beam delivery that is) or dose repainting. This process involves delivering say 90% of the dose to a target volume in a single or perhaps several beam-on phases. Then, by processing a log file of the beam properties and comparing against the known patient anatomy (from real-time images), it would be possible to generate an optimised final dose pattern that patches up the errors of the first 90% of the dose delivered. Conventional image guidance methods would most likely provide limited data on the patient anatomy over the fraction such as implanted markers or bony anatomy shifts observed using on-board kV x-ray systems. With real-time MR images, ideally in 4D, of the patient anatomy over the fraction, it would then possible to provide a more robust understanding of any dose discrepancies between the ideal and calculated.

Figure 13.1 provides a summary of a possible workflow for the delivery of particle therapy inside an integrated MRI-proton therapy system. The main elements of this workflow are described in the following sections:

(a) *Initial planning derived from CT and/or MRI-only dataset*: Conventional CT-based planning with MRI fusion to delineate soft tissues will be the expected method for contouring in the early stages. The treatment plan will be optimised for the default patient anatomy. In the case of tumours that move with the breathing cycle, a gated treatment, or treatment window, would be the natural choice.
(b) *Pre-fraction MRI*: This scan is designed to detail any significant anatomy changes as compared to the planning stage. If the patient anatomy is close or very similar to that of the planning dataset, then the fraction dose can be delivered as normal. If significant change to the anatomy is observed, then an adaptive replan would be initiated. In this process a new plan is generated on the new anatomy observed. Then the typical quality assurance processes would be invoked for the new plan. Overall this, similar to MRI-guided x-ray treatments, would take considerable time. The benefit is clearly the new adapted plan which meets the original dose requirement constraints.
(c) *Beam delivery*: For static tumour sites, the entire fraction dose could be delivered at this point. Real-time monitoring would ensure the PTV is always located inside a treatment window. In the case where a significant, unexpected patient movement occurs, the real-time images could be used to trigger a pause in the beam delivery. Such movements could be slow, for example, relaxation of the patient posture over minutes, or fast such as swallowing, coughing or movement of bowel gas. For dynamic tumours, such as thoracic and abdominal, the most natural choice may be gated delivery or delivery when the planning target volume is within a treatment window. The typical expected motion of the PTV would be known from the pre-fraction MRI scan, and the real-time 2D cine MR images would guide the beam delivery.
(d) *Offline dose assessment*: From the real-time anatomy information, an offline dose recalculation can be performed which would detail any deviations to the planned dose per fraction. This would then be merged and/or registered to the total dose delivered so far (if beyond the first fraction). If significant dose deviations are observed, then a new adaptive replan can be created and proposed for the next and remaining fractions to correct for the errors.

This process of daily adaptive replanning (when required) continues until all fractions are completed.

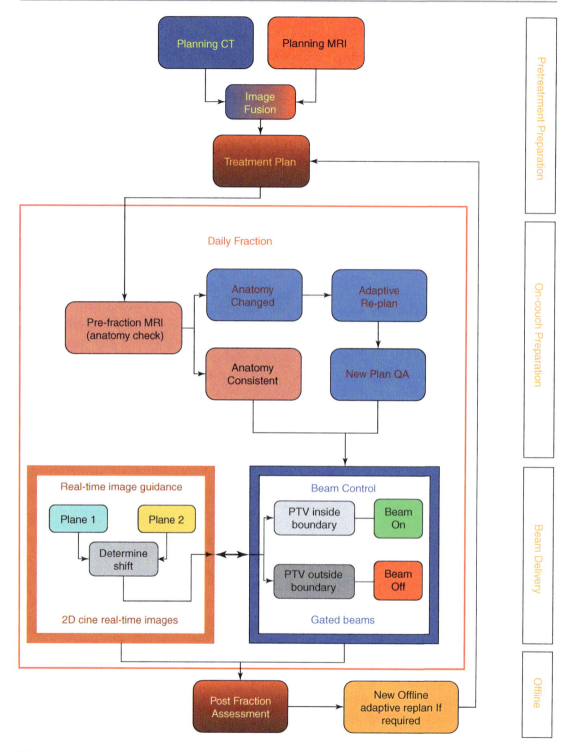

Fig. 13.1 Proposed workflow in MRPT. At the start of each treatment fraction, a daily MRI scan would detail the patient anatomy. If required, a new adaptive replan would be initiated

13.4 Dose Planning for MRPT

There will be some unique challenges in performing dose planning for MRPT. The major elements are discussed below:

(a) *Particle beam planning along the beamline in the MRI fringe field*: In order to transport a proton or other particle therapy ion to the centre of an MRI scanner requires passing the beam through the MRI fringe field. All current MRI-linac systems have some form of active or passive shielding to reduce the MRI fringe field. However there is still the requirement that the magnetic field must change from almost zero to full MRI isocentre strength and direction over some volume around the imaging isocentre. As a charged particle moves through this volume of changing magnetic field (towards the MRI isocentre), it will experience a deflection force according to the Lorentz force. Because the magnetic field direction and strength changes dramatically over the MRI fringe field, the resultant path of the charged particles may become also non-trivial. This effect has been modelled previously for protons incident upon the 1 T MRI scanner of the Australian MRI-linac system (Oborn et al. 2015). The general observed result was that protons fired down the MRI bore direction will rotate around the MRI axis, whilst those fired towards the isocentre through the split-bore magnet gap became deflected away from the isocentre. The important point to note is that each different MRI scanner will have a unique fringe field, and the deflection of the particle beams needs to be accurately modelled and accounted for in the beam delivery process.

With regard to dose planning, an accurate knowledge of the particle pencil beams is required as they enter the volume surrounding the patient. This includes both the direction vector and positions, for each pencil-beam energy. This is a unique requirement of MRPT as the deflection process is energy dependent. Without an MRI fringe field, the direction vector and positions of scanned beams (as they pass into the volume around a patient) is simply related via a straight line projection to their deflection origin within the PBS assembly. Perhaps the best way to determine this information will be through extensive commissioning of an integrated system with specialised detectors that can provide information on the trajectory of pencil beams as they cross a plane in space entering the patient treatment volume. The data would be stored in lookup tables (LUTs) and used as inputs for the next stage of dose planning, as outlined below.

(b) *Particle beam planning in B-fields inside the patient or imaging volume*: Once inside the patient treatment volume, the MRI field is highly uniform in both direction and magnitude. Thus dose planning can be optimised using calculations that have an external magnetic field that is independent from the MRI fringe field. This task has already been studied successfully by several groups (Hartman et al. 2015; Moteabbed et al. 2014; Kurz et al. 2017). The only extension required on these works is the requirement to use pencil-beam properties that start with realistic positions and direction vectors, i.e. from the LUTs, as described in the previous section. This would add some complexity to the process and further require careful verification in the quality assurance process.

(c) *Adaptive replanning in real-time*: Similar to MRI-guided x-ray therapy, an online adaptive replan, when required, will be a time-constrained process. Minimising the duration of the patient waiting on the treatment couch is a high priority. This process involves various steps including recontouring or registration, contour QA, replanning and plan optimisation and then replan QA. For x-ray therapy, this adaptive replan process is proving successful with a median time of 26 min for a sample of 20 patients treated in this way (Acharya et al. 2016). For particle therapy, an almost identical process will be required, and so at a first estimate, similar times would be expected for an adaptive replan in MRPT. This does make the assumption that the optimised replanning dose calculation for particle therapy is similar to that of x-ray methods. With x-ray dose calculations, fast Monte Carlo-based dose engines are routinely used for the MRI-linac systems. Thus it would be expected that particle beam replanning could be similarly successful in a short time frame. An important point to note that is different from x-ray therapy is the potential ability to optimise dose constraints through simple weighting of pencil beams, rather than generation of entirely new IMRT fields. Perhaps this process is simpler in both calculation times and quality assurance checking.

13.5 Beam Delivery and MRI Requirements for MRPT

The most concerning element with regard to hardware will surely be the integration of a particle therapy beamline and a split-bore or open MRI scanner. There cannot be significant crosstalk between the systems; otherwise the modality is compromised. In the first case, the MRI must contain the ideal magnetic field distribution for accurate imaging. This can be affected by the ferromagnetic components of the particle beamline nearby. Further to this, the dynamic nature of pencil-beam scanning must not interfere dynamically with image quality. Complete integrated modelling of the PBS and MRI will provide valuable information on the potential influence each system has on one another. As prototype systems become available, experimental measurements will be the obvious method to deduce the performance of each component. Beyond delivering a predictable dose to a patient with concurrent accurate real-time MRI images, the major hardware challenges would likely be that of beam monitoring in the presence of magnetic fields.

13.6 Beyond Real-Time MRI Guidance for Anatomy Delineation

Ideally we could envisage the integration of an MRI with particle therapy to offer more than just real-time anatomical information. Biologically guided particle therapy, where the daily pre-fraction MRI scan is able to detail some tumour changes at the biological level, would be a first thought. This could lead to further optimisation of the dose during an adaptive replan or initiate dose escalation to biological "hot spots" that are detailed in dedicated and novel MRI sequences. Such directions are already proposed in at least an offline workflow using MRI (Dewhirst and Birer 2016; O'Connor et al. 2016).

Another direction that pushes the novel concepts would be to somehow use the MRI to indirectly verify the dose distribution. Observing functional changes in the tumour volume in the seconds to minutes following irradiation may provide a link to the actual dose deposited by the particle beams. This could be related to both physical dose and biological dose. Perhaps even shedding imports light on the ever contentious topic of the radiobiological effectiveness (RBE) of particle beams. A final discovery could go a step further and aid the quality assurance of the pencil-beam scanning process, namely, identifying the location of individual Bragg peaks. Novel MRI sequences may discover a property that reveals where a Bragg peak has just occurred. This would offer superior 3D spatial information on the beam delivery, a large improvement over the current prompt gamma or acoustic methods.

13.7 MRPT Concept Design

To better appreciate the complexities of an integrated MRI-guided proton therapy system, two concept designs are presented in Fig. 13.2. A generic split-bore MRI system is used, to allow for a proton beam to reach a patient without obstruction from an MRI cryostat vessel. In part (a) an inline system is shown where the beam reaches the patient through the bore of the MRI. In this case the patient is positioned between the MRI halves and further may be axially rotated to allow for treatments from multiple angles. In (b) the perpendicular approach for the particle beam is shown, including a gantry. The split-bore nature of the MRI may also allow for a generic gantry ring support option. This may be in fact a method

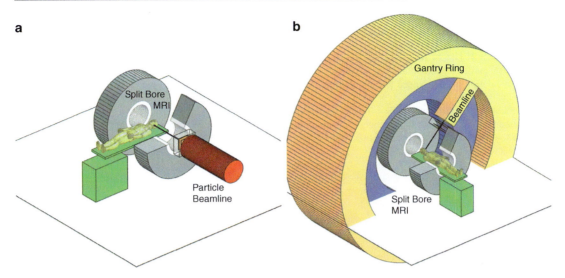

Fig. 13.2 Concept MRI-guided particle therapy systems. (**a**) An inline system which allows for axial rotation of the patient to treat from multiple angles. (**b**) A full gantry design with beam approaching from the perpendicular direction. In this design the particle beamline is supported via a gantry ring that surrounds the MRI system

to reduce the overall mass of a particle therapy gantry; current gantries are designed to allow for a full range of movement of the treatment couch, similar to conventional x-ray-based radiotherapy from a bunker with a gantry-based linear accelerator. This means large diameter gantries with large structures to maintain rigidity of the gantry. In MRPT, the split-bore magnet requirement reduces the couch range, and so this space can be utilised for gantry support instead.

Not shown in the figure is the requirement for radiofrequency (RF) decoupling between the MRI and particle beamline. Typically this is performed by using 1 mm of copper sheeting or similar, applied to an MRI room walls.

In the case of MRPT, the integrated system adds complexity in how this would work. For MRI-linac systems, the treatment room is RF shielded and so is the x-ray beam system. X-ray beams are minimally perturbed by 1 mm of copper, and so complete isolation of the linac source is feasible. A particle beamline is more sensitive to being fired through a thin copper layer, and so the expected solution would be to fire the beam, just above the patient, through a long copper tube (i.e. RF filter or waveguide) that allows a hole in the RF shielding around the treatment head. This would allow RF decoupling without degrading the particle beam.

Acknowledgements The author acknowledges funding from NHMRC Programme Grant No. 1036078 and ARC Discovery Grant No. DP120100821. The author also acknowledges a research agreement with Ion Beam Applications (IBA) and helpful discussions with P. J. Keall and P. E. Metcalfe regarding the content of this chapter.

References

Acharya S, Fischer-Valuck BW, Kashani R, Parikh P, Yang D, Zhao T, Green O, Wooten O, Li HH, Hu Y, Rodriguez V, Olsen L, Robinson C, Michalski J, Mutic S, Olsen J. Online magnetic resonance image guided adaptive radiation therapy: First clinical applications. Int J Radiat Oncol Biol Phys. 2016;94(2):394–403.

Allen AM, Pawlicki T, Dong L, Fourkal E, Buyyounouski M, Cengel K, Plastaras J, Bucci MK, Yock TI, Bonilla L, Price R, Harris EE, Konski AA. An evidence based review of proton beam therapy: the report of astros emerging technology committee. Radiother Oncol. 2012;103(1):8–11.

Bucholz R, Miller D. System combining prootn beam irradiation and magnetic resonance imaging. Patent number US 6725078b2. April 20, 2004.

Dewhirst MW, Birer SR. Oxygen-enhanced MRI is a major advance in tumor hypoxia imaging. Can Res. 2016;76:769–72.

Fallone BG, Carlone M, Murray B. Integrated external beam radiotherapy and MRI system. Patent number US 946777b2. October 18, 2016.

Fuchs H, Moser P, Grschl M, Georg D. Magnetic field effects on particle beams and their implications for dose calculation in MR guided particle therapy. Med Phys. 2017;44(3):1149–56.

Han D, Siebers JV, Williamson JF. A linear, separable two-parameter model for dual energy ct imaging of proton stopping power computation. Med Phys. 2016;43(1):600–12.

Hartman J, Kontaxis C, Bol GH, Frank SJ, Lagendijk JJW, van Vulpen M, Raaymakers BW. Dosimetric feasibility of intensity modulated proton therapy in a transverse magnetic field of 1.5 t. Phys Med Biol. 2015;60(15):5955.

Hoffmann A, Gantz S, Grossinger P, Karsch L, Pawelke J, Serra A, Smeets J, Schellhammer S. Characterization of in-beam mr imaging performance during proton beam irradiation. Radiother Oncol. 2018;127(Suppl 1):S548.

Koivula L, Wee L, Korhonen J. Feasibility of mri-only treatment planning for proton therapy in brain and prostate cancers: dose calculation accuracy in substitute ct images. Med Phys. 2016;43(8):4634–42.

Kruip MJM. Particle radiation therapy equipment. Patent number US 8838202b2. Sept 16, 2014.

Kurz C, Landry G, Resch AF, Dedes G, Kamp F, Ganswindt U, Belka C, Raaymakers BW, Parodi K. A monte-carlo study to assess the effect of 1.5 t magnetic fields on the overall robustness of pencil-beam scanning proton radiotherapy plans for prostate cancer. Phys Med Biol. 2017;62(21):8470.

Liao Z, Lee JJ, Komaki R, Gomez DR, O'Reilly MS, Fossella FV, Blumenschein GR Jr, Heymach JV, Vaporciyan AA, Swisher SG, Allen PK, Choi NC, TF DL, Hahn SM, Cox JD, Lu CS, Mohan R. Bayesian adaptive randomization trial of passive scattering proton therapy and intensity-modulated photon radiotherapy for locally advanced non-small-cell lung cancer. J Clin Oncol. 2018;36:1813–22.

Maspero M, van den Berg CAT, Landry G, Belka C, Parodi K, Seevinck PR, Raaymakers BW, Kurz C. Feasibility of mr-only proton dose calculations for prostate cancer radiotherapy using a commercial pseudo-ct generation method. Phys Med Biol. 2017;62(24):9159.

Moteabbed M, Schuemann J, Paganetti H. Dosimetric feasibility of real-time MRI-guided proton therapy. Med Phys. 2014;41(11):111713.

Oborn BM, Dowdell S, Metcalfe PE, Crozier S, Mohan R, Keall PJ. Proton beam deflection in mri fields: implications for mri-guided proton therapy. Med Phys. 2015;42(5):2113–24.

Oborn BM, Dowdell S, Metcalfe PE, Crozier S, Mohan R, Keall PJ. Future of medical physics: real-time mri-guided proton therapy. Med Phys. 2017;44(8):e77–90.

OConnor JP. System for combining magnetic resonance imaging with particle-based radiation systems for image guided radiation therapy. Patent number US 8427148b2. April 23, 2013.

O'Connor JPB, Boult JKR, Jamin Y, et al. Oxygen-enhanced MRI accurately identifies, quantifies, and maps tumor hypoxia in preclinical cancer models. Can Res. 2016;76:787–95.

Odei BCL, Boothe D, Keole SR, Vargas CE, Foote RL, Schild SE, Ashman JB. A 20-year analysis of clinical trials involving proton beam therapy. Int J Part Ther. 2016;3(3):398–406.

PadillaCabal F, Georg D, Fuchs H. A pencil beam algorithm for magnetic resonance imageguided proton therapy. Med Phys. 2018;45(5):2195–204.

Raaijmakers AJE, Raaymakers BW, Lagendijk JJW. Magnetic-field-induced dose effects in MR-guided radiotherapy systems: dependence on the magnetic field strength. Phys Med Biol. 2008;53(4):909–23.

Raaymakers BW, Raaijmakers AJE, Lagendijk JJW. Feasibility of MRI guided proton therapy: magnetic field dose effects. Phys Med Biol. 2008;53(20):5615–22.

Rank CM, Hnemohr N, Nagel AM, Rthke MC, Jkel O, Greilich S. Mri-based simulation of treatment plans for ion radiotherapy in the brain region. Radiother Oncol. 2013a;109(3):414–8.

Rank CM, Tremmel C, Hnemohr N, Nagel AM, Jakel O, Greilich S. Mri-based treatment plan simulation and adaptation for ion radiotherapy using a classification-based approach. Radiat Oncol. 2013b;8(1):51.

Schellhammer SM, Hoffmann AL. Prediction and compensation of magnetic beam deflection in MR-integrated proton therapy: a method optimized regarding accuracy, versatility and speed. Phys Med Biol. 2017;62(4):1548.

Schellhammer S, Karsch L, Smeets J, LAbbate C, Henrotin S, van der Kraaij E, Lhr A, Quets S, Pawelke J, Hoffmann A. First in-beam mr scanner for image-guided proton therapy: beam alignment and magnetic field effects. Radiother Oncol. 2018;127.(Suppl 1:S315–6.

Taasti VT, Petersen JBB, Muren LP, Thygesen J, Hansen DC. A robust empirical parametrization of proton stopping power using dual energy ct. Med Phys. 2016;43(10):5547–60.

Wilson RR. Radiological use of fast protons. Radiology. 1946;47:487–91.

Wolf R, Bortfeld T. An analytical solution to proton Bragg peak deflection in a magnetic field. Phys Med Biol. 2012;57(17):N329–37.

Yu JB, Soulos PR, Herrin J, Cramer LD, Potosky AL, Roberts KB, Gross CP. Proton versus intensity-modulated radiotherapy for prostate cancer: patterns of care and early toxicity. J Natl Cancer Inst. 2013;105(1):25–32.

Zhu J, Penfold SN. Dosimetric comparison of stopping power calibration with dual-energy ct and single energy ct in proton therapy treatment planning. Med Phys. 2016;43(6):2845–54.